T0313166

Analyzing Health Data in R for SAS Users

Monika Wahi
Peter Seebach

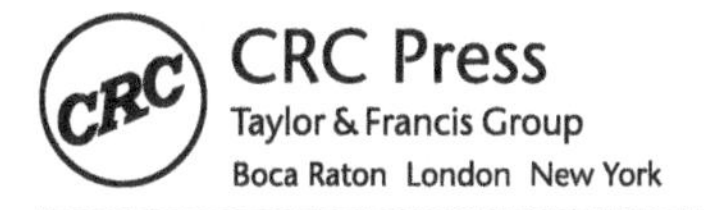

CRC Press is an imprint of the
Taylor & Francis Group, an informa business

CRC Press
Taylor & Francis Group
6000 Broken Sound Parkway NW, Suite 300
Boca Raton, FL 33487-2742

Printed on acid-free paper

International Standard Book Number-13: 978-1-4987-9588-3 (Hardback)

Library of Congress Cataloging-in-Publication Data

Names: Wahi, Monika, author. | Seebach, Peter, author
Title: Analyzing health data in R for SAS users / Monika Wahi and Peter Seebach
Description: Boca Raton : CRC Press, 2017. | Includes bibliographical
References, Identifiers: LCCN 2017021131 | ISBN 9781498795883 Subjects: LCSH: Bioinformatics. | Medical informatics. | R (Computer program language) | SAS (Computer file) Classification: LCC QH324.2 .W34 2017 | DDC 610.285--dc23
LC record available at https://lccn.loc.gov/2017021131

Visit the Taylor & Francis Web site at
http://www.taylorandfrancis.com

and the CRC Press Web site at
http://www.crcpress.com

Contents

Preface

When I, Monika Wahi, gave a presentation at the *Effective Applications of the R Language* (*EARL*) *Conference* in Boston in November 2015, there I attended a panel discussion of the event leaders, although it was a very open discussion, with the audience enthusiastically participating. The goals of the R Consortium were delineated, which led to the consideration of how to promote the increased usage of the R language by statisticians. After all, R is open source software, so it does not have a *marketing department* per se. Someone in the audience brought up with the specific topic of healthcare analytics, asking the attendees why R is not used more often in healthcare. After a pause, someone pointed out the domination of SAS in the industry, which crowds out R. But then, another person speculated that the Food and Drug Administration (FDA) would only accept analysis in SAS (a myth which we debunked in Chapter 1). It became clear that there seemed to be many barriers to promoting R among healthcare analysts.

After further consideration, this was ironic, because both R and SAS are very extensive languages, but what we do in healthcare analytics on a day-to-day basis is relatively straightforward. We are not modeling any spaceship trajectories, or building complex economic models, or predicting weather or the outcome of sports games. It occurred to me that as we generally do the same things over and over again in healthcare analytics, and because most people in healthcare analytics do these things in SAS, a book that focuses only on explaining how to do what we normally do in SAS in R would help healthcare analysts who may want to use R also.

Therefore, this book is aimed at the healthcare analyst who is a SAS user looking to learn R. Chapter 1: "Differences between SAS and R" is written mainly for those who are interested in the backstory of how SAS and R are run differently. Readers who want to get immediately to coding should skip to Chapter 2: "Preparing Data for Analysis," which describes editing and validating an analytic dataset in R rather than using SAS data steps. Chapter 3: "Basic Descriptive Analysis" will explain how to use the analytic dataset developed to produce a basic descriptive analysis (often presented as *Table 1* in manuscripts). Finally, Chapter 4: "Basic Regression Analysis" covers linear and logistic regression and basic survival analysis. As R produces such lovely plots, an insert with 16 color plots is included in the center of this book.

We hope this book encourages you to try R for some healthcare analysis tasks.

Monika Wahi and Peter Seebach

Acknowledgments

The number of people who have helped us with this book is large, and we are eternally grateful. But after controlling for age, relevant skills, and education, it turns out that specifically no one individual contributed significantly more to help us with this book than another. Our conclusion is that you are all amazing, and we thank you very much for your support!

Authors

Monika Wahi, MPH, CPH obtained a bachelor of science in costume design and textiles and clothing (with a concentration in Journalism) from the College of Human Ecology, University of Minnesota, St. Paul, Minnesota, and, then went on to complete her masters in public health from the University of Minnesota School of Public Health, Minneapolis, Minnesota. After serving in several different scientific and administrative roles at Hennepin County in Minnesota, a nonprofit Alzheimer's research institute in Florida, and at the U.S. Army at a site in the Greater Boston area, she struck out on her own to build her consulting business, DethWench Professional Services (DPS). Since 2012, she has been serving as a lecturer at the Labouré College, Milton, Massachusetts, teaching classes in the U.S. healthcare system and statistics. Monika has also led to the expansion of DPS to serving an international clientele through providing online educational material and services as well as public health research consulting.

Peter Seebach was raised by mathematicians, and never fully recovered. He earned his bachelor's degree in psychology from St. Olaf College, Northfield, Minnesota, and then went on to apply it to a career as a software developer and writer. He enjoys computers, writing, and writing about computers. He is an outlier, and therefore tends to throw off the average.

1

Differences between SAS and R

This chapter is meant to help the SAS user conceptualize the important differences between R and SAS that will affect the work of the healthcare analyst who knows SAS but is looking to learn how to use R. The first section describes important differences in the structures of the SAS and R programs. This leads to the discussion in the second section, which focuses on how these differences in structure affect the differences in data handling between the two programs. The third section of this chapter contextualizes the choice between using R versus SAS for a healthcare analytics project and provides a guide for selecting which software to use. Optional practice exercises are included in the fourth section.

Structure of Program

Perhaps the most important difference between SAS and R is the structure of how the program is built and maintained. To begin to explain this difference, we will start with considering how different the download and install process is between PC SAS and R. Next, we will cover how these differences are also reflected in the differences in the way licensing is maintained in the two programs. Third, the differences between SAS components and their parallel in R, called R packages, will be discussed, and after that, differences between SAS and R in approach to maintaining the most current version in a production environment will be explained. The differences between the activities of SAS and R user communities will be described, followed by the differences between the SAS and R user interfaces. Finally, some thoughts on the principles of organizing code, metadata, and documentation in SAS and R are presented.

Installation of PC Version: SAS versus R

When using a typical PC SAS license from a university, the data analyst has to download and install the program on his or her Windows personal computer (PC), as the current operating system (OS) for Macintosh is not supported.* To do this, the analyst is provided access to either many CDs that her computer will tell you to put in or take out of her CD/DVD drive during the installation process, or alternatively, an extremely large setup file that takes a very long time to download (plan for hours, not minutes). The analyst is also provided a small text file with unique license information for her institution's license.

Once the analyst has access to these setup files, a setup file is run on the analyst's PC, and this setup file takes a while to extract. The installation must be monitored because the user has to click through many menus. This is because these SAS institutional licenses are very extensive and include many add-ons and components. This heavy-handed installation process is designed to make sure the analyst has access to all the components to which she is entitled under the license (which, at a university, tends to be a large volume).

However, when working in SAS, the analyst may encounter the rare case in which she is using an analytic function that is not included in the SAS license components, and this throws up an error message. This is a confusing situation because the error message does not usually point to a missing component; it simply rejects the code as being incorrect in some way, so troubleshooting can be challenging.

Because R is open source, meaning that R developers are volunteers and make the code and documentation for how R runs readily available on the Internet, there is no need for the advanced functions to control licensing that SAS employs. This makes the way R is distributed different from SAS. Anyone can go to the public website called "The Comprehensive R Archive Network" (CRAN) (https://cran.r-project.org) [1] and download the latest version of R for Mac or Windows and install the core program. The user interface (UI) looks slightly different on Mac versus Windows, but the differences are minor.† The R installation file is small relative to the SAS installation file, and once the user downloads this file and runs it, the setup wizard is clear and easy, making for a quick installation process.

* Per SAS, SAS versions developed since Macintosh OS X came out are not supported on OS X. A modification of SAS called JMP (pronounced "jump") has been developed for Mac and Windows users alike, although it has greatly reduced functionality. SAS also has a web-based version that can run in Mac and Windows browsers which is mainly used in teaching rather than production environments.

† The examples given in this book refer to the Windows version of R.

Licensing Differences: SAS versus R

The exact components of the SAS institutional license make are communicated to SAS during the installation process at the step where the user is asked by the setup wizard to reference the small text file provided with the setup files. As stated earlier, the list of components included in a SAS institutional license are usually large. When SAS negotiates enterprise licenses with universities, they are set up such that a large volume of components is included, and the student or faculty pays only a negligible fee or nothing to obtain this licensed version, provided they can prove their status with the university. This is because SAS wants to promote use and learning of all its components at universities.

Importantly, SAS prices their licenses for non-university businesses differently. As an example, an independent nonprofit research institute on the campus of a state university in Florida contacted SAS and asked if the research institute could use the university license. SAS did not agree, and instead, prepared a license for PC SAS strictly for the research institute. This license only had one seat, and only had the base component of SAS ("base SAS") and the basic engine that runs regression functions ("SAS STAT"). This one-seat license cost the nonprofit approximately $10,000 per year in 2007, so the nonprofit could not add extra seats. Hence, researchers who learned SAS at the university and then went on to be hired as scientists at the nonprofit research institute were not able to use their extensive knowledge of all the components of SAS due to the prohibitively expensive licensing approach.

Because R is open source, there is no licensing fee, so R is perfectly suited for public health work in low- to middle-income (LME) countries, nonprofits, and businesses with a low profit margin. This book can hopefully help bridge the gap between SAS and R for SAS-experienced healthcare analysts who are priced out of the market by this situation.

SAS Components versus R Packages

Base SAS, the core of SAS, is a rather large program. As mentioned before, the main R program that is downloaded from CRAN is much smaller than the SAS setup program, and therefore, downloading it is fast and installing it is very easy. The drawback is that just about anything the user tries to do once installing R will require an outside component not in the base program, called an R "package."

Because R is not licensed for purchase, it is much more efficient for each user to simply build their version of R by installing the packages needed. Admittedly, this can be a daunting task, as some packages are based on other packages, so these all need to be installed. For example, to make a Kaplan–Meier plot in R, the user must install the "`survival`" package, as well as the "`KMSurv`" package [2]. More recently, packages are designed to automatically install packages on which they are dependent, so this problem does not occur as frequently anymore.

Luckily, as with the base R program, all the packages are free and are easy to install from within the program. In the native R UI, there is a menu with only seven selections, and "packages" is one of them. If the user chooses the "packages" menu and selects "load package," the UI presents a list of packages that can be installed, and the user just needs to select the correct ones and install them. Packages can also be installed using commands, but the load package menu makes the process extremely easy.

What is RStudio?

This book gives guidance on using the PC version of R in Windows as it appears with its native UI. R's native UI is typically sufficient to be used by healthcare analysts to develop statistical models. However, there is also an integrated development environment (IDE) that can be used called RStudio. This is supported by the R Consortium, which is a collaboration between the R Foundation (which maintains CRAN), RStudio (a collection of R developers working on the IDE), and other big tech companies such as Microsoft and Google [3]. Like R, RStudio is also open source and free to individual users.

RStudio is different than R in that it is an IDE and includes a source code editor, build automation tools, and a debugger. RStudio can be run as a desktop or server version, so it is used at universities in programs that teach programming in IDEs [4]. It is an excellent tool for deploying Shiny, which is an R package that interfaces R with the web and turns R analyses into web applications [5].

Generally, the capabilities afforded by RStudio are required for deploying web applications, but for hypothesis-driven healthcare analytics, RStudio can be overkill. For example, RStudio has several windows that are associated specifically with the IDE, and would not appear in R. Therefore, unless the analyst needs an IDE, using R rather than RStudio is preferred.

Maintaining Current Versions in SAS versus R

When using a university SAS license, there is a month in the year that the license expires because these are set up as yearly licenses. When the license expires, the user can still open the SAS program, but it throws up an error message indicating the user will need an updated text file with a new license, and does not let the user unlock the program until this is loaded. At this point, the user must obtain the new text file from the university, and from within SAS, load this license, thus unlocking the program. Although SAS does update its base program with new version from time to time, it does not do it often, so renewing the license is much more common than installing a new version of SAS.

Part of the reason SAS does not update its base program often has to do with how it determines what to put in updates. Independent SAS programmers typically develop macros (canned code procedures) in SAS macro language and make these available on the Internet. These are not held in a central repository but posted all over the Internet, and are also highlighted in SAS white papers presented for regional as well as national and international user groups [6–8], which are also not available in a central indexed repository (although they are posted on SAS-sponsored websites and are easy to find through a search on the web).

If a particular macro becomes popular with SAS users, some may choose to write a peer-reviewed article about it [9], fostering discussion of the macro in the SAS community. If SAS receives enough requests to include the macro as a main function in SAS, and can verify the functioning of the macro, SAS may choose to include it in its next build. This is a decision made by SAS on a business level, not by the SAS user community, so opinions may differ between the user community and the business as to what macros should be included as procedures, or "`PROC`s," in new versions of SAS.

R does not have the constraints SAS has with respect to innovation and change management. First, its base program is very lean, which means it is not difficult to update and disseminate. For this reason, new versions of R can be released quite often (at least once per year). The penalty for the R user is that if she wants to update her core version of R, she will have to reload all the R packages she has been using to carry on with her analysis. An advantage is that the newest version is always available on the CRAN site for free, as are the packages, and this means that the only loss in efficiency is through time required to update the R core program and reload the packages. Also, R developers have created packages available on CRAN that can be loaded and configured to run automated functions to help R shops keep their base R and all its packages updated on a regular basis.

SAS macros that are not available within the program are documented all over the Internet by individual programmers, just like R packages that are not official or are under development. However, macros built into SAS as commands or "`PROC`s" are well-documented in SAS's online and paper help files. Similarly, R's published packages are well-documented on the CRAN website [10], as standardized comprehensive documentation is required to be approved to have a package published to CRAN.

When SAS updates its program, it includes updates to its core, new macros built in as `PROC`s, and updates to old PROCs and functions as well. This means that production operations dependent on SAS can effectively plan for change management. Conversely, because R updates its core regularly, and the authors of their packages also update their packages idiosyncratically, maintaining the most up-to-date version of R is actually rather challenging in a production environment. Independent tools, functions, and routines have been developed to assist with this task [11], but it is important to emphasize that those running R in production must be proactive in maintaining the most up-to-date versions of R and packages being used in production.

It must be noted that R has a different method than SAS in deciding what packages to include on CRAN. Like with SAS, R users can prepare and publish unverified packages for R online [12,13], and adventurous R users can test them. If the package is deemed worthy by many, the author may apply to have the package included on the CRAN site (and thus have it show up in the "load package" menu). But depending upon the package, installing a new package may effectively require devoting 15 min or more to loading different packages on which a new package might be based, and testing the results to make sure the new package can actually run. When this happens, the R user may nostalgically muse about how easy it is to run macros and PROCs in SAS by comparison, but once the packages are sufficiently loaded in R and running well, this nostalgia generally passes.

SAS versus R User Communities

SAS is known for its expansive support for its user community. SAS organizes "SUGs," or SAS User Groups, and provides logistic and financial support for conferences requested by user groups [6–8,14,15]. These conferences produce an extensive set of non-peer-reviewed white papers that promote the use of all of SAS's various components by helping the user deal with the unnecessary complexity of SAS. These white papers are unfortunately of varying quality; some are well-written and helpful, whereas others are poorly written and confusing, and there seems to be little in the way of consistent standards as to what is accepted as a SAS white paper. Nevertheless, SAS users are provided a fertile opportunity to thrive academically with SAS given the many opportunities offered to publish white papers and present them at meetings of SUGs, as well as the vast amount of documentation available online that results from the publication of these white papers, which effectively facilitates the adoption of SAS's more complex functions.

On the other hand, R, which is an open-source software and therefore does not have a conference or marketing department, has a different landscape when it comes to user groups and community gatherings. Meetup.com, an online platform designed with tools meant to be used to build communities through the scheduling of informal meetings or "Meetups," has been used extensively by the R community to gather old hands as well as early adopters together informally for mutual presentations [16]. Unlike with SUGs, these Meetups are community-initiated and supported, so they are held in cheaply available spaces, and often garner little or no industry financial support.

Happily, this trend is changing, as R is piquing interest with big players, most notably Microsoft, which purchased Revolution Analytics in 2015. Revolution Analytics was an R shop that specialized in improving data handling in R so as to enable it to process larger datasets [17]. In addition, larger scale gatherings, such as the Effective Applications of the R Language (EARL) conference, which is now held twice per year on two different continents, is sponsored by various members of industry, including Mango Solutions, a long-time big-ticket R analytics consulting group founded in 2002, as well as Microsoft itself [18].

SAS versus R User Interfaces

The PC SAS interface provides a birds-eye-view of many of SAS's functions all at once. On the left panel, the user can toggle between a list of results (output) and an explorer window that will show the contents of "work" (the temporary directory where SAS puts datasets while it is running) as well as other libraries mapped with the `LIBNAME` statement. Through this panel, the user can easily open and view the datasets (in *.sas7bdat format) in the mapped libraries.

In the main panel, users can display multiple windows at once. The user can open multiple code windows (which can be saved as *.sas files), display the log window (which shows the log of executed statements as well as error messages, and can be saved as a *.log file), as well as view an output file that can be displayed in hypertext markup language (HTML) and saved separately.

R's interface runs differently. Like SAS, the R PC interface allows for multiple windows to be opened at once, but the function of the windows is different. When R is launched, only one window is opened automatically, and this is called the R console. This window is where statements will be executed, log statements will be recorded, and tabular and numeric output will appear.

Next, the user can open one or more code editing windows. R has a menu with only five choices: File, Edit, Packages (described earlier), Windows, and Help. Choosing File—New Script from the menu will open a new code editing window. If the users saves a file from this window (Choose File—Save As when the code window is selected), it will be saved as an *.R file.* Please note that it is easy to open *.R files in Notepad or another word processing program without needing to load R.

Once the user has a code window open, she can prepare code and run it in the console by either copy/pasting it from the code editing window into the console and pressing "enter," or by highlighting the code in the code window, right-clicking and choosing "Run line or selection" (also Control-R), and this will transfer the code to the console and run it. Or, she can simply type code directly into the console and hit "enter," and the code will run.

An important point to be made here is that although R has an extensive array of statements that could be used to do the equivalent of mapping a `LIBNAME` in SAS, probably the easiest way to set a singular default directory

* Our experience is that occasionally, the *.log extension used in SAS is already designated to default to another application in Windows (thus prompting a dialogue box during installation). So far, we have not encountered extension conflicts in R.

is to run the R program, select the console, then using the menu, choose File—Change Dir. This will allow the user to navigate to the directory on her PC or server where most of her R project is stored, and this will make loading code from that directory much simpler throughout the session. Please note that this designation will end at the end of the R session. Also, please take notice of the fact that if the code window is selected and the user chooses File—Open Script, the browser will default to the last code directory used, but if the console is selected, the same operation will bring the user to the directory designated during the File—Change Dir function.

The console is the place where the following appear: log messages, error messages, and non-graphical output. For example, if the user requests a frequency table, or conducts a calculation, or asks for the number of observations in a dataset, after the line of code is run in the console (displayed in red text), this information will be reported subsequent to the code (displayed in blue text). The console will continue to fill up with a history unless the user chooses Edit—Clear Console. Clearing the console from time to time may be helpful for the user involved in a large project, and might be seen as equivalent to clearing the log file in SAS.

Because so many different types of messages appear in the console when R code is run, saving "log files" is not as straightforward in R as it is in SAS. (Please notice that the menus change depending upon whether the console or the code window is highlighted.) Other options exist in the console's set of menus, but it may serve the user best if the user wants to save elements of the session (such as error messages for later troubleshooting, spontaneously formed code in the console, or log messages) to select the console window and choose Edit—Select All, and then choose Edit—Copy.* Next, the user can switch to a word processing environment (such as Notepad or Microsoft Word) and choose Paste or Control–V.

At this point, it is important for the user to edit the pasted text to remove the elements of the output not wanted to be saved in the manually edited "log file."† Because the R log files require some hand-editing, there are both pros and cons. An advantage in R, unlike in SAS, is that the user can easily remove parts of the text that are unimportant to her (such as confirmation of reading in a data file, or reports of successful execution of simple commands). It is also easy to annotate these parts to provide insight into the documentation being kept. The disadvantage is that this effort constitutes work that is generally not done when SAS log files are saved. In reality, however, anyone who has dug through SAS log files to troubleshoot the execution of a large batch of code might not consider this feature of R a disadvantage!

* Please note that the menu must be used to execute the Select All command, but after that, Control-C can be used in lieu of Edit – Copy command.

† Users familiar with SPSS will consider this reminiscent of the output window in SPSS, which is easy to save in an SPSS analysis, but hard to understand after the fact if the file is not somehow reduced, rearranged, or annotated.

This is because actually organizing a log file into what is important and annotating it builds in efficiency later when troubleshooting may be necessary, especially when a programming team is involved. Otherwise, it may not be helpful to save the log file in the first place.

Finally, R handles graphical output files somewhat similarly to PC SAS in that it opens and displays graphics in a separate window. The window automatically opens when graphics requests are run in the console, and the window is titled R Graphics. Once this window is open, the user can select it (which changes the menu options) and choose Save As, where the user is presented a list of formats to choose from, including the popular *.pdf, *.png, and *.jpg. If *.jpg is chosen, the user is offered the selection between 50%, 75%, and 100% quality.

R's handling of graphics represents a strong advantage over SAS, because in SAS, the output function for graphics always involves the rigid and complex "output delivery system," or ODS, which produces files that generally need to be post-processed in another program to be made even minimally presentable for journal publication or even presentation in an informal meeting. In SAS, the alternative to this requires advanced expertise on the part of the programmer to set options in SAS to modify the output as SAS commands are executed so the resulting graph does not need extensive post-processing.

With R, this entire complexity is avoided, and even a basic graphics editor such as Paint can be used to manually add detail to *.png and *.jpg graphics files saved from R in this way. Further, as will be demonstrated later in this book, but most specifically in Chapter 2, little expertise is required to add elements through programming code to graphical output in R, such as adding labels to x and y-axes, whereas these functions require much more programming ability when done in SAS.

Code Documentation and Metadata: SAS versus R

A classic common challenge in any statistical program when working with large datasets to complete a complex, long-term health data analytics project involving an interdisciplinary team, a lot of data, a lot of code, and a lot of time, is entropy.* A part of this entropy that can drive the programmer to distraction is having trouble keeping track of the meaning, content, and method of generation of both the native variables (the variables present in the original data file used in the analysis) and the new variables the programmer creates through code that edits data. For this reason, *in both SAS and R as well as any other statistical program,* the following modern process for maintaining code files is recommended:

1. Code files should be relatively short and focused on only one function (e.g., reading in a dataset, running histograms, running frequencies, running regressions).

* A close colleague has referred to this phenomenon as "biostatistics paper hell."

2. Code files should have a numerical prefix that causes the code files to line up in the order in which they should be run, followed by a shorthand label indicating the function of that code (e.g., 100_Read in data, 105_Run summary statistics, 110_Create age group variable).
3. Advanced users can designate logic and naming conventions with respect to these prefixes (code starting with 00n indicates pre-processing, code starting with 10n indicates code that edits data, code starting with 20n indicates analytic code that does not edit data, code starting with 70n indicates exploratory code).
4. Prefixes should not be named in increments of 1 to allow for insertion of code in between code files at a later date (e.g., naming code "100_read in data," with the next code being named "105_create age group variable" will allow for the possibility of insertion of code "103_*" after the fact, in case minor post-processing is found to be required after reading the data in).

An analogy can be made to making a movie. Although viewers perceive the movie as happening in chronological order, the director and actors are aware that the scenes are actually not shot in chronological order. As a data "director," the programmer may develop "scenes" (programming commands) for later in the "movie" (such as regression code), only to find that to make the story straight and clear, she has to redo scenes from earlier in the movie (such as generating a new variable in the analytic dataset). This way, if the age group variable she created has an error or needs to be changed, she can go back to the code earlier in the "movie," edit this code properly, then start from the beginning and run the whole "movie" of code from the beginning to the present state to make sure the story hangs together after the edit.

Along with this principle, the importance of prolific and well-organized comments in code, *in both SAS and R as well as any other statistical program*, cannot be overstated. In SAS, commenting is done in between bookends of /* and */ (e.g., /***This is a comment***/) or by simply using * at the beginning of the line (e.g., ***This is a comment**). R uses the second approach to commenting (e.g., #**This is a comment**), but not the first. Therefore, although old hands at SAS might be familiar with SAS banners that precede the code in code files, these are not used in R.

This discarding of banners before code actually represents an innovation; modernly, SAS banners (as well as banners in other statistical code) are to be strongly discouraged in health data analysis. Instead, the information that would have belonged in the SAS banners of the 1980s and 1990s programming styles should now be placed instead in an outside program that is more accessible (such as Microsoft Word or Excel) and follow an organized standard. Banners contain information that is human-generated, such as notes on interpretation of variables or variances from standards in programming, not information that can be automatically generated, such as a list of field names and attributes.

Many long-term SAS programmers have not learned this new principle, and this inhibits clear communication and discussion about the nature of the data, code, and analysis, as non-programmer managers and subject matter experts in other fields in healthcare and science cannot easily view this metadata reported in the SAS banners. Hence, today, SAS banners should be avoided in code, and R code should also not include banners, and should only include prolific, carefully-worded and carefully-placed comments. While some programmers shun excessive commenting, given the modular approach recommended to developing code files, many code files are short, so the comments do not complicate comprehension of the code.

Additionally, datasets themselves should not be documented in actual code anymore, and all dataset metadata should be developed and made available in easily accessible word processing and spreadsheet applications (such as Microsoft Word and Excel) or else in the less-recommended PDF format.* This means that SAS "labels" and "formats" should no longer be used, and instead, this information should appear in a data dictionary document, preferably in a spreadsheet format. An excellent example of publicly available metadata that is presented in optimal format is the set of metadata developed for the US Military Health System Data Repository, the MDR [19].† The MDR's use of this approach to metadata ensures that those receiving MDR data files can study them adequately before attempting to read them into any statistical software. This excellent set of metadata also provides researchers from all fields necessary documentation to aid them in developing intelligent and informed data requests prior to receiving the data.

SAS programmers have historically embedded the metadata of variable meanings, meanings of various categories in categorical variables, or information about complex code functions that require explanation in their actual SAS files, not in external metadata. This means that the actual file of SAS code that assigns labels to variables in a dataset, and SAS `FORMAT` code that labels the meanings of various levels of a categorical variable, would sometimes be the only documentation of what these variables mean. This effectively limits the ability of an interdisciplinary team to use the metadata and complicates the interdisciplinary communication required to complete a health analytics project successfully. It also essentially quashes the prospect of group troubleshooting if multiple programmers are using different types of statistical software.

On the other hand, using the methods described here of code organization, naming conventions, and metadata maintained external to the statistical program, the programmer can not only reduce the time and complexity associated with troubleshooting but also make sure that such a "movie" can

---

* PDF format is harder to navigate, copy, and paste, compared to Microsoft Word and Excel.

† For an excellent example, the reader is encouraged to download the M2 data dictionary from the MDR web site, which is formatted in Microsoft Excel, and browse the different tabs to better understand the optimal format of metadata described in this section.

be watched and understood by an outside programmer. This is especially important for scientific writers who may be lucky enough to have their work accepted in a top-tiered journal, such as the *Journal of the American Medical Association* (JAMA) or the *New England Journal of Medicine* (NEJM). If this occurs, the journal requests the code and data from the analyst and hires an independent statistician to verify the results from the analysis. Following these coding and documentation conventions can make this transfer of knowledge accurate and easy. If the programmer finds herself is such a situation, without much complexity, she can provide the metadata files as well as an organized compendium of code to the verifying statistician with an air of professionalism while leaving little room for miscommunication during the transfer process.

Handling of Data

This section begins with a short description of some issues with SAS data handling that must be understood to make an informed comparison with R data handling. Next, features of R data handling will be described and contrasts between SAS and R data handling will be highlighted. Third, basic differences in SAS and R code syntax will be explained, followed by a discussion about how to approach the thought of SAS macros when developing code in R. Finally, an explanation of approaches in R equivalent to SAS labels and SAS formats will be described.

A Focus on SAS Data Handling

In order to effectively contrast SAS data handling with R data handling, it is extremely important to gain at least a working knowledge of the issues inherent in SAS data handling. This is because SAS data handling is particularly complex, and therefore is the topic of many SUG-initiated white papers [6,14].

The main reason SAS data handling is so commonly discussed that it is more complex than that of other modern programs, and relies on the user developing extremely efficient code using SAS's commands. SAS's current yet historical "data step" language (which is used for data editing in SAS) is unnecessarily restrictive and complex simply due to lack of modern innovation which is now possible.* Even in the current version, SAS executes data

* The monopoly status of SAS has relieved much pressure on the company to improve the product in this way. Also, those who are data step masters may feel their positions threatened by users of simpler data editing software, so they inadvertently collude with SAS by continuing to study, receive certifications in, and promote the use of SAS data step language.

steps by reading row by row (observation by observation) and executing code in the data step to that particular row. SAS then walks to the next qualifying row and performs the set of code again, being stuck in an implied loop [20]. This means that any indexing in SAS is most efficiently done by simply sorting the SAS dataset by the indexing variable before executing a function. In other words, when executing data step code on records where a field is a certain value, sorting by that field will make the execution of the SAS code go faster. Sorting may seem easy, but the sort function itself is inefficient and can take enormous amounts of time depending on the dataset and SAS implementation [21].

Aside from the complexity of the data step code, the second main reason that data step functions are discussed *ad nauseum* in SAS white papers is that to overcome the inefficiency of these data step functions, the programmer needs to craft optimal code to ensure data management functions execute in a reasonable timeframe as is generally required of a "procedural" language.* Crafting this optimal code requires much study of data step language and function. Compare this situation to that with structured query language (SQL), which is a "declarative" rather than "procedural" language. This means that the user declares what she wants returned in her query output with relatively simple code, and a query optimizer running in the background automatically generates an evidence-based optimized execution plan based on known dataset information such as the performance of prior, recent queries. Thus, the query executes according to an optimal plan developed on-the-fly as a custom algorithm from the query optimizer, taking into account all information known by the optimizer about the query at the time (such as location of certain types of data within the dataset being queried).

When the process is described this way, one does not need to make a leap to realize how much more efficient developing data editing code is in SQL, which relies on a well-designed optimizer, when compared to programmer-developed data step language in SAS, which is more prone to inefficiencies. In reaction to this expanding realization among SAS users, SAS developed `PROC SQL`, which is not really a `PROC` but a "language within a language." While adopting the characteristics of SQL and being much more intuitive and easier to use than SAS data step language, SAS `PROC SQL` is prohibitively inefficient in processing and cannot be used on large datasets. This is due to an inefficient optimizer that results in extremely slow-executing queries, leading disappointed SAS users back to the data step drawing board [22].

Comparison to R Data Handling

Before making a direct comparison between R's and SAS's handling of datasets, it is necessary to take one step back and look at the "forest" of R and SAS

* Note that the nomenclature of "PROCs" in SAS point to its procedural processing feature.

rather than the "trees" of specific functions in R and SAS. SAS was developed expressly for data analysis, meaning importing large datasets and running statistical analyses on them. SAS has certainly developed other functions—such as data editing commands, commands to execute calculations, and commands to set global variables—but these were all developed with the endgame of a statistical analysis in mind. For this reason, although SAS can execute functions like defining global variables, SAS's core processes largely revolve around the manipulation of datasets and executing statistical calculations on them.

R, on the other hand, was not designed expressly to handle datasets. Although it is excellent at this function, it is also used for complex mathematical calculations, and is deployed extensively in the field of engineering. Instead of having the separate, specially-designed functions expressly for handling datasets that SAS has—data steps, `PROC`s, macros, and other SAS functions—R has generic functions for handling not only datasets but also all the other types of objects in R [20]. Although SAS users tend to think of programming in terms of dataset editing and analysis, it is important to adopt a different perspective when approaching R for these functions. It is more useful to consider R as a multifaceted program with an extensive set of functions for the user to apply, and the health data analyst chooses to use the functions helpful for dataset editing and analysis. This book is a guide to choosing these functions.

Here are examples as to where this difference plays out. In SAS, health analysts work with datasets and also arrays—which are a defined group of columns in a SAS dataset. In R, there are other objects. The main R object data analysts use is a "data frame," which is similar to a SAS dataset. However, in R, it is possible to make a "vector," which is a single column of variables all of the same type, a "matrix," and a "list" (collection of objects) [20]. This ultimately is an advantage if the R user learns how to make use of these other objects to assist in data analysis, as they are not available to the SAS user.

SAS can be used in an object-oriented way, but this is not typically done in health analytics. However, R is completely object-oriented—which is why it is so much easier to create and invoke objects in R compared to SAS [20]. This difference also sheds light on how R processes indexes differently than SAS. When R is used for data analysis, the main object is a dataset—which should be coerced to be a "data frame" object in R. The first column of the R data frame needs to be a primary key, or a column where all the numbers are unique. This column is designated as the "row.names" column in R. In a published dataset, there is usually a column already existing that has this attribute that can be used as the row.names column. However, if there is not one, R generates one on loading, which is similar to the OBS or observation count generated by SAS when loading a dataset.

These differences are reflected in basic differences in how code is formed in R versus SAS, and those impact how the programmer should approach designing code. The next sections will describe some high-level differences in thought that need to be applied while designing a project in R versus SAS.

Basic Differences in Code Syntax: R versus SAS

As SAS users know well, SAS's functions revolve around two main areas: `PROCs`, for running procedures, and data steps, for editing data. These different functions are each complex, but they are necessary to use for completing even a basic statistical analysis. The data step code is a language unto itself, whereas the `PROCs` tend to use similar syntax (call procedure, set arguments). In SAS, data steps are what are typically used to create dataset objects for analysis. However, for outputting results from data analysis, such as a frequency table resulting from running a `PROC FREQ`, the ODS must be used. Therefore, to leverage all of SAS's functionality, ODS syntax must also be learned by the programmer. SAS also offers the ability to make macros using "macro language," which is very similar to data steps and `PROCs`, but there are nuances that can create troubleshooting headaches [23]. This means that for building code for analyses that will be repeated regularly, the programmer must also master SAS macro language. In addition, graphing and other non-analytic `PROCs` in SAS tend to have extremely complex arguments (such as `PROC TABULATE`, which is intended for designing nicely formatted tables in SAS [24]). This complexity of the various functions needed from SAS to complete a statistical analysis can pose challenges even for a relatively fluent programmer.

In contrast to SAS, R really only has two basic syntax approaches: one used for making objects and the other used for analysis. The syntax used for making objects is basic. First, a string is stated (the name of the object the programmer wants to create), followed by the less-than sign and a dash, which form an arrow visually (<-).* Finally, the argument of what should be copied into the object is stated. This is illustrated below.

```
SexVetFreq <- table(BRFSS_a$SEX, BRFSS_a$VETERAN3)
```

In this code, the table command is used to create a frequency table between two variables, `BRFSS_a$SEX` and `BRFSS_a$VETERAN3`. The arrow command is used to create the resulting object, `SexVetFreq`.

In the second case, if the goal is not to make an object but just to view the results of a calculation, the arrow is not used. This happens in the example below, where the frequency table above is run without making an object.

```
table(BRFSS_a$SEX, BRFSS_a$VETERAN3)
```

The best way to demonstrate this difference is using a short example that will explain the variables used in the example code above. If the user reads in the 2014 Behavioral Risk Factor Surveillance System (BRFSS) dataset

* In some cases, a = can replace the <-, but this format of code is discouraged and the arrow preferred.

(named BRFSS_a in the code) [25], she will find that each respondent has a variable for sex (SEX, 1=male, 2=female) and veteran status (VETERAN3, 1=yes, 2=no, 7=don't know/not sure, 9=refused). Note that the directory containing the SAS dataset referred to in the code below has been mapped to the LIBNAME r. In SAS, if the programmer wanted a frequency table to appear on the screen, the following code could be used:

```
Proc freq data=r.BRFSS_a;
        tables SEX*VETERAN3;
run;
```

But to output the resulting frequency dataset, the programmer is faced with different choices of how to invoke the ODS. The method below uses a version of code described by Myra A. Oltsik in her SAS white paper on ODS and output datasets [26].

```
ods listing close;
ods output CrossTabFreqs=SexVetFreq;
proc freq data=r. BRFSS_a;
       tables SEX*VETERAN3;
run;
ods listing;
```

The output from ODS is admittedly suboptimal. Using this code, SAS outputs dataset SexVetFreq (into the work directory in SAS), which has a predefined structure where each row in the table represents a unique combination of rows and column values (e.g., SEX=1 and VETERAN3=1) and has a fixed set of attributes reported, such as percent of row and percent of column. A table of this structure is hard to utilize in subsequent processing.

Compare the same code in R, which was shown earlier. The frequency table command is output to the console using this code:

```
table(BRFSS_a$SEX, BRFSS_a$VETERAN3)
```

Note that this table just has the raw frequencies. SAS users may be more accustomed to also seeing row percentages, column percentages, and other items that come with the default output in SAS from PROC FREQ. Other SAS users may be adept at using PROC FREQ's options to reveal or suppress certain calculations on the output, or to request a particular type of output on screen.

In R, obtaining more information from this frequency table is handled differently than in SAS. The first step is to make an object out of the raw frequency table. Unlike with the SAS ODS, the way to turn this table into an object in R is to use the arrow and name the resulting object, as was demonstrated earlier.

```
SexVetFreq <- table(BRFSS_a$SEX, BRFSS_a$VETERAN3)
```

The raw frequency table is now saved as an object named `SexVetFreq`. Users who want to see the row percentages can run the prop.table function on the new object, the `SexVetFreq` table, and it will output the row percentages:

```
prop.table(SexVetFreq, 1)
```

The argument in the prop.table command "1" indicates that the row percentages should be output. Using the "2" argument will output column percentages, and leaving this argument out of the code will output cell percentages.

There are cases where the programmer needs to refer to proportions in subsequent code. In that case, it would be useful to create an object from the results of the `prop.table` command that can be referred to in other code. We will use the same strategy to output this table with row percentages, naming it `RowPctTbl`:

```
RowPctTbl <- prop.table(SexVetFreq, 1)
```

Hence, for the data analyst working with data frames, much of the work in R can be conceptualized as either running functions on objects that report to the screen (usually raw datasets or summary datasets), or running functions on objects that result in making other objects.

One last note on programming differences: comments are formatted differently in R and SAS. In SAS, banners usually use the commenting approach where /* opens the comment and */ closes the comment.

```
/*A comment in a SAS banner*/
```

Also, SAS users sometimes just use * to open a comment on the fly, and this will be closed automatically at the end of the line if ; is added.

```
Proc freq data=r. BRFSS_a; *comment;
        tables SEX*VETERAN3; *another comment;
run;
```

In R, comments start with # and do not require a close.

```
#row percentages
prop.table(SexVetFreq, 1)
#make row percentage table
RowPctTbl <- prop.table(SexVetFreq, 1)
```

SAS Formats and Labels versus R Approaches

As described before, relying on metadata that cannot be easily read by commonly available software or easily understood by non-statisticians can readily result in inefficiency and miscommunication on a multidisciplinary team when completing a hypothesis-driven health analytics project. Therefore, the practice of using SAS format code as the metadata to define categorical levels in dataset variables, as well as using SAS label code as the metadata to define the meaning of variables, should be avoided. This is because the main function of formats and labels is to make SAS output clear to the non-user, and because there are better ways currently of presenting tables and graphs that are clearer, those on the team who are not SAS users should not be exposed to SAS output. Instead, clearly formatted journal-ready tables in word processing or spreadsheet programs should be presented, as well as journal-ready figures, when the statistician approaches the research team with the results of her analysis. Given these new standards, the use of SAS format code and SAS label code should be sunsetted.

There are not only penalties to using SAS formats and labels as metadata, but their use also introduces problems in using SAS itself. The modular code approach can be difficult as datasets are remade in different code files, making the application of formats and labels a set of code that is difficult to run in the middle of the "movie." Format and label files require updates and maintenance, and each new variable generated needs these items to be applied.

Another problem is that once formats and labels are applied in a SAS dataset, it is difficult to access the actual fieldnames or values in fields for programming purposes except to look them up in metadata, as they generally do not display in SAS after formats and labels are applied, with the label text or format text being what is displayed. Programmers historically used these devices not only for their explanatory function but also because formats and labels can be used in workarounds designed to make SAS run faster [27]. However, outside SAS, format and label files are almost useless. Even as documentation, they are not in a user-friendly format.

If the information that would normally go in SAS labels and formats were instead stored in metadata in a data dictionary format in a spreadsheet similar to the MDR documentation described earlier [19], then this metadata would be sufficient for the R user as well. This means that R would need no equivalent of SAS labels and formats, and this is generally true. However, R does have the capability of reproducing something like SAS labels and formats.

First, R's equivalent of labels can be attached to variables most easily using the `Hmisc` package [28]. After loading the `Hmisc` package, we start by calling up the `Hmisc` library.

```
library(Hmisc)
```

Using the BRFSS 2014 dataset, we will subset it into a dataset called `BRFSShtwt` by just taking four fields to use as examples so it is easier to demonstrate the label and format functions.

```
BRFSShtwt <- BRFSS_a[, c('HEIGHT3','WEIGHT2','SEX',
     'VETERAN3')]
```

Using the label function in `Hmisc`, we will add a label to each of the fields.

```
label(BRFSShtwt$HEIGHT3) <- "Height in inches"
label(BRFSShtwt$WEIGHT2) <- "Weight in pounds"
label(BRFSShtwt$SEX) <- "Respondent's Sex"
label(BRFSShtwt$VETERAN3) <- "Veteran Status"
```

Unfortunately, the only way to make use of these labels is to use other commands in the `Hmisc` package, like describe.

```
describe(BRFSShtwt)
```

Typing this will result in the following output:

```
4  Variables      464664  Observations
--------------------------------------------------------------------------------
HEIGHT3 : Height in inches
      n missing  unique  Info    Mean  .05  .10  .25  .50  .75  .90
 458948    5716     151     1  671.7  500  502  504  506  510  600
   .95
   602

lowest : 207 209 300 302 303, highest: 9196 9197 9200 9204 9999
--------------------------------------------------------------------------------
WEIGHT2: Weight in pounds
      n missing  unique  Info    Mean  .05  .10  .25  .50  .75  .90
 459354    5310     527     1  581.6  118  127  147  175  206  250
   .95
   330

lowest : 50 51 52 57 59, highest: 9248 9260 9280 9300 9999
--------------------------------------------------------------------------------
SEX
      n missing  unique
464664        0       2

Male (192970, 42%), Female (271694, 58%)
--------------------------------------------------------------------------------
VETERAN3
      n missing  unique
464075      589       4

Yes (62120, 13%), No (401561, 87%), Refused (100, 0%)
Dont Know (294, 0%)
--------------------------------------------------------------------------------
```

However, unlike with SAS labels, these will not show up on functions outside of the Hmisc packages, like the table function, for making frequency tables. Consider the output of the following code after adding Hmisc labels:

```
table(BRFSShtwt$SEX, BRFSShtwt$VETERAN3)
```

The output is as follows:

```
         1        2    7     9
1    56596   135840   68   213
2     5524   265721   32    81
```

Unlike in SAS PROC FREQ, after applying the labels using Hmisc functions in R, a table function will not display the names of the fields. So, the Hmisc label function is not really useful for labeling fields within objects.

Unlike with equivalent of "SAS labels" in R, the equivalent of "SAS formats" in R can be added more easily. First, the variable must be converted to a "factor" class, one of the data types in R. Next, label text for the various levels of the categorical variable are attached to each factor level. The factor class is used in R for categorical variables. If values corresponding to the different levels of the categorical variable are stored as integers in an R column designated as a factor column and later used in a regression, the regression will treat it as a categorical variable.

Here is an example of a code that attaches text for the various levels of the SEX and VETERAN3 categorical variables:

```
BRFSShtwt$SEX <- factor(BRFSShtwt$SEX,
       levels = c(1,2),
       labels = c('Male','Female'))

BRFSShtwt$VETERAN3<- factor(BRFSShtwt$VETERAN3,
       levels = c(1,2,7,9),
       labels = c('Yes','No','Refused','Dont Know'))*
```

Unlike with the field labels as demonstrated using the Hmisc package earlier, these labels on variable levels (equivalent to SAS formats), after being attached, show up in basic functions in R run afterward, such as the table function, which now will produce the following output:

```
           Yes       No   Refused   Dont Know
Male     56596   135840        68         213
Female    5524   265721        32          81
```

As a final note on trying to do the equivalent of SAS labels and formats in R, one place where this concept can be useful is in terms of labeling graphics that output in R. As is the pattern with R, this maneuver is done through

* Please note that the apostrophe was left out of the "Don't Know" level label because including it would throw an error in R.

objects and functions. For example, in making a histogram, options in the `hist` function are set to label the histogram, *x*-axis, and *y*-axis. Here is an example of code that will make a histogram for the continuous variable, age:

```
hist(BRFSS_a$X_AGE80,
        main = "Histogram of Age",
        xlab = "Class Age",
        ylab = "Frequency",
        xlim=c(18,80),
        ylim=c(0,50000),
        border = "red",
        col= "yellow",
        las = 1,
        breaks = 100)
```

Please see Figure 1.1. This code will be revisited later, in Chapter 2, but for now, please notice that the xlab and ylab options are where the user can place text to label these axes. In SAS, these labels are often facilitated through first running code that places labels and formats on the variables. In R, these are typically placed when actually running the plot by setting options.

Note that R also has the flexibility of adding text through a text statement immediately after running the plot. This next code will place text on the plot at the x-coordinate of 30 (`X_AGE80=30`) and the y-coordinate of 20,000 (frequency = 20,000)

```
text(30, 20000, "This is added text")
```

As will be demonstrated in Chapter 2, legends can also be added in a `legend` statement after the statement that generates the plot.

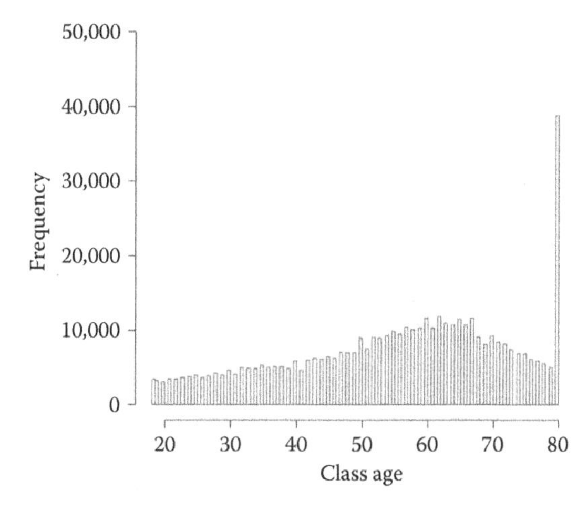

FIGURE 1.1
(See color insert.) Histogram of Age.

In summary, although the equivalent of SAS labels and formats are possible to mimic in R, they are probably not worth the trouble, just as they are usually not worth the trouble in SAS. First, labels on R variables will not work outside of the `Hmisc` package. Next, the equivalent of SAS formats have the same problem in R—they clutter up output with long names as shown above and are only accessible to the R user, leaving users of other software in the dark about the definitions of the various levels of categorical variables. More importantly, the value that can be gained in efficiency in SAS processing by using labels and formats is unnecessary in R, so there is little need to use them.

SAS versus R—What to Choose?

This section will begin with a narrative about weighing the pros and cons of choosing R rather than SAS for public health efforts. At the end, a summary comparison table will be presented.

Why R Can Be a Difficult Choice for Public Health Efforts

R has several main limitations for application to public health efforts. First, probably the most important limitation R has when compared to SAS is that it cannot handle the large datasets that can be quickly processed by PC SAS, not to mention server SAS. SAS data processing is not especially efficient, so much of the gain in speed over the years has been a result of improvements in other technology on which SAS runs. R is efficient, but unable to read in and process extremely large datasets without enhancements such as those provided by Revolution Analytics [17]. As an example, a monthly file from the Defense Management Data Center (DMDC) of the US military of active duty Army soldiers typically contains between 500,000 and 1,000,000 records [29–31]. Hence, a yearly dataset could be as large as 12 million records, and this would be prohibitive for R to process. As with other challenges presented by R, independent developers have created workarounds and enhancements to improve the ability of R to process larger datasets [17], but this main functional limitation still exists and can be prohibitive for some analyses.

A second limitation of R with respect to the field of public health is that SAS has essentially a monopoly on the industry, and this has several ramifications that inhibit the use of R in both obvious as well as clandestine ways. SAS has unfortunately proudly established itself as a particularly expensive monopoly, boasting surpassing $3 billion in revenue in 2013, representing a 5.2% growth compared to 2012 [32]. Due to lack of competitive pressure, rather than using this revenue to prioritize improving the efficiency and reducing the complexity of its product, SAS instead employs a large support team and provides them an exceedingly healthy environment in which to work, while encouraging customers who are facing problems to call and get custom tech support free as part of their licenses [33].

SAS has been a monolith in public health data analytics since its founding, so the US government has typically maintained a relationship with SAS such that government-level datasets released for public consumption are typically available in two formats: ASCII and SAS's dataset transport format (currently *.xpt, which is unpacked using SAS into a *.sas7bdat file). A typical example is the BRFSS data, published by the US Centers for Disease Control and Prevention (CDC), which are published in both a SAS *.xpt and an ASCII file [25].

Of course, reading the ASCII format into any software (including SAS) will require some troubleshooting, so the publication of datasets in SAS transport format essentially guarantees a smoother analysis using SAS than any other program, leading health analysts to lean heavily toward choosing SAS as their software. In fact, code for unpacking the *.xpt file, code for attaching appropriate SAS labels, and code for attaching appropriate SAS formats are provided by the CDC on the data download page [25], thus further encouraging the use of SAS in analysis. As the BRFSS data are pre-processed at the CDC in SAS, documentation of pre-processing also is provided with a reprinting of the exact SAS code used for the pre-processing steps.

In addition to these obvious efforts by SAS to promote the use of its software over others, there are other, more sinister approaches SAS takes to ensure the ubiquity of its software's use in public health. The extensive university license that is available cheaply for students and faculty but creates prohibitive costs for a non-profit if used outside that setting is part of this strategy. Although SAS is glorified for its unique ability to analyze large datasets, the many other functions in SAS, such as the clumsiness of its data handling [6,14] and its unattractive graphing and other output display processes that require much detailed and obscure knowledge to make presentable (compounded by the use of a complicated ODS) [7,8], are often derided by those who are otherwise SAS disciples.

Rightfully, due to the ubiquity of SAS, there can be some apprehension on the part of health data analysts to begin to use R as their predominant software and to put SAS on the back burner. For example, a kerfuffle in the R and SAS communities about whether the US Food and Drug Administration (FDA) would accept drug trial data analyzed in R was put to rest in 2012 by an FDA statistician who reiterated that sponsors may use R in their FDA submissions [34]. This apprehension has been effectively cultivated by SAS over the years and continues to succeed at leading health data analysts away from R. The constant warnings from university statistics professors that R cannot handle large datasets feed this apprehension of switching to R, although most biostatisticians admit they rarely have such large analytic datasets such that they encounter this limitation.

Further, the overall promotion in universities for students to use all components of SAS for all their work, including data management and graphing functions, which are done more effectively in other programs, serve to scare students away from attempting to use other software for the same functions, such as Microsoft Excel for graphing, or SQL for data management. Professors pacify students who are exasperated with SAS's complexity by reminding them that SAS provides access to an extensive and expert support team students can call at any time. Please note that this is in stark contrast to the situation with R, which, due to its open source status, only provides online documentation, thus rendering R users as chronic "do-it-yourselfers," where prohibitive problems require obtaining real-time help from actual R programmers through personal networking or through hiring R consultants to troubleshoot.

These amplified warnings from professors and industry against using R as the main analytic software when there is no readily available tech support team is compounded by the fact that public health data analysts generally enter graduate school without a background in programming, as they are typically biologists, healthcare providers, chemists, or engineers. Thus, SAS becomes their first exposure to the world of computer programming. Hence, the experienced programmer's comfort zone with the principle of "same tasks, different syntax" as they experiment with different types of software aimed at accomplishing the same functions is missing from these public health trainees.

Another more subtle strategy SAS uses to ensure the ubiquity of their software in public health can be found in SAS's extensive, expensive, formalized global certification program that insists the student master the most complex details of the more poorly functioning components as well as the classically excellent ones [35], and consequently, high-profile and prestigious workplaces demand these certifications of their analysts. All of these pressures serve to scare the typical healthcare analyst away from R, and artificially increase adoption of SAS even when other software programs might be more appropriate.

But there is hope. In Bob Muenchen's thoughtful blog post, "The Popularity of Data Analysis Software," which was originally published in 2012 but continues to be updated, the author analyzes and graphs several indicators of the popularity of various data analysis software overall [36]. Muenchen is a well-known expert in the field of data analytics software, and the author of the book "R for SAS and SPSS Users" [37]. As of this writing, his analysis of online job posting data on Indeed.com demonstrates that the percentage of postings mentioning R rose steadily from about 2.5% in 2010 to just over 5% in 2014, and this appears to be trending upward, whereas during the same time, those mentioning SAS fell from approximately 11%–10%, and this appears to be trending downward [36]. Other results presented in the article suggest that R is establishing a stronger presence in not only the job market but also in the fields of big data analytics and academic research [37].

Considerations When Choosing R versus SAS

Table 1.1 summarizes the considerations described in this chapter in the selection of using R versus SAS for a public health data analysis effort.

TABLE 1.1

Considerations in Using R versus SAS for a Public Health Data Analysis Effort

Consideration	SAS	R
Cannot afford cost of non-university license	–	+
Project requires professional graphics	–	+
Programming team is new to both SAS and R	–	+
Project requires efficient coding to be developed in a very short amount of time	–	+
Project involves extensive data editing	–	+
Legacy code is in SAS	+	–
Metadata only exists in SAS files	+	–
Project requires extensive tech support	+	–
Project requires extremely large datasets	+	–
Supporting files published with dataset are in SAS	+	–
Programming team includes experts in SAS who do not know R	+	–
Workplace culture not supportive of use of R or other open source software	+	–

Optional Exercises

All Sections

Questions

1. How does one load a package into R?
2. What is the difference between R and RStudio?
3. How much does an R license cost, and how often is R updated?
4. What are ways to interact with the R community?
5. What are the two basic approaches to syntax in R?
6. How can the equivalent of SAS labels be applied in R?
7. How can the equivalent of SAS formats be applied in R?
8. Even though SAS is standard to use in health analytics, are the results produced by R equivalent?
9. What is the most important functional limitation of R compared to SAS with respect to health analytics?

Answers

1. To load a package in R, choose "load package" from the "packages" menu from within the R UI, and select the package from the list.
2. R has a basic UI, and RStudio is an IDE. The IDE is useful for deploying R-based applications on the web.

3. R licenses are free because R is open source software. For this reason, R is updated frequently. It is not unusual for R to upgrade several times over the course of a year.
4. Attend Meetups on R, as well as R conferences. Unlike with SAS, these are arranged by users as well as companies that use R.
5. Using the <- for creating objects, and not using the arrow when doing calculations that will output to the console.
6. Labels similar to SAS labels can be applied in R using the `Hmisc` package, but they are not accessible outside of the `Hmisc` package.
7. The equivalent of SAS formats can be applied in R through converting the variable to factor class and labeling the various levels as part of the arguments in the command.
8. The results of health analyses in both SAS and R are equally acceptable to journals and government agencies.
9. The most important functional limitation of R compared to SAS with respect to health analytics is R's inability to read extremely large datasets without assistive modifications.

2

Preparing Data for Analysis

This chapter covers all the steps normally followed in SAS to prepare health data for analysis. The first section of this chapter covers reading data into R, and the second section will cover checking the data as would normally be done using SAS PROC UNIVARIATE and PROC FREQ. The third section is very extensive and covers data editing in R. Procedures covered are those typically followed in SAS data steps, and they include removing rows and columns from datasets, creating grouping variables, creating indicator variables, using plots to guide data editing decisions, creating survival analysis variables, dealing with dates, and recoding continuous variables. The last section discusses the last steps in preparing an analytic dataset, including examining bivariate relationships between the variables retained in the analytic dataset. It also discusses power calculations, and reading out the final analytic dataset.

Reading Data into R

This section covers two main tasks associated with writing data into R. The first part covers how to import data into R. The second part explains how to use R to obtain the information reported in a PROC CONTENTS command in SAS as that is generally the first procedure conducted after reading data into SAS.

Importing Data

SAS users are generally familiar with the challenges associated with reading data into SAS that is not already in the *.sas7bdat format. Datasets in the *.sas7bdat format are easily read into SAS by setting a LIBNAME mapping to where the dataset resides and conducting a simple data step. Imagine a dataset named BRFSS in the *.sas7bdat format. We can set the LIBNAME as a folder where this SAS dataset is stored, and then easily read it in with a data step.

```
Libname r "D:\Dropbox\Dropbox\R Stats Book\Analytics\Data";
data BRFSS;
   set r.BRFSS;
run;
```

However, if the SAS dataset is not in the *.sas7bdat format, reading it in gets more involved. Large datasets like the Behavioral Risk Factor Surveillance System (BRFSS) dataset from the Centers for Disease Control and Surveillance (CDC) are stored in the *.xpt format, which is essentially equivalent to a "zipped" version of a *.sas7bdat file, and needs to be unpacked using commands aimed at converting a *.xpt file into a *.sas7bdat file [25]. Datasets in the *.txt and *.csv formats, as well as in other formats, can also read into SAS, but different coding is needed for each. The `PROC IMPORT` function in SAS helps, but even this needs to be configured properly [38].

As mentioned in Chapter 1, R users generally do not set the equivalent to a `LIBNAME` using code. Instead, once the R session is running, users choose File—Change Dir, and browse to the directory holding their data files. This sets a default directory for the session. In this case, we would choose the directory containing the *.xpt file so that when we run R commands to read in the data, R will look in that directory.

The commands for reading various data formats into R are much more straightforward, thanks to the "`foreign`" package [39]. Not only will commands from the foreign package easily help read in a SAS *.xpt or *.sas7bdat file, but the package can also help the user read in data in SPSS's *.sav format, STATA's *.dta format, as well as other software formats.

Here is an example of reading in the BRFSS 2014 dataset stored in the *.xpt format to R (naming it `BRFSS_a`) as mentioned earlier using the foreign package:

```
library(foreign)
BRFSS_a <- read.xport("D:/Dropbox/Dropbox/R Stats Book/
Analytics/Data/LLCP2014.xpt")
```

It is worth pointing out that there are other methods to use to read data into R, such as the read.table method [40]. However, these tend to be fraught with errors and challenges similar to those experienced by SAS users importing data through a data step. For this reason, the foreign package is highly recommended for reading data into R.

Checking the Dataset after Reading It in

In SAS, after reading in a dataset, it is typical to check the contents of the dataset (meaning the names of the columns) using a `PROC CONTENTS` command, and it is also typical to check the log file to see if the number of observations read in matches what is expected, or else, to see if there are any errors. As an example, we will show the code to unpack the BRFSS *.xpt file in SAS:

```
/*libnames r and target point to the same location, but are
named differently to make it easier to explain the coding.*/
/*libname xportin points to the specific XPT file to be
unpacked.*/
```

```
Libname r "D:\Dropbox\Dropbox\R Stats Book\Analytics\Data";
Libname target 'D:\Dropbox\Dropbox\R Stats Book\Analytics\
Data';
libname xportin xport 'D:\Dropbox\Dropbox\R Stats Book\
Analytics\Data\LLCP2014.XPT';

/*data step reads it in and unpacks it into libname mapped
to r*/
/*the native file is called LLCP2014.xpt*/

data target.xpt_infile_2014;
   set xportin. LLCP2014;
     run;
```

This operation registers the following in the SAS log file:

```
NOTE: There were 464664 observations read from the data set
XPORTIN.LLCP2014.
NOTE: The data set TARGET.XPT_INFILE_2014 has
464664 observations and 279 variables.
```

Next, we will run a `PROC CONTENTS` command to see the field names in the dataset:

```
Proc contents data = r.Xpt_infile_2014;
   run;
```

The output from this command is two different headers followed by a long table with all of the fields listed in alphabetical order by default. This list includes the data type and length of the field, as well as any labels attached. Table 2.1 shows an example with only certain fields reported for brevity.

Please notice that BRFSS has fields that begin with an underscore (indicating by the dataset authors that these are calculated fields). This fact will become important later when we try to do the same operation in R.

TABLE 2.1

Example of `PROC CONTENTS` Output

Alphabetic List of Variables and Attributes				
#	**Variable**	**Type**	**Len**	**Label**
37	ADDEPEV2	Num	5	Depressive disorder
70	ALCDAY5	Num	5	Days in past 30 had alcoholic beverage
141	ASACTLIM	Num	5	Activities limited due to asthma during
...	...	...	...	...
201	_AGE80	Num	8	Imputed age value collapsed above 80
233	_AGE65YR	Num	8	Reported age in two age groups calculate
232	_AGEG5YR	Num	8	Reported age in 5-year age categories

Before we continue, let us choose some naming conventions. Let us start with renaming our new SAS dataset from xpt_infile_2014 to BRFSS_a. The "a" indicates that the dataset is in memory, not written out to disk. As the dataset is updated, we will increment this suffix up one letter (e.g., the next one will be called BRFSS_b). That way, if the update fails, we can easily roll back to earlier versions of the dataset.

Note that in R, we already named the dataset BRFSS_a as we read it in, but we did not do that in SAS because of the complexity of the commands associated with reading in an *.xpt file. In SAS, copying the dataset to a new dataset with the name BRFSS_a is accomplished with a data step:

```
data r.BRFSS_a;
     set r.Xpt_infile_2014;
run;
```

Since we already have run the PROC CONTENTS command on this file in SAS, we need to now accomplish the same work in R. Unlike in SAS, in R, the number of observations is not reported in the console when the read.xpt code is run. Therefore, after reading in the file, we need to use the nrow command to see the number of rows. Here is an example of running the nrow command on BRFSS_a and seeing the results that show up in the console:

```
nrow(BRFSS_a)
```

Output:

```
[1] 464664
```

When using the nrow command, we do not see the same output as we would see in a SAS PROC CONTENTS command. We only see the resulting number of rows.

PROC CONTENTS also gives us a list of column names. We can obtain a list of column names in R using the colnames command. Here is an example of the colnames command, and a subset of the output in the console window, again, shortened for brevity:

```
colnames(BRFSS_a)
```

Output:

```
   [1] "X_STATE" "FMONTH" "IDATE" "IMONTH" "IDAY" "IYEAR"
   [7] "DISPCODE" "SEQNO" "X_PSU" "CTELENUM" "PVTRESD1"
"COLGHOUS"
  [13] "STATERES" "LADULT" "NUMADULT" "NUMMEN" "NUMWOMEN"
"GENHLTH"
...
```

```
[193] "HHADULT" "QSTVER" "QSTLANG" "MSCODE" "X_STSTR"
"X_STRWT"
[199] "X_RAWRAKE" "X_WT2RAKE" "X_AGE80" "X_IMPRACE" "X_IMPNPH"
"X_CHISPNC"
```

First, it is important to notice that the default in R has the columns reported in the order they are in the dataset, not in alphabetical order like SAS's `PROC CONTENTS` default. A second important thing to notice is that R does not like it when fields start with an underscore, so instead, it adds an X before the field name. Notice how `_AGE80` in the SAS `PROC CONTENTS` output has turned into `X_AGE80` in the R output. Also, observe how R numbers the columns in the output. You can see [1] at the beginning of the list, and then [7] on the next line, indicating that line is starting with the seventh column name.

Also, unlike SAS, R does not automatically report the field type and the field length with the `nrow` and `colnames` commands after a dataset is read in. To find the field type of a column, the `class` command is used. For example, we will look at the class of `X_AGE80`:

```
class(BRFSS_a$X_AGE80)
```

Output:

```
[1] "numeric"
```

Note that if we use the command `class(BRFSS_a)` (without a field name specified), the answer will be "`data.frame`," as that is the type of object `BRFSS_a` is.

We can also look at the length of a field in R, which is another element that gets output in `PROC CONTENTS`. The length reported in `PROC CONTENTS` refers to the numeric constant that is the number of bytes used for storing the variable values [41]. This is a technical point, because calculating variable length in R will take a different approach.

One might assume that to obtain the same measurement in R, we could use the length command. However, "`length`" does not work that way in R. The code `length(BRFSS_a$X_AGE80)` would give us, the number of observations in that field, which is (as we know from our count of observations) 464,664.

We instead use the `nchar` command which is designed for counting the number of characters (or bytes) [42]. The `nchar` command is meant to be run on character fields (meaning they are in the character class), not ones that are factors, are numeric, or are in any other class. Because of this, the `as.character` function is used to have the `nchar` command consider the field numeric for the purposes of counting the length, as shown in the following code. Because there are so many rows in this dataset, we can use the "`head`" command to request just showing the first 10 rows, so we can provide a succinct example:

```
head(nchar(as.character(BRFSS_a$X_AGE80)), n=10)
```

Output:

```
[1] 2 2 2 2 2 2 2 2 2 2
```

Because we are aware of the dataset structure, and that each field has a maximum length that is the field length reported in the SAS PROC CONTENTS command, a workaround is just to request the maximum nchar of the field to know the field's length:

```
max(nchar(as.character(BRFSS_a$X_AGE80)))
```

Output:

```
[1] 2
```

From this, we know that the field BRFSS_a$X_AGE80 is two characters long, and from running the class command earlier, we know this field is numeric.

Admittedly, R does not really give the same kind of the PROC CONTENTS output we are used to seeing in SAS. The examples given here are piecemeal ways to try to generate the same information in R that is normally reported with an SAS PROC CONTENTS. However, there is a package named Hmisc that has a contents command that works something like PROC CONTENTS [28]. Previously, we used the Hmisc package in Chapter 1 to demonstrate attaching labels to R variables. Now, we will call up the Hmisc library and use the contents command.

```
library(Hmisc)
contents(BRFSS_a)
```

Here is the beginning of the output from this command:

```
Data frame:BRFSS_a   464664 observations and 279 variables
Maximum # NAs:464664

         Levels Storage  NAs
X_STATE          double    0
FMONTH           double    0
IDATE       399 integer    0
IMONTH       12 integer    0
IDAY         31 integer    0
IYEAR         2 integer    0
DISPCODE         double    0
SEQNO            double    0
```

Notice that the variable is listed on the left along with the number of levels (such as 12 for IMONTH, which is the month of the year in which the interview took place in BRFSS), the type of storage used for the variable, and the number of NAs (missing). Unfortunately, when the variable is stored as "double" instead of "integer," the number of levels in the categorical variable is not displayed (note DISPCODE versus IMONTH).

The output above continues for all variables, and after that, output in the following format appears (note that IDATE, the first variable with levels, was removed for brevity from the following output):

```
|Variable|Levels                                              |
+--------+----------------------------------------------------+
|IMONTH  |01,02,03,04,05,06,07,08,09,10,11,12                 |
+--------+----------------------------------------------------+
|IDAY    |01,02,03,04,05,06,07,08,09,10,11,12,13,14,15,16,
          17,18,19,20,21,22,23,24,25,26,27,28,29,30,31       |
+--------+-----------------------------------------------------
-------------------------------------------------------------+
|IYEAR   |2014,2015                                           |
```

At first glance, these levels seem very useful for profiling the dataset. After all, levels do not print out in SAS PROC CONTENTS. However, as noted before, only those variables stored as integer and not double will produce this output from the contents command in Hmisc, and since very few of those exist in the BRFSS dataset, this feature is not particularly useful.

In reality, whether using SAS or R, it is typically necessary to run checks on each field that will be used in an analysis individually, especially when preparing to recode or transform a variable. The next section covers doing these operations.

Checking Data in R

This section will cover checking our raw variables in R. First, we will review how to check continuous variables in R the way we would normally do in SAS using PROC UNIVARIATE and how to generate plots to reveal data distributions. Next, we will discuss how to check categorical variables in R the way we would do in SAS with PROC FREQ—first as single variables and next as a crosstab.

Statistics on Continuous Data in R

In the BRFSS dataset, most continuous variables have some categorical coding. For example, the answers to the survey question "On average, how many hours of sleep do you get in a 24-hour period?" is associated with variable SLEPTIM1, which is coded as 1–24 hours, 77 for don't know/not sure, and 99 for refused. This coding means that this variable would have to be recoded before looking at distributions or any other summary operations would make any sense.

However, the variable talked about previously, `_AGE80` (named `X_AGE80` once read into R), is a calculated variable, and is defined as "Imputed Age value collapsed above 80" in the codebook. It takes on the real values of 18–99, so we can use this native variable to demonstrate checking a continuous data field before diving into describing recoding, which we will cover in the next section.

In SAS, with continuous variables, our first instinct is typically to run a `PROC UNIVARIATE`:

```
proc univariate data = r.BRFSS_a;
   var _AGE80;
   run;
```

The default output to `PROC UNIVARIATE` is organized into five sections. The first reports "moments," which includes summary statistics such as mean and standard deviation, as well as sums of squares. The second reports "basic statistical measures"; this includes the mean and standard deviation as well as other summary statistics such as median and mode. The third reports "Tests for Location: Mu0=0," meaning it reports test statistics and *p*-values for testing whether the mean of the variable is 0, something that is rarely needed in healthcare analytics. By contrast, the fourth reports output that is particularly useful for healthcare analytics, and those are "`quantiles`," including percentiles 0, 1, 5, 10, 25, 50, 75, 90, 95, 99, and 100. Finally, the last section of the default output of `PROC UNIVARIATE` lists the lowest and highest observed values.

As was seen with the `PROC CONTENTS` example, all of the default `PROC UNIVARIATE` outputs can be made available through R commands, but there is not one overarching function that will provide everything. This is not a particularly bad problem, because, as noted before, default `PROC UNIVARIATE` sometimes provides duplicate output for the same metric (such as mean, standard deviation, and median), and also provides output that is not needed (such as the tests for location where μ is hypothesized to be 0).

One command that is particularly useful in R to get summary statistics of a continuous variable is "`summary`." See the results of running the summary command on the `X_AGE80` field:

Code:

```
summary(BRFSS_a$X_AGE80)
```

Output:

```
 Min.   1st Qu.   Median    Mean    3rd Qu.    Max.
18.00    44.00     58.00    55.49     69.00   80.00
```

As seen from the output, the minimum (`Min.`), 25th percentile (`1st Qu.`), median, mean, 75th percentile (`3rd Qu.`), and maximum (`Max.`) are reported. To report only one of these items, the label can be added in quotes and brackets after the `summary` command.

Code:

```
summary(BRFSS_a$X_AGE80)["Mean"]
```

Output:

```
Mean
55.49
```

If requesting one of the items with a different label, make sure to include the label in quotes exactly as it is written. For example, in requesting the maximum, we need to make sure that we include the period in the request.

Code:

```
summary(BRFSS_a$X_AGE80)["Max."]
```

Output:

```
Max.
   80
```

Noticeably, while the summary command provides quartiles (including median) and mean, it does not include standard deviation, as well as many other metrics provided in `PROC UNIVARIATE`. It also does not provide some of the percentiles, such as the 99th, the way `PROC UNIVARIATE` does. We can remedy this by using the `quantile` command where we can request exactly which percentiles we want.

First, let us run the `quantile` command on the field `BRFSS_a$X_AGE80` and see what defaults we get. We set the `na.rm` option to `TRUE` meaning that we want the NAs removed from the consideration of `quantiles` (although technically, since there are no NAs in `BRFSS_a$X_AGE80`, we would not have to do that anyway).

```
quantile(BRFSS_a$X_AGE80, na.rm=TRUE)
```

Output:

```
0%  25%  50%  75%  100%
18   44   58   69    80
```

Using the quantile command and the "prob" option, we can request the same probabilities that PROC UNIVARIATE provides us:

```
quantile(BRFSS_a$X_AGE80, na.rm=TRUE, prob = c(0.00, 0.01, 0.05,
   0.10, 0.25, 0.50, 0.75, 0.90, 0.95, 0.99, 1.00))
```

Output:

```
0%   1%   5%   10%   25%   50%   75%   90%   95%   99%   100%
18   19   24    30    44    58    69    78    80    80     80
```

The quantiles that were helpful in PROC UNIVARIATE are available under the quantile command using the prob option, but we still have not generated the other useful metrics that come out of PROC UNIVARIATE—namely, the summary statistics.

R without packages can produce these in various ways. For example, the mean command will produce the mean:

```
mean(BRFSS_a$X_AGE80, na.rm=TRUE)
```

Output:

```
[1] 55.49154
```

Similarly, we can use the sd command for calculating standard deviation:

```
sd(BRFSS_a$X_AGE80, na.rm=TRUE)
```

Output:

```
[1] 16.85709
```

But again, this is piecemeal and not very convenient. A lot of R programmers noticed this, and they developed packages that will output batches of summary statistics, such as Hmisc [28], pastecs [43], and psych [44]. In terms of summary statistics, the package psych's "describe" command probably comes closest to what would be seen in PROC UNIVARIATE [44]*:

```
library(psych)
describe(BRFSS_a$X_AGE80)
```

* Each package has its own set of commands, and several packages have specified a "describe" command. This command will be executed according to the package most recently loaded (the one most recently placed in the "library" command before the "describe" command).

Output:

```
  vars      n  mean    sd median trimmed   mad min max range skew kurtosis   se
X1    1 464664 55.49 16.86     58   56.38 17.79  18  80    62 -0.4    -0.77 0.02
```

These commands and packages can be used in R to provide the same info as the `PROC UNIVARIATE` output. However, we also usually want to visualize continuous variables in R, which will be covered in the next section.

Visualizing Continuous Data in R

There are many ways continuous data are visualized in SAS. An easy way that can be used is by simply calling a `PROC UNIVARIATE` and requesting the "`normal plot`" option.

```
proc univariate data = r.BRFSS_a normal plot;
   var _AGE80;
   run;
```

Adding "`normal plot`" after the data argument in `PROC UNIVARIATE` adds on three plots to the summary statistics output: a histogram on its side, a box plot, and a quantile–quantile (QQ) plot. While these plots are nice, any modifications to them can be challenging in SAS, and also exporting and manipulating them can be a challenge as well.

As shown in Chapter 1, in R, we can already make a histogram of this variable, and easily set some parameters for customization:

```
hist(BRFSS_a$X_AGE80,
   main = "Histogram of Age",
   xlab = "Class Age",
   ylab = "Frequency",
   xlim=c(18,80),
   ylim=c(0,50000),
   border = "red",
   col= "yellow",
   las = 1,
   breaks = 100)
```

Please refer to Figure 1.1 in the color inset for the plot. As can be seen, the `hist` command is used to visualize the variable, and options are easy to set. The option `main` sets the title, while `xlab` and `ylab` set the x-axis and y-axis labels, respectively. Options `xlim` and `ylim` set the limits, which might take some trial and error, but can be informed by the previous descriptive statistic output. The `border` option allows for setting a color for the border, and the `col` option allows for setting a color for the bars.*

* R has a large selection of colors, all of which can be referred to by number or a name [45].

The `las` option is not as obvious; this sets the orientation of the number labels on both the axes. We chose `las=1`, which made the *y*-axis labels perpendicular to the axis, and the *x*-axis labels parallel to the axis—meaning that all the labels look "right-side-up." To make the *y*-axis labels parallel to the *y*-axis but keep the *x*-axis labels as they are in `las=1`, we can set `las=0`. To make the *x*-axis labels perpendicular to the axis and leave the *y*-axis labels as they are in `las=1`, we can set `las=2`. Most histograms, though, would use labels in the orientation of `las=1`.

Finally, breaks sets how many `breaks` there are in the data, meaning how many bars get graphed in the histogram. There are other options that can be set, but for the purposes of observing the distribution of a continuous variable, this histogram plot is sufficient.

Next, we can use the `boxplot` command. Let us try some different colors—blue for the border and green for the interior—this time.

```
boxplot(BRFSS_a$X_AGE80,
   main = "Box Plot of Age",
   ylab = "Age in Years",
   border = "blue",
   col= "green")
```

The inset in Figure 2.1 shows the results of this box plot. Often, we like to compare distributions in groups, and because the native `SEX` variable in BRFSS has complete values, and either `MALE=1` or `FEMALE=2`, we can demonstrate a box plot where the SEX groups are plotted separately.

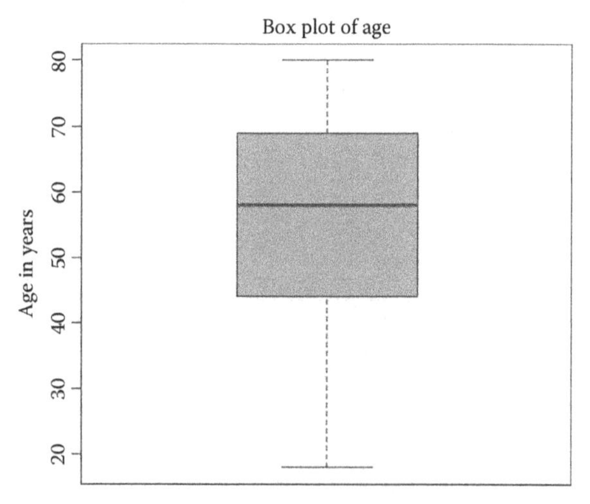

FIGURE 2.1
(See color insert.) Box plot of age.

```
boxplot(BRFSS_a$X_AGE80~BRFSS_a$SEX,
        main = "Box Plot of Age by Sex",
        ylab = "Age in Years",
        xlab = "Sex",
        names = c("Men", "Women"),
        border = "black",
        col=(c("gold","darkgreen")))
```

The resulting plot is not shown, but you can see examples in Figures 2.8 and 2.9, and box plots by groups will be covered more extensively in Section 3. Notice that how we got R to produce separate box plots of age by sex was by using a tilde (~) between the variable being graphed, `BRFSS_a$X_AGE80`, and the grouping variable, which is `BRFSS_a$SEX`. Another nuance is that we used the `names` command to designate that the left plot was for men and the right one was for women—otherwise, the values of 1 and 2 would have been printed. Also, notice how we designated the color so that the plot for men was gold, and the plot for women was dark green.

Finally, we can make an attractive QQ plot using the following code:

```
qqnorm(BRFSS_a$X_AGE80,
       main = "Q-Q Plot of Age",
       col= "pink")
qqline(BRFSS_a$X_AGE80,
       col = "purple")
```

Please see the color inset for the plot, which is Figure 2.2. As you can see, for the QQ part of the plot, we use the `qqnorm` function. Again, `main` puts a title

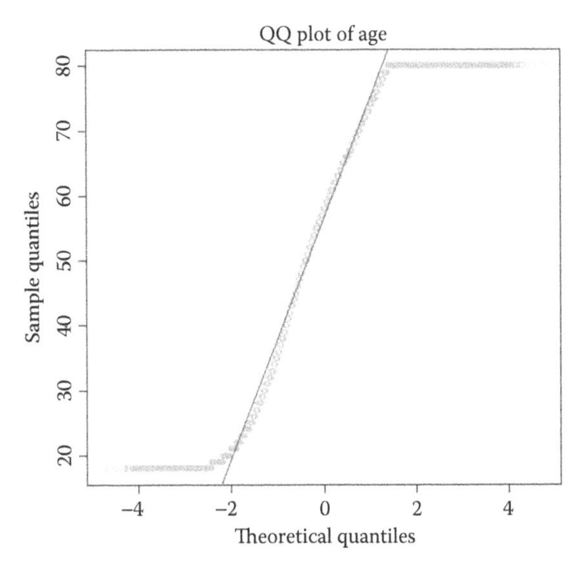

FIGURE 2.2
(See color insert.) QQ plot of age.

on the plot, and col determines the color. Typically, however, the QQ plot is hard to interpret without a line as a reference. Hence, the qqline command is called right after the qqplot command, thus placing the line on top of the QQ plot.

Now that we have covered how to do data-checking approaches we typically do in SAS in R for continuous variables, we can move on to looking at categorical variables.

Statistics on Categorical Data in R: One Variable

In SAS, when it comes to categorical data, PROQ FREQ is your friend, although the default PROC FREQ output is admittedly quite cumbersome. This is because it reports a huge pile of numbers crushed into a small, tabular format. Default PROC FREQ output reports row frequencies and percentages, column frequencies and percentages, marginal frequencies and percentages, and total frequencies and percentages. Also, the default in SAS PROC FREQ is to ignore the missing values, so without using the "missing" option, it is not possible for these percentages to include the missing variables in the denominator.

Because default PROC FREQ output is so cumbersome, analysts typically use options whenever they run PROC FREQ. An easy solution to reducing the output to something visually manageable and to include the missing values in the denominator of percentages is to include the /list missing options in the tables command. This can be demonstrated with the variables VETERAN3, which is veteran status (1=Yes, 2=No, 7=Don't know/Not sure, 9=Refused, Blank=Missing):

```
proc freq data = r.BRFSS_a
     tables VETERAN3 /list missing;
     run;
```

This output lists each level (including missing), the frequency at each level, the total percentage of rows in the dataset in that level, the cumulative frequency as the levels advance, and the cumulative percentages. Admittedly, this is not the most useful output; row percentages and column percentages are often also needed. Reporting those along with these metrics requires setting more options in the PROC FREQ command. Also, it is important to acknowledge that outputting the table displayed would require an output delivery system (ODS) call, and the resulting table would not be in the same format (meaning it would not have the same rows and columns).

It is a little easier to customize frequency output in R. First, we will use the table command to demonstrate the simplest version of a frequency in R, as we mentioned in Chapter 1. We will add the useNA = c("always") option to make sure the missings come out in the output.

```
table(BRFSS_a$VETERAN3, useNA = c("always"))
```

Output:

```
    1       2    7    9  <NA>
62120  401561  100  294   589
```

While the output is much simpler than PROC FREQ, it leaves much to be desired, in that all the percentages are missing, and there is no other information that comes out by default besides the frequencies. The package `summarytools` includes a `freq` command that approximates the output of `PROC FREQ` with the `/list missing` option, and this can be useful [46]:

```
library(summarytools)
freq(BRFSS_a$VETERAN3)
```

Output:

```
Frequencies

Dataframe name: BRFSS_a
 Variable name: VETERAN3

              N    %Valid    %Cum.Valid    %Total    %Cum.Total
-----    ------   -------    ----------   -------    ----------
    1     62120     13.39         13.39     13.37         13.37
    2    401561     86.53         99.92     86.42         99.79
    7       100      0.02         99.94      0.02         99.81
    9       294      0.06           100      0.06         99.87
 <NA>       589        NA            NA      0.13           100
Total    464664       100           100       100           100
```

In healthcare analytics, we are often asked to visualize data in a pie chart, although critics have written *ad nauseum* about how bad it is to use pie charts for the visualization of data, mainly because they lend themselves to error in visual interpretation [47]. Nevertheless, those who are unaware of the debate often request pie charts, and they expect the analyst to supply them. For this reason, we present a way of visualizing the distribution of levels in `VETERAN3` in a pie chart format here.

Referring back to our output from the `table` command, the order in which the levels were reported was numerical, with the NAs being last. This means that we can create a vector with the labels in it, so long as it is the same length (has five entries, one for each level), and that the entries are in the same order that the levels are reported. This vector will come in useful for labeling any plots we make of `VETERAN3`.

```
VetLabels <- c("Yes","No","Don't Know", "Refused", "Missing")
```

Because we are using the arrow symbol to make an object, no output is reported in the console. But if we want to see what the vector looks like, we can simply type the name of it, `VetLabels`, into the console.

Code:

```
VetLabels
```

Output:

```
[1] "Yes"  "No"  "Don't Know" "Refused"  "Missing"
```

Now, let us turn our table from the `table` command into an object called `VetFreq`. This is the object we are going to plot in subsequent commands.

```
VetFreq <- table(BRFSS_a$VETERAN3, useNA = c("always"))
```

Again, nothing is reported to the console because we made an object, but we already know what it looks like from when we ran the `table` command earlier without the arrow, which produced output to the screen.

Next, we can use the `pie` command to make the plot. Please notice, though, that the frequencies of the last three levels are so small that the labels for those pieces of the pie will overlap. To remedy this, we have suppressed the labels by telling R to print nothing for the labels, and we follow this up by a legend command that will place a `legend` on the pie chart using the label vector we made.

```
pie(VetFreq,
        col = rainbow(5),
        main = "Pie Chart of VETERAN3",
        label = "")
legend("topleft",
        VetLabels,
        cex=0.8,
        fill=rainbow(5))
```

See Figure 2.3 (top) in the inset for the plot. In our code, the first argument is the table we made called `VetFreq`. Since we want it to graph five levels, if we have no particular preferences for color, we can set color to the rainbow palette—the five in the parentheses specifies to use five colors.* As before, `main` sets the title of the plot, and as described before, setting the label to `""` will prevent the labels from being printed next to each pie piece (which would have been the actual value of VETERAN3).

Next, the `legend` command is called to place a legend on the plot. The first argument, `topleft`, says where to put the legend, and the next command tells the legend to use our vector, `VetLabels`. The `cex` option says how large to scale the legend. The default is `cex=1`. As an experiment, change 0.8 to 1, and it is easy to observe the legend be scaled up from 80% to 100%. To scale

* There are five color palettes in R: rainbow, heat.colors, terrain.colors, topo.colors, and cm.colors [48].

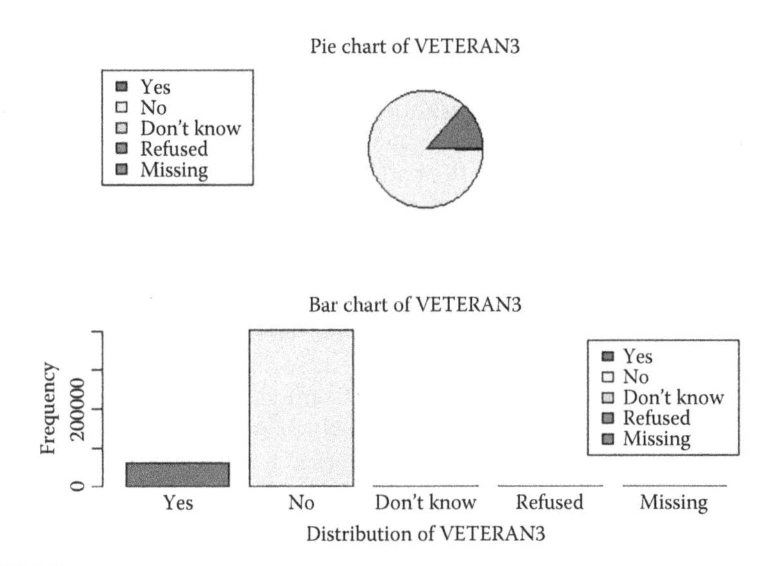

FIGURE 2.3
(See color insert.) Pie and bar chart example from R.

the legend larger, set the `cex` to larger than 1. Finally, we designate the fill to be `rainbow(5)` to match the same colors we used in the pie chart.

Please note that the following SAS code achieves a similar pie chart:

```
TITLE 'Pie Chart of VETERAN3';
PROC GCHART DATA=r.BRFSS_a;
      PIE VETERAN3/ DISCRETE VALUE=INSIDE
                 PERCENT=INSIDE SLICE=OUTSIDE;
RUN;
```

For those who avoid pie charts and would prefer a bar chart, we include this barplot code:

```
barplot(VetFreq,
      col = rainbow(5),
      xlab = "Distribution of VETERAN3",
      ylab = "Frequency",
      yaxt = "n",
      main = "Bar Chart of VETERAN3",
      names = VetLabels,
      legend = VetLabels,
      args.legend=list(cex = 0.8))
axis(2,
      axTicks(4),
      format(axTicks(4),
      scientific = F),
      las=0,
      cex=.5)
```

See Figure 2.3 (bottom) for the inset of this bar chart. Notice that like with the pie command, the barplot command's first argument is the frequency table we made. The xlab option determines what the *x*-axis will be labeled, and main is the title of the chart. The yaxt = "n" suppresses printing the y-axis; we will make a custom axis at the end of the barplot command to prevent the numbers on the axis labels from being printed with scientific notation. The names command is used to label the bars, and again we use our VetLabels vector for that; otherwise, the raw values would be reported. Unlike pie, barplot includes a legend option, so we set that to VetLabels and our legend matches our barplot. We want to make the legend a little smaller, but in order to add arguments to the legend we are calling as part of the barplot code, we need to use the args.legend option. Inside the args.legend option, we list the arguments we will set – which in this case is only cex = 0.8, to make the legend only 80% of the size it would normally be. In the code after this starting with axis, we add the y axis we suppressed with the yaxt option in the barplot code. The first argument, 2, says we are drawing a y-axis (vertical and on the left). axticks(4) and format(axticks(4)) set that there will be four tickmarks, and scientific = F sets scientific notation to false, so the labels will not print in scientific notation. Finally, las=0 sets the orientation of the label on the axis, and cex=.5 makes the label 50% of original size.

To make the pie chart and barplot appear side by side, we precede the plotting with the par command:

```
par(mfrow=c(2,1))
```

The par command indicates how many rows of figures (we designate two), and how many columns of figures (we designate one, to make them appear on top of each other). Par(mfrow=c(1,2)) would make them appear side by side.

SAS code to produce a similar bar chart is given here:

```
TITLE 'Bar Chart of VETERAN3';
PROC GCHART DATA=r.BRFSS_a;
       VBAR VETERAN3/ DISCRETE;
RUN;
```

Statistics on Categorical Data in R: Crosstabs

Once the data are read in, not only is it necessary to check each individual categorical variable, but the analyst should also examine the crosstabs, especially for identifying small cells. The simplest way to perform a crosstab in R is by adding a column to the table command. We will demonstrate this by adding the variable ASTHMA3, which is whether or not the respondent has ever been told that he or she has asthma, and is coded using the same values as VETERAN3.

```
table(BRFSS_a$VETERAN3, BRFSS_a$ASTHMA3, useNA = c("always"))
```

Output:

```
              1       2      7     9   <NA>
  1        5693   56213    171    43      0
  2       55660  344636   1059   206      0
  7          10      85      5     0      0
  9          34     240      3    17      0
  <NA>       75     513      1     0      0
```

The output is problematic because it is unclear which axis is which. For the record, whichever variable is listed first will be the rows (in this case, `VETERAN3`), and the one listed second will be the columns (in this case, `ASTHMA3`). Again, this problem can be solved by using a package. SAS users who like the default `PROC FREQ` output will enjoy using the package `gmodels`, which has a `CrossTable` command that approximates the `PROC FREQ` output [49].

```
library(gmodels)

CrossTable(BRFSS_a$VETERAN3, BRFSS_a$ASTHMA3)
```

Output:

```
   Cell Contents
|-------------------------|
|                       N |
| Chi-square contribution |
|           N / Row Total |
|           N / Col Total |
|         N / Table Total |
|-------------------------|


Total Observations in Table: 464075

                 | BRFSS_a$ASTHMA3
BRFSS_a$VETERAN3 |        1|        2|      7|        9| Row Total|
-----------------|---------|---------|-------|---------|----------|
               1 |     5693|    56213|    171|       43|     62120|
                 |  776.051|  117.580|  0.168|    1.535|          |
                 |    0.092|    0.905|  0.003|    0.001|     0.134|
                 |    0.093|    0.140|  0.138|    0.162|          |
                 |    0.012|    0.121|  0.000|    0.000|          |
-----------------|---------|---------|-------|---------|----------|
               2 |    55660|   344636|   1059|      206|    401561|
                 |  120.826|   17.964|  0.140|    2.538|          |
                 |    0.139|    0.858|  0.003|    0.001|     0.865|
```

```
                |    0.907|    0.859| 0.855|    0.774|          |
                |    0.120|    0.743| 0.002|    0.000|          |
----------------|---------|---------|------|---------|----------|
               7|       10|       85|     5|        0|       100|
                |    0.789|    0.024|83.981|    0.057|          |
                |    0.100|    0.850| 0.050|    0.000|     0.000|
                |    0.000|    0.000| 0.004|    0.000|          |
                |    0.000|    0.000| 0.000|    0.000|          |
----------------|---------|---------|------|---------|----------|
               9|       34|      240|     3|       17|       294|
                |    0.616|    0.788| 6.260|1681.141|          |
                |    0.116|    0.816| 0.010|    0.058|     0.001|
                |    0.001|    0.001| 0.002|    0.064|          |
                |    0.000|    0.001| 0.000|    0.000|          |
----------------|---------|---------|------|---------|----------|
    Column Total|    61397|   401174|  1238|      266|    464075|
                |    0.132|    0.864| 0.003|    0.001|          |
----------------|---------|---------|------|---------|----------|
```

Noting the key to the cells at the top, SAS users will find this output familiar. But admittedly, we generally do not want all of this info in our crosstab output. Usually, when doing an analysis, we are concerned with the proportions of one variable as they relate to another. For example, we may be concerned that veterans have a higher proportion of asthmatics compared to nonveterans. In this case, veteran status is the denominator, and asthma status would be the numerator.

This issue can be dealt with by turning the table into an object, and then running the `prop.table` command on it (with different options). Let us first create the table as an object called `VetAsthmaFreq`.

```
VetAsthmaFreq <- table(BRFSS_a$VETERAN3, BRFSS_a$ASTHMA3,
useNA = c("always"))
```

If we want to know what proportion of veterans are asthma sufferers (meaning we want to use the row as the denominator), we can run `prop.table` on `VetAsthmaFreq` with the 1 option:

```
prop.table(VetAsthmaFreq, 1)
```

Output:

```
                1            2            7            9         <NA>
1    0.0916452028 0.9049098519 0.0027527366 0.0006922086 0.0000000000
2    0.1386090781 0.8582407156 0.0026372083 0.0005129980 0.0000000000
7    0.1000000000 0.8500000000 0.0500000000 0.0000000000 0.0000000000
9    0.1156462585 0.8163265306 0.0102040816 0.0578231293 0.0000000000
<NA> 0.1273344652 0.8709677419 0.0016977929 0.0000000000 0.0000000000
```

As we can see, among veterans (row 1), the proportion with asthma (column 1) is about 0.0916, and the proportion without asthma (column 2) is about 0.9049. On the other hand, if we want to see what proportion of asthma sufferers are veterans, we can run the same command, only with the 2 option.

```
prop.table(VetAsthmaFreq, 2)
```

Output:

```
                1            2            7            9 <NA>
1    0.0926112702 0.1399422934 0.1380145278 0.1616541353
2    0.9054528891 0.8579715052 0.8547215496 0.7744360902
7    0.0001626757 0.0002116075 0.0040355125 0.0000000000
9    0.0005530973 0.0005974801 0.0024213075 0.0639097744
<NA> 0.0012200677 0.0012771138 0.0008071025 0.0000000000
```

Now, we see that the proportion of those with asthma (column 1) who are veterans (row 1) is about 0.0926, and the proportion of those without asthma (column 2) who are veterans is about 0.1399.

Let us assume that we care more about the proportions of veterans versus non-veterans with asthma (row proportions), and we want to visualize this in a stacked bar chart. We can use the `barplot` command again and reuse our `VetLabels` vector. However, we need to make a vector for labeling the asthma levels also; this will be named `AsthmaLabels`.

```
AsthmaLabels <- c("Yes","No","Don't Know", "Refused", "Missing")

barplot(VetAsthmaFreq,
        col=terrain.colors(5),
        xlab="Veteran Status",
        main="Asthma Status by Veteran Status",
        names = VetLabels,
        legend = AsthmaLabels)
```

The resulting plot is not shown, but stacked barplots are shown in Figure 2.10 and are discussed at length in the third section. Notice how this time, instead of using the rainbow palette, we use the `terrain.colors` palette (specifying five colors, one for each level of `ASTHMA3`). The `names` command refers to the labels on the x-axis, so we used our `VetLabels` vector for this, and the legend describes the asthma levels, so we use our `AsthmaLabels` vector for this.

Once we have a chance to take a look at the distribution of all of the variables we contemplate using in our analysis, we find that we generally need to edit them. Editing the `data.frame` will be covered in the next section.

Editing Data in R

This section explains how to perform data editing tasks normally done in an SAS data step. First, removing columns from datasets, and then subsetting datasets by applying inclusion and exclusion criteria will be covered. Next, methods to create categorical variables will be covered, including creating new grouping variables, indicator variables for different types of categorical variables, missing flags, and a binary outcome variable for logistic regression or survival analysis. Third, how to prepare time-to-event times will be demonstrated, with a short discussion of dealing with dates. Finally, this section will end with a demonstration on how to recode and classify continuous variables.

Trimming off Unneeded Variables

Earlier in the chapter, we read in the entire BRFSS 2014 data file, but the reality is that we will only need to use a small set of these variables in our analysis. When doing an epidemiologic analysis, we hypothesize that a particular *x*, or independent variable, is associated (possibly causally) with a particular *y*, or dependent variable. We call the *x* an "exposure" and the *y* the "outcome."

For example, we may hypothesize that alcohol consumption (exposure) is associated with average hours of sleep per night (continuous outcome), or alcohol consumption is associated with having asthma (categorical outcome that can be collapsed into a binary variable of "yes" and "not yes"). Regardless of whether we are predicting an association between the exposure and a continuous outcome, or the exposure and a categorical outcome, we acknowledge that the outcome can be caused by other factors. For example, hours of sleep per night have been shown to be influenced by age, and asthma status has been shown to be influenced by whether or not a person smokes cigarettes.

This brings up a discussion of confounding variables, also known as "confounders." As a quick review, the definition of a true confounding variable is one that meets three criteria: (1) is associated with the exposure, (2) is associated with the outcome, and (3) is not on the causal pathway between the exposure and outcome [50]. The confounding variable also cannot be a "surrogate" for the outcome, meaning that it cannot be a characteristic that always or almost always accompanies with the outcome.

How to tell if a variable needs to be included in the analytic dataset to see if it indeed confounds the relationship between the exposure and outcome during multivariate regression is not straightforward. That is because it is often not known if the variable meets the criteria for a confounding variable. How analysts choose variables as potential confounders to include in their analytic datasets is often not described in reports [51,52]. For the purpose of the demonstrations in this book, the potential confounding variables to include in the analytic dataset were guided by a review of the scientific literature for the decisions made by other analysts using BRFSS data or analyzing similar hypotheses [53,54].

We ultimately will want our regression models to control confounders, so that they will appear as other x's in our model along with the exposure. Hence, our dataset at this point only needs to contain the native variables that we will need to determine the exposure, the outcomes, and the confounders. Our first step should be to trim off the variables we do not need.

For our example analysis, imagine that we selected the following factors as candidate confounding variables: age, smoking status, sex, ethnicity, race, marital status, general health status, health insurance status, highest education level, household income level, obesity status, and exercise status. In addition to the raw variables needed for us to identify our exposure and our two outcomes, we will also need to keep in our dataset the raw variables needed to classify our potential confounders.

In SAS, that would typically be done by incrementing our dataset from `BRFSS_a` to `BRFSS_b` in a data step, and using a long keep statement:

```
data r.BRFSS_b;
      set r.BRFSS_a (keep =
                VETERAN3
                ALCDAY5
                SLEPTIM1
                ASTHMA3
                _AGE_G
                SMOKE100
                SMOKDAY2
                SEX
                _HISPANC
                _MRACE1
                MARITAL
                GENHLTH
                HLTHPLN1
                EDUCA
                INCOME2
                _BMI5CAT
                EXERANY2);
run;
```

This is somewhat simplified in R, where we can choose our keep variables and put them in a vector object called `BRFSSVarList`*:

```
BRFSSVarList <- c("VETERAN3",
                  "ALCDAY5",
                  "SLEPTIM1",
                  "ASTHMA3",
```

* Please remember that X's are prepended to the beginning of the names of variables that begin with _ in R.

```
                              "X_AGE_G",
                              "SMOKE100",
                              "SMOKDAY2",
                              "SEX",
                              "X_HISPANC",
                              "X_MRACE1",
                              "MARITAL",
                              "GENHLTH",
                              "HLTHPLN1",
                              "EDUCA",
                              "INCOME2",
                              "X_BMI5CAT",
                              "EXERANY2")
```

Then, this BRFSSVarList can be used to generate BRFSS_b with only the variables in the list:

```
BRFSS_b <- BRFSS_a[BRFSSVarList]
```

Notice that the brackets are used around the vector name to indicate the list of variables we want to keep.

In SAS, this would typically be followed by a PROC CONTENTS of BRFSS_b to verify that the correct variables were kept. In R, the colnames command could be used to verify this.

Applying Qualification Criteria through Subsetting Datasets

Before we proceed with our analysis, we need to make sure that we know to whom our findings will apply. Generally, the hypothesis of the exposure being associated with the outcome is limited to a particular demographic group, so that the results can be externally valid to that group. In this case, let us assume our two hypotheses, that drinking alcohol is associated with average hours of sleep per night, or sleep duration, and that drinking alcohol is associated with asthma status, apply only to veterans. This means that we will have to limit our dataset to veterans only before we proceed with our analysis.

Also, since our dataset is relatively complete, to prevent any issues with our analysis, we should only keep rows in our dataset where the exposure (alcohol status) has a valid entry, and where both of our outcomes (sleep duration and asthma status) also have valid entries.

In SAS, this is typically done in a series of data steps. Each data step applies one criterion, and the output command is used to create two datasets—one containing the records that will be kept and be the subject of the application of the next criterion, and another containing the rows that are removed.

Let us apply our veteran criterion first. This analysis will only be done on veterans (VETERAN3=1), and all other records will be removed. This is code in SAS that would produce BRFSS_c (dataset with only veterans) and BRFSS_b_out (dataset with all other records).

```
data r.BRFSS_c r.BRFSS_b_out;
       set r.BRFSS_b;
       if VETERAN3=1 then output r.BRFSS_c;
       else output r.BRFSS_b_out;
run;
```

After running this code, the log file will report the following:

```
NOTE: The data set R.BRFSS_C has 62120 observations and
17 variables.
NOTE: The data set R.BRFSS_B_OUT has 402544 observations and
17 variables.
```

Doing the same operation in R uses the subset command. First, we will create `BRFSS_c` from `BRFSS_b` using the subset command and keeping only those who have `VETERAN3=1`.

```
BRFSS_c <- subset(BRFSS_b, VETERAN3==1)
```

Please observe that we need to use a double equal sign for equals. The reason why will become apparent when we run our next subset command that will create `BRFSS_b_out` to represent the records removed from `BRFSS_b` to make `BRFSS_c`:

```
BRFSS_b_out <- subset(BRFSS_b, VETERAN3!=1 | is.na(VETERAN3))
```

Notice that the criterion is expressed as `VETERAN3!=1`, with the `!=` meaning "not equal to." The `!` is often used in R preceding an operation to negate it.* Please notice that in R, the expression "`!=` to a particular value" (in this case, 1) does not include the NAs, or missing records. In order to include them, we add a pipe for the "or," and then use the `is.na` command. If, for a row, `is.na(VETERAN3) = TRUE` (meaning `VETERAN3` has NA in it), the row will be added to the `BRFSS_b_out` dataset along with records where `VETERAN3` is set to some other value than 1.

We can verify that we get the same results as SAS by using the `nrow` command on `BRFSS_c` and `BRFSS_b_out`:

```
nrow(BRFSS_c)
nrow(BRFSS_b_out)
```

Output:

```
[1] 62120
[1] 402544
```

* Later in this section, we will cover `!is.na()` for use in identifying where values "are not missing".

Since we just split BRFSS_b into two pieces, BRFSS_c and BRFSS_b_out, theoretically, the number of rows in BRFSS_c added to the number of rows in BRFSS_b_out should total the number of row in BRFSS_b. If not, we made a mistake with our coding. To make sure we really did split the dataset properly, we can use the identical command to test this. The identical command compares two objects, and if they are identical, then it returns a TRUE; otherwise, it returns a FALSE. Here, we use it to see if the number of rows in BRFSS_b is identical to the sum of the number of rows in BRFSS_c and BRFSS_b_out.

```
identical(nrow(BRFSS_b), nrow(BRFSS_c) + nrow(BRFSS_b_out))
```

Output:

```
[1] TRUE
```

R returned a TRUE, so we know that we split the dataset properly.

The example exposure we will be demonstrating in this book, alcohol consumption, is the variable ALCDAY5, and is the answer to the question, "During the past 30 days, how many days per week or per month did you have at least one drink of any alcoholic beverage such as beer, wine, a malt beverage or liquor?" The possible values the answer can take on are 101 to 199 (the leading 1 indicating "per week" and 1–99 indicating how many drinks), 201 to 299 (the leading 2 indicating "per month" and 1–99 indicating how many drinks), 777 (meaning Don't know/Not sure), 888 (meaning "no drinks in the last 30 days"), 999 (meaning Refused), and missing.

As described earlier, it is important to remove all records with no value in the exposure. This means that we should remove all of the records that are coded with a 777, a 999, or missing. Here is some example code followed by our identical test:

```
BRFSS_d <- subset(BRFSS_c, ALCDAY5 < 777 | ALCDAY5==888)
BRFSS_c_out <- subset(BRFSS_c, ALCDAY5 == 777 | ALCDAY5 == 999 |
is.na(ALCDAY5))
identical(nrow(BRFSS_c), nrow(BRFSS_d) + nrow(BRFSS_c_out))
```

Output:

```
[1] TRUE
```

The continuous outcome we will be using for demonstration in this book is SLEPTIM1, which is the answer to the question, "On average, how many hours of sleep do you get in a 24-hour period?" Possible values are 1–24 (meaning number of hours of sleep), 77 (meaning Don't Know/Not Sure), and 99 (meaning Refused). Again, we should remove all records with no value for the outcome, and in this case all records coded with 77 or 99. Also, it is prudent to include a code to remove all records coded as missing.

```
BRFSS_e <- subset(BRFSS_d, SLEPTIM1 < 77)
BRFSS_d_out <- subset(BRFSS_d, SLEPTIM1 == 77 | SLEPTIM1 == 99 |
is.na(SLEPTIM1))
```

Because this operation passes our identical test (not shown), we will move on to the categorical outcome we will demonstrate, which is `ASTHMA3`, where we will remove records with the values 7, 9, and missing.

```
BRFSS_f <- subset(BRFSS_e, ASTHMA3 < 7)
BRFSS_e_out <- subset(BRFSS_e, ASTHMA3 == 7 | ASTHMA3 == 9 |
is.na(ASTHMA3))
```

This passes our identical test, so our working analytic dataset is `BRFSS_f`. In the next section, we will cover editing data to calculate the variables needed for our analysis.

Creating Grouping Variables

Categorical variables with two or more levels can serve as grouping variables, but in most datasets, these need to be created based on calculations from raw data variables. For example, imagine that we wanted a grouping variable for our alcohol exposure that was in three levels: 1=drink weekly (meaning the respondent answered in "drinks per week," or some value 101–199), 2=drink monthly (meaning the respondent answered in "drinks per month," or some value 201–299), and 3=nondrinker (meaning the respondent answered "no drinks in the last 30 days," which was coded as 888). We would need to create a variable in our dataset that was coded this way based on the raw variable `ALCDAY5`. Please recall that we removed all the records with Don't know/Not sure, Refused, and missing because we want to use this factor for our exposure.

We can create a new variable for alcohol grouping (`ALCGRP`) and populate it with the various levels described previously. In SAS, this is often done in a data step where we create the variable by causing it to equal what we would use for a code that indicates an "unknown" level (such as 9), and then editing it on the basis of criteria in the raw variable from which it is derived using if-then statements. Our working dataset is `BRFSS_f`, so if we were using SAS, we would be reading `BRFSS_f` into the data step and outputting `BRFSS_g`. The following SAS code would accomplish creating the recoded variable as described previously.

```
data r.BRFSS_g;
     set r.BRFSS_f;

     ALCGRP = 9;
     if ALCDAY5 <200
          then ALCGRP = 3;
     if ALCDAY5 ge 200 and ALCDAY5 < 777
          then ALCGRP = 2;
```

```
        if ALCDAY5 = 888
               then ALCGRP = 1;

run;
```

In SAS, this data step should be followed by a PROC FREQ examining a cross-tab of ALCDAY5 and our new variable, ALCGRP, to make sure that the recoding was done properly.

In R, before manipulating the dataset, we should copy it to a new dataset so that we can roll back if we encounter problems. In SAS, this is accomplished as a side effect of the data step, but in R, we need to explicitly copy the dataset before manipulating it.

```
BRFSS_g <- BRFSS_f
```

Next, we can follow our approach in SAS by first creating the variable with a value indicating unknown, which is 9. Since we have already removed all of the unknown records for ALCDAY5, this 9 should get entirely overcoded in a subsequent code, but for instantiating the variable and later checking, it is useful.

```
BRFSS_g$ALCGRP <- 9
```

Just as we used the arrow to copy the entire dataset, now we use the arrow to populate a new field entirely with the value 9. Then, we execute the code to repopulate the variable if ALCDAY5 meets certain criteria, as we did in SAS:

```
BRFSS_g$ALCGRP[BRFSS_g$ALCDAY5 < 200]<- 3
BRFSS_g$ALCGRP[BRFSS_g$ALCDAY5 >=200 & BRFSS_g$ALCDAY5 < 777]
<- 2
BRFSS_g$ALCGRP[BRFSS_g$ALCDAY5 == 888] <- 1
```

Notice that the criteria go to the left of the arrow in brackets, not the right. Notice also the "and" operator used in updating the "drink monthly" level. After running this code, just like with SAS, it is important to check to see if the variable is recoded properly. This can be done with a simple table command between the two variables.

```
table(BRFSS_g$ALCDAY5, BRFSS_g$ALCGRP, useNA = c("always"))
```

The output is very long, because there are many levels of the variable, but here is an example of the beginning of the output.

```
          1       2     3 <NA>
    101   0       0  2454    0
    102   0       0  1888    0
    103   0       0  1334    0
```

```
104  0     0  634    0
105  0     0  686    0
106  0     0  309    0
107  0     0 2011    0
201  0  4353    0    0
202  0  3271    0    0
203  0  1890    0    0
204  0  1576    0    0
205  0  1431    0    0
206  0   564    0    0
```

As can be seen by the beginning of this output, our coding appears accurate, as those with a value in ALCDAY5 of 101-199 are coded asbeing in level 3 of ALCGRP, and those with an ALCDAY5 of 201 or more are coded as level 2 of ALCGRP. Observing the rest of the output confirms a successful recode.

Regrouping grouped categorical variables is typically necessary in healthcare analytics, mainly to collapse levels. However, it should also be used to populate all fields so as to remove any missing (NA) values. In continuous variables, having an NA can be advantageous because summary operations such as "average" and "sum" will ignore NA values and records. But in categorical variables, we want to make sure that nothing is ignored and that records with no value recorded are somehow recorded as having a value (such as "unknown").

An example of this in the BRFSS dataset is the variable _BMI5CAT (or, as read into R, X_BMI5CAT). This categorizes weight status as 1=Underweight, 2=Normal, 3=Overweight, 4=Obese, and missing=no information. We want to create a categorical grouping variable that places an actual value (such as 9) in the rows that currently have an NA in X_BMI5CAT. We create BMICAT with the same values as X_BMI5CAT, but with NAs replaced with 9s:

```
BRFSS_g$BMICAT<- 9
BRFSS_g$BMICAT[BRFSS_g$X_BMI5CAT ==1] <- 1
BRFSS_g$BMICAT[BRFSS_g$X_BMI5CAT ==2] <- 2
BRFSS_g$BMICAT[BRFSS_g$X_BMI5CAT ==3] <- 3
BRFSS_g$BMICAT[BRFSS_g$X_BMI5CAT ==4] <- 4

table(BRFSS_g$X_BMI5CAT, BRFSS_g$BMICAT, useNA = c("always"))
```

We include the table command to check the code, but do not provide the output. In a similar way, we recode a grouping variable for general health status, GENHLTH, coded as 1=Excellent, 2=Very Good, 3=Good, 4=Fair, 5=Poor, 7=Refused, 9=Unknown, missing=Unknown. Our new variable is called GENHLTH2, and changes the NAs to 9s, but also adds 9s and 7s into the Unknown category.

```
BRFSS_g$GENHLTH2 <- 9
BRFSS_g$GENHLTH2[BRFSS_g$GENHLTH == 1] <- 1
BRFSS_g$GENHLTH2[BRFSS_g$GENHLTH == 2] <- 2
```

```
BRFSS_g$GENHLTH2[BRFSS_g$GENHLTH == 3] <- 3
BRFSS_g$GENHLTH2[BRFSS_g$GENHLTH == 4] <- 4
BRFSS_g$GENHLTH2[BRFSS_g$GENHLTH == 5] <- 5

table(BRFSS_g$GENHLTH, BRFSS_g$GENHLTH2, useNA = c("always"))
```

Because BRFSS and other datasets tend to code unknowns with higher values (such as 77 or 99), sometimes operations can be used for recoding a multilevel variable just to collapse unknown values into one category. The variable `INCOME2` is the respondent's annual household income from all sources. The variable is divided into eight groups (1 = < \$10,000, 2 = \$10,000–14,999, 3 = \$15,000–19,999, 4 = \$20,000–24,999, 5 = \$25,000–34,999, 6 = \$35,000–49,999, 7 = \$50,000–74,999, and 8 = \$75,000 or more). Imagine that we want to recode this variable into `INCOME3` with the same coding, except where we have 77 (DK), 99 (Refused), or missing in `INCOME2`, we will place a 9 in `INCOME3`. This can be done relatively easily with this code:

```
BRFSS_g$INCOME3 <- BRFSS_g$INCOME2
BRFSS_g$INCOME3[BRFSS_g$INCOME2 >=77] <- 9

table(BRFSS_g$INCOME2, BRFSS_g$INCOME3, useNA = c("always"))
```

Notice how the variable was first copied and then updated where `INCOME2` was >= 77, meaning coded with a 77 or 99. Had there been any NAs, we would have had to add an "or" clause handling this criterion.

Our exposure, `ALCGRP`, is also ordinal. We will choose nondrinkers as our reference category and create the indicator variables for `DRKMONTHLY` and `DRKWEEKLY`:

```
BRFSS_h$DRKMONTHLY <- 0
BRFSS_h$DRKMONTHLY[BRFSS_h$ALCGRP == 2] <- 1
table(BRFSS_h$ALCGRP, BRFSS_h$DRKMONTHLY, useNA = c("always"))
BRFSS_h$DRKWEEKLY <- 0
BRFSS_h$DRKWEEKLY [BRFSS_h$ALCGRP == 3] <- 1
table(BRFSS_h$ALCGRP, BRFSS_h$DRKWEEKLY, useNA = c("always"))
```

Collapsing categories into only three levels, mainly for the purposes of grouping the unknown values together, is simple using this approach. BRFSS variable `EXERANY2` is the answer to the question, "During the past month, other than your regular job, did you participate in any physical activities or exercises such as running, calisthenics, golf, gardening, or walking for exercise?" and is coded as 1=Yes, 2=No, 7=Don't know/Not sure, and 9=Refused/missing. `HLTHPLN1`, which is the answer to the question, "Do you have any kind of healthcare coverage, including health insurance, prepaid plans such as HMOs, or government plans such as Medicare, or Indian Health Service?" is coded the same way. This code generates new grouping variables EXERANY3 and HLTHPLN2 which collapse the 7 and 9 categories.

```
BRFSS_g$EXERANY3<- 9
BRFSS_g$EXERANY3[BRFSS_g$EXERANY2 ==1] <- 1
BRFSS_g$EXERANY3[BRFSS_g$EXERANY2 ==2] <- 2

table(BRFSS_g$EXERANY2, BRFSS_g$EXERANY3, useNA = c("always"))

BRFSS_g$HLTHPLN2 <- 9
BRFSS_g$HLTHPLN2[BRFSS_g$HLTHPLN1 == 1] <- 1
BRFSS_g$HLTHPLN2[BRFSS_g$HLTHPLN1 == 2] <- 2

table(BRFSS_g$HLTHPLN1, BRFSS_g$HLTHPLN2, useNA = c("always"))
```

Before collapsing categories in a grouping variable where there are multiple levels, it is helpful to make some documentation. Table 2.2 proposes collapsing the marital status variable MARITAL into the grouping variable MARGRP:

TABLE 2.2

Plans for Collapsing Marital Status Variable

MARITAL	Description	MARGRP
1	Married	1
2	Divorced	2
3	Widowed	2
4	Never married	3
5	A member of an unmarried couple	1
9	Refused	9

Note that this grouping arrangement places "Married" with "A member of an unmarried couple" in the same category ("Living as married"), and "Divorced" and "Widowed" into the same category ("Formerly married"). Making this table first can guide the development of code:

```
BRFSS_g$MARGRP <- 9
BRFSS_g$MARGRP[BRFSS_g$MARITAL == 1 | BRFSS_g$MARITAL == 5] <- 1
BRFSS_g$MARGRP[BRFSS_g$MARITAL == 2 | BRFSS_g$MARITAL == 3]<- 2
BRFSS_g$MARGRP[BRFSS_g$MARITAL == 4] <- 3

table(BRFSS_g$MARGRP, BRFSS_g$MARITAL, useNA = c("always"))
```

The results from the table command confirm the correct recoding of the new variable MARGRP. Race (_MRACE1 or X_MRACE1 in R) in BRFSS is another example of a difficult variable to collapse. It is helpful again to make a table first (Table 2.3):

TABLE 2.3

Plans for Collapsing Race Variable

X_MRACE1	Description	RACEGRP
1	White only	1
2	Black or African American only	2
3	American Indian or Alaskan Native only	3
4	Asian only	4
5	Native Hawaiian or other Pacific Islander only	5
6	Other race only	6
7	Multiracial	6
77	Don't Know	9
99	Refused	9
Null	Missing	9

Notice how this plans for a grouping variable `RACEGRP` that groups together "Other race only" and "Multiracial," as well as grouping together all the unknowns. Coding and checking the variable against the table become easy with the table as a guide.

```
BRFSS_g$RACEGRP <- 9
BRFSS_g$RACEGRP[BRFSS_g$X_MRACE1 == 1] <- 1
BRFSS_g$RACEGRP[BRFSS_g$X_MRACE1 == 2] <- 2
BRFSS_g$RACEGRP[BRFSS_g$X_MRACE1 == 3] <- 3
BRFSS_g$RACEGRP[BRFSS_g$X_MRACE1 == 4] <- 4
BRFSS_g$RACEGRP[BRFSS_g$X_MRACE1 == 5] <- 5
BRFSS_g$RACEGRP[BRFSS_g$X_MRACE1 == 6 | BRFSS_g$X_MRACE1 == 7]
<- 6

table(BRFSS_g$X_MRACE1, BRFSS_g$RACEGRP, useNA = c("always"))
```

Another example is collapsing groups for the variable representing respondent's highest level of education, `EDUCA` (Table 2.4):

TABLE 2.4

Plans for Collapsing Education Variable

EDUCA	Description	EDGROUP
1	Never attended school or only attended kindergarten	1
2	Grades 1–8 (Elementary)	1
3	Grades 9–11 (Some high school)	1
4	Grade 12 or GED (High school graduate)	2
5	College 1 to 3 years (Some college or technical school)	3
6	College 4 years or more (College graduate)	4
9	Refused	9

EDGROUP represents a recode that collapses all with less than a high school education together into one group. Note that this means that where EDUCA equals 1, 2, or 3, EDGROUP is equal to 1. EDUCA provides an excellent situation to introduce using "in". In SAS, we might recode EDUCA the following way:

```
data r.BRFSS_g;
      set r.BRFSS_g;

      EDGROUP = 9;
      if EDUCA in (1,2,3)
            then EDGROUP = 1;
      if EDUCA = 4
            then EDGROUP = 2;
      if EDUCA = 5
            then EDGROUP = 3;
      if EDUCA = 6
            then EDGROUP = 4;
      run;
```

Note that the first condition uses the SAS "in" statement. There is an equivalent "in" statement in R.

```
BRFSS_g$EDGROUP <- 9
BRFSS_g$EDGROUP[BRFSS_g$EDUCA %in% 1:3] <- 1
BRFSS_g$EDGROUP[BRFSS_g$EDUCA == 4] <- 2
BRFSS_g$EDGROUP[BRFSS_g$EDUCA == 5] <- 3
BRFSS_g$EDGROUP[BRFSS_g$EDUCA == 6] <- 4

table(BRFSS_g$EDUCA, BRFSS_g$EDGROUP, useNA = c("always"))
```

For the recode for EDGROUP=1, the argument %in% 1:3 is used to indicate having a value in the sequence from 1 to 3. The %in% argument can also refer to a vector. In this alternative way to recode EDGROUP, we start by making a vector with the three values for the lowest education group, and call it LowEdValues. Then, we refer to this vector after the %in% statement.

```
LowEdValues <- c(1,2,3)

BRFSS_g$EDGROUP <- 9
BRFSS_g$EDGROUP[BRFSS_g$EDUCA %in% LowEdValues] <- 1
BRFSS_g$EDGROUP[BRFSS_g$EDUCA == 4] <- 2
BRFSS_g$EDGROUP[BRFSS_g$EDUCA == 5] <- 3
BRFSS_g$EDGROUP[BRFSS_g$EDUCA == 6] <- 4
```

At this point, it may be helpful to consider all the operations in R that could be used as criteria for subsetting and updating data. These appear in Table 2.5.

As a final example of editing data to produce grouping variables, we will consider the smoking variables in BRFSS. Our goal is to develop the variable SMOKGRP, where 1=current smoker, 2=current nonsmoker, and

TABLE 2.5

Operators and Examples

Operator	What it Means	Example in Subsetting Data	Example in Editing Data
`==`	Is equal to	`Subset(BRFSS_c, ALCDAY5 == 777)`	`BRFSS_c$NOALC[BRFSS_c$ALCDAY5 == 888] <- 1`
`!=`	Is not equal to	`Subset(BRFSS_c, ALCDAY5 != 777)`	`BRFSS_c$ALCVAL[BRFSS_c$ALCDAY5 != 888] <- 1`
`<`	Is less than	`Subset(BRFSS_c, ALCDAY5 < 777)`	`BRFSS_c$DRINKER[BRFSS_c$ALCDAY5 < 888] <- 1`
`!<`	Is not less than	`Subset(BRFSS_c, ALCDAY5 !< 777)`	`BRFSS_c$DRKUNK[BRFSS_c$ALCDAY5 !< 888] <- 1`
`<=`	Is less than or equal to	`Subset(BRFSS_c, ALCDAY5 !<= 777)`	`BRFSS_c$DRKVAL[BRFSS_c$ALCDAY5 <= 888] <- 1`
`>`	Is greater than	`Subset(BRFSS_c, ALCDAY5 > 777)`	`BRFSS_c$DRKUNK[BRFSS_c$ALCDAY5 > 888] <- 1`
`!>`	Is not greater than	`Subset(BRFSS_c, ALCDAY5 !> 777)`	`BRFSS_c$DRKVAL[BRFSS_c$ALCDAY5 !> 888] <- 1`
`>=`	Is greater than or equal to	`Subset(BRFSS_c, ALCDAY5 >= 777)`	`BRFSS_c$DRKNOUNK[BRFSS_c$ALCDAY5 >= 888] <- 1`
`&`	And	`Subset(BRFSS_c, ALCDAY5 > 100 & ALCDAY5 < 777)`	`BRFSS_c$DRKVAL[BRFSS_c$ALCDAY5 >100 & BRFSS_c$ALCDAY5 < 777] <- 1`
`|`	Or	`subset(BRFSS_c, ALCDAY5 == 777|ALCDAY5 == 999)`	`BRFSS_c$DRKUNK[BRFSS_c$ALCDAY5 == 777|BRFSS_c$ALCDAY5 == 999] <- 1`

9=Don't know/Not sure/Refused/missing. However, the smoking information in BRFSS is split into two questions. The first, `SMOKE100`, is the answer to, "Have you smoked at least 100 cigarettes in your entire life?," with the answer options the same as for `EXERANY3`. A 1=Yes does not necessarily mean that the person is a current smoker, because he or she could have quit after the first 100 cigarettes (which is equal to five packs of cigarettes). However, 2=No definitely means the person should be classified as a current nonsmoker, because s/he has never smoked more than 100 cigarettes. Using this information, we start by creating a `NEVERSMK` field, setting it to 0, and then updating it to 1 if the respondent answers 2 for `SMOKE100`.

```
BRFSS_g$NEVERSMK <- 0
BRFSS_g$NEVERSMK [BRFSS_g$SMOKE100 == 2] <- 1

table(BRFSS_g$SMOKE100, BRFSS_g$NEVERSMK, useNA = c("always"))
```

If the respondent says 1=Yes to `SMOKE100`, s/he is asked, "Do you now smoke cigarettes every day, some days, or not at all?" and this variable is called `SMOKDAY2`. The respondent's choices are 1=Every Day, 2=Some Days, 3=Not at All, 7=Don't know/Not sure, 9=Refused, and missing. In our new grouping variable, SMOKGRP, we want those who said 1 or 2 to SMOKDAY2 to be classified as 1 (current smokers), and those who said either 3 to SMOKDAY2 (former smokers) or 2 to SMOKE100 (meaning they have never smoked, or NEVERSMK=1) to be classified as 2 (current nonsmokers), and everyone else classified as 9 (unknown, refused, missing). Our NEVERSMK variable helps us with this classification.

```
BRFSS_g$SMOKGRP <- 9
BRFSS_g$SMOKGRP[BRFSS_g$SMOKDAY2 == 1 | BRFSS_g$SMOKDAY2 == 2]
<- 1
BRFSS_g$SMOKGRP[BRFSS_g$SMOKDAY2 == 3 | BRFSS_g$NEVERSMK == 1]
<- 2

table(BRFSS_g$SMOKDAY2, BRFSS_g$SMOKGRP, useNA = c("always"))
table(BRFSS_g$SMOKE100, BRFSS_g$SMOKGRP, useNA = c("always"))
```

Grouping variables are useful for conducting chi-squared tests and for providing descriptive statistics. However, two-state flag variables are particularly useful as independent variables in regression. The next section will describe preparing two-state flag variables, also known as indicator variables.

Creating Indicator Variables for Two-Level Categories

Indicator variables are two-state flag variables, meaning they take on one of two values—1 or 0. This section will talk about preparing indicator variables for later use as independent variables in regression. Before more demonstration, let us copy the dataset so that we can more easily roll back if we find problems with our recoded variables.

```
BRFSS_h <- BRFSS_g
```

The reason the two-state indicator variable is so useful in regression is that the slope that is printed for that variable in the output clearly indicates the magnitude of impact that state has on the outcome (compared to the other state). For example, imagine that we wanted to know the impact of being male on the outcome (compared to all other sexes—which for BRFSS is only female). Rather than using the SEX variable from the BRFSS dataset (coded as 1=male and 2=female, with no other values), for regression, it would be more intuitive to recode it as an indicator variable named MALE:

```
BRFSS_h$MALE <- 0
BRFSS_h$MALE[BRFSS_h$SEX == 1] <- 1

table(BRFSS_h$MALE, BRFSS_h$SEX, useNA = c("always"))
```

But there are few two-level categories in the native BRFSS dataset. Most have more levels to indicate unknown, refused, and missing, and some have a lot of levels, such as INCOME2. Considerations need to be made when selecting which levels of categorical variables should be reflected as indicator variables in a regression.

Creating Indicator Variables for Three-Level Categories

Because MALE is coded with a 1 if the person is a male and 0 if the person is a female, the slope on the output will clearly indicate the impact of being a male (compared to a female) with respect to the outcome. This approach is similarly helpful in using three-level variables in a regression, where the third level is unknown, and there are not that many. For example, the number of respondents who did not report their Hispanic ethnicity status was 607, which represents approximately 1% of the dataset of 58,131 veterans. Therefore, coding them into the 0 category with an indicator variable named HISPANIC is not an unreasonable choice:

```
BRFSS_h$HISPANIC <- 0
BRFSS_h$HISPANIC[BRFSS_h$X_HISPANC == 1] <- 1

table(BRFSS_h$HISPANIC, BRFSS_h$X_HISPANC, useNA = c("always"))
```

Only 299 in our dataset did not report their smoking status, so unknowns will get coded as 0 with our new indicator variable named SMOKER:

```
BRFSS_h$SMOKER <- 0
BRFSS_h$SMOKER[BRFSS_h$SMOKGRP == 1] <- 1

table(BRFSS_h$SMOKGRP, BRFSS_h$SMOKER, useNA = c("always"))
```

It is intuitive to select the flags for HISPANIC and for SMOKER. After all, we can imagine that being Hispanic may confer either protection or risk, depending upon the outcome, and we imagine that being a smoker would confer risk (although sometimes reverse relationships are found, depending upon the outcome being modeled). Perhaps it is less intuitive to choose how to code an indicator variable for the exercise grouping variable or the health plan status grouping variable.

In the cases where an intuitive level that should be coded as 1 does not jump out, an easy rule of thumb is to code the state that is predicted to be the most risky with respect to the outcome as a 1. It is intuitive to predict not exercising and not having a health plan would be two risky states to be in, no matter what the outcome. Therefore, coding a flag as 1 indicating not exercising and not having a health plan may be the best choice, because it will lead to a more intuitive interpretation. Here, we code flags NOEXER for "no exercise" and NOPLAN for "no health plan."

```
BRFSS_h$NOEXER <- 0
BRFSS_h$NOEXER[BRFSS_h$EXERANY3 ==2] <- 1
```

```
table(BRFSS_h$NOEXER, BRFSS_h$EXERANY3, useNA = c("always"))

BRFSS_h$NOPLAN <- 0
BRFSS_h$NOPLAN [BRFSS_h$HLTHPLN2== 2] <- 1

table(BRFSS_h$NOPLAN, BRFSS_h$HLTHPLN2,useNA = c("always"))
```

These examples show how to code indicator variables for categorical variables that have the answers "yes," "no," and various codes meaning "unknown." The next section will describe creating indicator variables for multilevel ordinal categories.

Creating Indicator Variables for Multilevel Ordinal Categories

Two examples of multilevel ordinal categorical variables include the BRFSS variable `X_AGE_G`, which is a six-level imputed age category (1 = 18–24, 2 = 25–34, 3 = 35–44, 4 = 45–54, 5 = 55–64, 6 = 65 and older), and the grouping variable we made, `INCOME3`, which classifies income into eight levels (with 9=unknown). The point of making indicator variables for levels of `X_AGE_G` and `INCOME3` is that each group may have its own unique relationship with the outcome. Entering `X_AGE_G` and `INCOME3` into a model as they assume a linear relationship between the levels of these variables and whatever outcome is being modeled.

That can be a big assumption to make. Allowing each level to take on its own slope will allow the data to show if that relationship is indeed linear. A dose-response effect in a model is where higher levels of an independent variable are associated with higher predicted variables of the dependent variable. A reverse or inverse dose-response effect is where higher levels of an independent variable are associated with lower levels of a dependent variable. These dose-response effects can be revealed if each level is modeled separately (and can convince the analyst that the relationship is indeed linear). Analysts who like to hunt for significant interaction terms in final models will find it easier to interact each level (of age, say, with `MALE`) using an indicator variable for each level. But this leads to the previous question—what level should be chosen as the overall reference level? As with the advice to choose the level hypothesized to have the most risk of the outcome in a two-state flag to set to 1, here, the advice is the opposite—choose the level hypothesized to have the least risk of the outcome, and choose that as the overall reference group.

With respect to `X_AGE_G`, the youngest group would be assumed to have the least risk of any bad outcome. Hence, indicator variables are created only for values 2–6 of this six-level variable (`AGE2-AGE6`), leaving the youngest category as the reference group:

```
BRFSS_h$AGE2 <- 0
BRFSS_h$AGE3 <- 0
BRFSS_h$AGE4 <- 0
```

```
BRFSS_h$AGE5 <- 0
BRFSS_h$AGE6 <- 0

BRFSS_h$AGE2[BRFSS_h$X_AGE_G == 2] <- 1
table(BRFSS_h$X_AGE_G, BRFSS_h$AGE2, useNA = c("always"))

BRFSS_h$AGE3[BRFSS_h$X_AGE_G == 3] <- 1
table(BRFSS_h$X_AGE_G, BRFSS_h$AGE3, useNA = c("always"))

BRFSS_h$AGE4[BRFSS_h$X_AGE_G == 4] <- 1
table(BRFSS_h$X_AGE_G, BRFSS_h$AGE4, useNA = c("always"))

BRFSS_h$AGE5[BRFSS_h$X_AGE_G == 5] <- 1
table(BRFSS_h$X_AGE_G, BRFSS_h$AGE5, useNA = c("always"))

BRFSS_h$AGE6[BRFSS_h$X_AGE_G == 6] <- 1
table(BRFSS_h$X_AGE_G, BRFSS_h$AGE6, useNA = c("always"))
```

`INCOME3`, which is in eight levels plus unknown, can be viewed similarly, but this has the added issue of having a large proportion of records without a value (n = 6,217, and of 58,131 records, that is about 10%). If we use the same logic to choose the top level (highest income group) as likely to be associated with the least risk, then we can code this set of indicator variables for seven of the levels (`INC1–INC7`), leaving the unknowns in the reference group along with the highest level of income:

```
BRFSS_h$INC1 <- 0
BRFSS_h$INC2 <- 0
BRFSS_h$INC3 <- 0
BRFSS_h$INC4 <- 0
BRFSS_h$INC5 <- 0
BRFSS_h$INC6 <- 0
BRFSS_h$INC7 <- 0

BRFSS_h$INC1[BRFSS_h$INCOME3 == 1] <- 1
table(BRFSS_h$INC1, BRFSS_h$INCOME3, useNA = c("always"))

BRFSS_h$INC2[BRFSS_h$INCOME3 == 2] <- 1
table(BRFSS_h$INC2, BRFSS_h$INCOME3, useNA = c("always"))

BRFSS_h$INC3[BRFSS_h$INCOME3 == 3] <- 1
table(BRFSS_h$INC3, BRFSS_h$INCOME3, useNA = c("always"))

BRFSS_h$INC4[BRFSS_h$INCOME3 == 4] <- 1
table(BRFSS_h$INC4, BRFSS_h$INCOME3, useNA = c("always"))
```

```
BRFSS_h$INC5[BRFSS_h$INCOME3 == 5] <- 1
table(BRFSS_h$INC5, BRFSS_h$INCOME3, useNA = c("always"))

BRFSS_h$INC6[BRFSS_h$INCOME3 == 6] <- 1
table(BRFSS_h$INC6, BRFSS_h$INCOME3, useNA = c("always"))

BRFSS_h$INC7[BRFSS_h$INCOME3 == 7] <- 1
table(BRFSS_h$INC7, BRFSS_h$INCOME3, useNA = c("always"))
```

Creating Indicator Variables for Multilevel Nominal Categories

Using the grouping variables we generated as guides, we now have to choose which levels of nominal categories we want to try to model as independent variables and which ones we want to keep in the reference group. A table can come in handy in deciding what indicator variables might be generated.

Table 2.6 proposes two marital status indicator variables: `NEVERMAR`, indicating never married, and `FORMERMAR`, indicating formerly married (divorced or widowed). This would place married and those with no marital status value (n = 1,010, almost 2%) in the reference group. This choice was made because many studies show that there is a positive effect of being married on health (although not every study shows this). Hence, married people were hypothesized to the least risky relationship with any health outcome compared to the other levels.

TABLE 2.6

Plans for Proposed Marital Status Indicator Variables

MARITAL	Description	MARGRP	NEVERMAR	FORMERMAR
1	Married	1	0	0
2	Divorced	2	0	1
3	Widowed	2	0	1
4	Never married	3	1	0
5	A member of an unmarried couple	1	0	0
9	Refused	9	0	0

For race, a shown in Table 2.7, three indicator variables are proposed: `BLACK`, flagging only those in the Black or African American category, `ASIAN`, flagging those in the Asian only category, and `OTHRACE`, which flags those in all the other race categories except White Only. Using this approach, those in the White Only or missing information group are placed in the reference group by default. This choice was made because many studies show that White race is associated with better outcomes (although not in all cases).

TABLE 2.7

Plans for Proposed Race Indicator Variables

X_MRACE1	Description	RACEGRP	BLACK	ASIAN	OTHRACE
1	White only	1	0	0	0
2	Black or African American only	2	1	0	0
3	American Indian or Alaskan Native only	3	0	0	1
4	Asian only	4	0	1	0
5	Native Hawaiian or other Pacific Islander only	5	0	0	1
6	Other race only	6	0	0	1
7	Multiracial	6	0	0	1
77	Don't Know	9	0	0	0
99	Refused	9	0	0	0
Null	Missing	9	0	0	0

Choosing educational indicator variables can also be helped by a table. As shown in Table 2.8, two indicator variables are planned. `LOWED` collapses together all levels below and through high school graduation, and `SOMECOLL` flags those who report attending some college. This approach places college graduates along with those in the unknown group (n = 106, < 1%) in the reference group.

TABLE 2.8

Plans for Proposed Education Indicator Variables

EDUCA	Description	EDGROUP	LOWED	SOMECOLL
1	Never attended school or only attended kindergarten	1	1	0
2	Grades 1–8 (Elementary)	1	1	0
3	Grades 9–11 (Some high school)	1	1	0
4	Grade 12 or GED (High school graduate)	2	1	0
5	College 1–3 years (Some college or technical school)	3	0	1
6	College 4 years or more (College graduate)	4	0	0
9	Refused	9	0	0

Choosing what to flag as indicator variables can be done empirically. For example, the BMI categories are labeled as 1=Underweight, 2=Normal, 3=Overweight, and 4=Obese (with `BMICAT`, our grouping variable, indicating 9=missing). The logical choices for indicator variables would be to include Normal and unknown (n = 870, 1.5%) in the reference group, and code `UNDWT`, `OVWT`, and `OBESE` for levels 1, 3, and 4, respectively.

```
BRFSS_h$UNDWT <- 0
BRFSS_h$OVWT <- 0
BRFSS_h$OBESE <- 0

BRFSS_h$UNDWT[BRFSS_h$BMICAT== 1] <- 1
table(BRFSS_h$UNDWT, BRFSS_h$BMICAT, useNA = c("always"))

BRFSS_h$OVWT[BRFSS_h$BMICAT== 3] <- 1
table(BRFSS_h$OVWT, BRFSS_h$BMICAT, useNA = c("always"))

BRFSS_h$OBESE[BRFSS_h$BMICAT== 4] <- 1
table(BRFSS_h$OBESE, BRFSS_h$BMICAT, useNA = c("always"))
```

Finally, considering the general health variable (we created grouping GENHEALTH2), research has shown that the "fair" and "poor" levels of self-reported health are associated with risk of many negative health outcomes. Therefore, we will create flags for just those levels.

```
BRFSS_h$FAIRHLTH <- 0
BRFSS_h$POORHLTH <- 0

BRFSS_h$FAIRHLTH [BRFSS_h$GENHLTH2 == 4] <- 1
table(BRFSS_h$FAIRHLTH, BRFSS_h$GENHLTH2, useNA = c("always"))

BRFSS_h$POORHLTH [BRFSS_h$GENHLTH2 == 5] <- 1
table(BRFSS_h$POORHLTH, BRFSS_h$GENHLTH2, useNA = c("always"))
```

Creating Missing Flags

We will copy BRFSS_a, the dataset with all the variables in it, to give an example of making a flag to indicate that a row is missing a value for a variable. The new dataset will be called Miss_example. The variable "number of adults in the household" (NUMADULT) is coded 1–99, but according to the BRFSS codebook, also a large proportion are missing there.

In SAS, we might create a missing flag called NUMADULT_MISS this way, followed by a check in PROC FREQ:

```
Data Miss_example;
        set r.BRFSS_a;

        NUMADULT_MISS = 0;
        If NUMADULT =.
              then NUMADULT_MISS = 1;

run;

procfreq data=Miss_example;

       Tables NUMADULT*NUMADULT_MISS/list missing;

run;
```

In R, to do the same thing, we would start by copying the dataset.

```
Miss_example <- BRFSS_a
```

To make a flag to indicate this variable is missing (called NUMADULT_MISS), we use the is.na command:

```
Miss_example$NUMADULT_MISS <- 0
Miss_example$NUMADULT_MISS[is.na(Miss_example$NUMADULT)] <- 1

table(Miss_example$NUMADULT, Miss_example$NUMADULT_MISS, useNA =
c("always"))
```

Conversely, we may want a flag indicating NUMADULT is populated (NUMADULT_POP). This could be accomplished using the !is.na command, with the preceding exclamation point making the statement mean "if not missing is true," then populate:

```
Miss_example$NUMADULT_POP <- 0
Miss_example$NUMADULT_POP[!is.na(Miss_example$NUMADULT)] <- 1

table(Miss_example$NUMADULT, Miss_example$NUMADULT_POP, useNA =
c("always"))
```

Preparing Binary Outcome Variable

Earlier, we chose to use having asthma (yes/no) as our binary outcome variable, and removed all the records in the dataset not coded with either a "yes" or a "no" to ASTHMA3. With binary dependent variables, it is easier to interpret if they are coded as binary flags, with 0 and 1. Hence, we code ASTHMA4 with 0 for no asthma and 1 for asthma:

```
BRFSS_i$ASTHMA4 <- 9
BRFSS_i$ASTHMA4[BRFSS_i$ASTHMA3 == 1] <- 1
BRFSS_i$ASTHMA4[BRFSS_i$ASTHMA3 == 2] <- 0

table(BRFSS_i$ASTHMA3, BRFSS_i$ASTHMA4)
```

The table command confirms that there are no records where ASTHMA4 = 9, so ASTHMA4 is indeed a binary flag that can be used as a dependent variable in a logistic regression or survival analysis.

Planning a Survival Analysis Dataset with Time-to-Event Variables

Later in this book, survival analysis will be demonstrated. Survival analysis is similar to logistic regression in that it depends on a binary dependent variable that indicates whether a person has had an "event" (set to 1) or not had an "event" (set to 0). In this demonstration, the event will be "being diagnosed with asthma," so that the ASTHMA4 variable can be used.

What's different between survival analysis and logistic regression is that survival analysis also has a measurement of "time-to-event." The BRFSS dataset has a variable, ASHTMAGE, which is the age in years that a person reports having gotten the event, or having been diagnosed with asthma. In other words, for those with asthma, the "time-to-event" variable is ASTHMAGE. The ASTHMAGE variable contains the answer to the question, "How old were you when you were first told by a doctor, nurse, or other health professional that you had asthma?" which is asked of respondents reporting an asthma diagnosis. The valid answers to this variable, ASTHMAGE, are 11–96 (meaning ages 11–96), 97 = 10 or younger, 98 = Don't know/Not sure, 99 = refused, and blank = missing.

ASTHMAGE, logically, would only be filled in if the respondent actually reporting having asthma, which would be ASTHMA4 = 1. If the respondent was never diagnosed with asthma (ASTHMA4 = 0), then they are considered "censored" in survival analysis—meaning that they did not get the event in the time period studied, which, in our case, are the lives of the respondents up to year 2014 when the BRFSS did this survey. For the censored, time-to-event is just "time to the end of the dataset." In this case, that would be their age at the time of the survey, or X_AGE80.

For demonstration purposes, we will form a survival analysis hypothesis which is similar to the hypothesis for a binary-dependent variable, but with a survival analysis twist. The survival analysis hypothesis will be: among BRFSS respondents, alcohol consumption is associated with the "survival experience" of being diagnosed with asthma. It is hard to explain what the "survival experience" is until we get to Chapter 3 and look at a descriptive survival analysis, but for now, this hypothesis will guide our development of a survival analysis dataset.

First, we want to think of the steps necessary for preparing a survival analysis dataset. Like with the other analytic dataset, we need to copy in the variables we need for survival analysis from BRFSS_a. In this case, we select ASTHMA3 (to generate ASTHMA4), ASTHMAGE (as just described), X_AGE80 (needed for the time-to-event in the censored respondents), ALCDAY5 (to generate the ALCGRP variable), and SEX and VETERAN3. SEX and veteran status will play the role of potential confounders in the descriptive and regression analysis demonstration.

Next, after trimming off unneeded variables, we want to generate and check ASTHMA4 and ALCGRP. After this, we want to subset the data, keeping only respondents with a valid veteran, asthma, and alcohol status.

After this, we need to look at ASTHMAGE in relation to ASTHMA4. If a respondent reports having asthma (ASTHMA4 = 1), then ASTHMAGE should be populated with a valid entry. If there are records where ASTHMA4 = 1 but ASTHMAGE is not populated, they should be removed from the dataset as well.

Finally, ASTHMAGE needs to be recoded. As stated earlier, only values of 11–96 are considered valid, but 97 was used to indicate "10 or younger," so we could recode these 97s to 10s and keep them in the dataset if we are willing to truncate the lower level of ASTHMAGE at 10. However, the other values of ASTHMAGE should not be in our recode, as they indicate "unknown." After ASTHMAGE is recoded, like with any continuous variable, distributions should be examined through summary statistics and plots to get a feel for the behavior of the variable.

In survival analysis, the time period examined matters. If we want to know if alcohol status is associated with the survival experience of being diagnosed with asthma by age 30, we are making the leap that the current alcohol consumption level reported by the respondent was the same her whole life—especially before age 30. That is probably a big leap to make, as people can change their alcohol consumption patterns over time. However, if we make this assumption that we would need two variables to address this specific hypothesis: ASTHMA30, which will be set to 1 if the respondent was diagnosed with asthma by age 30 (ASTHMAGE < = 30), and 0 for everyone else. Those who were not diagnosed with asthma by age 30 will be coded as 0, even if they were eventually diagnosed with asthma at a later age (ASTHMA4 = 1 but ASTHMAGE is greater than 30), because the later age of diagnosis is not in our window of study. In the case of ASTHMA30, we declare our study period to be the first 30 years of the respondent's life.

After making ASTHMA30, then, for those who have a 1 in ASHTMA30, ASTHMAGE will be their time-to-event variable, and for those with a 0, X_AGE80, or their current age, will be their time-to-event variable. The trick is to make one variable called TIME30 that is filled in this way: for those with ASTHMA30 = 1, it is filled in with ASTHMAGE, and for those with ASTHMA30 = 0, it is filled in with X_AGE80. And, in both cases, if the ASTHMAGE or X_AGE80 is greater than 30, we cap it at age 30, since we are only interested in the first thirty years of life.

But as we reviewed earlier, assuming that a person's ALCGRP as reported at the time of the survey was their ALCGRP before our censoring year, especially if we are talking about the young age of 30. It might be fairer to look at age 50 or age 80. If we wanted to do that, we would need two more sets of time-to-event variables. For age 50, we would need the set ASTHMA50, coded as 1 if they got asthma by age 50 and 0 if they did not, and TIME50, coded as ASTHMAGE for ASTHMA50 = 1 and as X_AGE80 for ASTHMA50 = 0, and for the final set, we would need the corresponding ASTHMA80 and TIME80.

Developing the Survival Dataset

As per our aforementioned plans, let us go back to BRFSS_a and make a new dataset just for the survival analysis demonstration (called SurvivalData_a) with just the variables we need, which, stated earlier, were ASTHMA3, ASTHMAGE, X_AGE80, ALCDAY5, SEX, and VETERAN3. In SAS, we will do this in a data step with a KEEP option.

```
data r.SurvivalData_a;
       set r.BRFSS_a (keep =
               ASTHMA3
               ASTHMAGE
               _AGE80
               ALCDAY5
               SEX
               VETERAN3);
run;
```

But in R, we will use our trick of making a "keep list" in a vector called `SurvivalVarList`, and using that vector to trim off unwanted columns to make the dataset smaller and easier to handle.

```
SurvivalVarList <- c("ASTHMA3", "ASTHMAGE", "X_AGE80",
"ALCDAY5", "SEX", "VETERAN3")
SurvivalData_a <- BRFSS_a[SurvivalVarList]
```

Our next step is to regenerate `ASHTMA4`, `ALCGRP`, and the alcohol and sex indicator variables in our survival dataset. In SAS, we create a dataset and increment the dataset to `SurvivalData_b`, followed by a check with `PROC FREQ`.

```
data r.SurvivalData_b;
      set r.SurvivalData_a;

      ALCGRP = 9;
      if (ALCDAY5 <200 & ALCDAY5 ne.)
             then ALCGRP = 3;
      if ALCDAY5 ge 200 and ALCDAY5 < 777
             then ALCGRP = 2;
      if ALCDAY5 = 888
             then ALCGRP = 1;

      DRKMONTHLY = 0;
      if ALCGRP = 2
             then DRKMONTHLY = 1;

      DRKWEEKLY = 0;
      if ALCGRP = 3
             then DRKWEEKLY = 1;

      ASTHMA4 = 9;
      if ASTHMA3 = 1
             then ASTHMA4 = 1;
      If ASTHMA3 = 2
             then ASTHMA4 = 0;
```

```
      MALE=0;
      if SEX=1
             then MALE=1;

run;

proc freq data=r.SurvivalData_b;
      table ALCGRP * ALCDAY5 / list missing;
      table ASTHMA4 * ASTHMA3 / list missing;
      table ALCGRP * DRKMONTHLY / list missing;
      table ALCGRP * DRKWEEKLY / list missing;
      table SEX * MALE / list missing;
run;
```

In R, we choose when we want a rollback, and we do that by incrementing the letter at the end of the dataset name. Let us choose to set a rollback here, and copy `SurvivalData_a` to `SurvivalData_b`. Next, we will add `ASTHMA4`, `ALCGRP`, and the alcohol and sex indicator variables, and check these with table commands.

```
SurvivalData_b$ASTHMA4 <- 9
SurvivalData_b$ASTHMA4[SurvivalData_b$ASTHMA3 == 1] <- 1
SurvivalData_b$ASTHMA4[SurvivalData_b$ASTHMA3 == 2] <- 0

table(SurvivalData_b$ASTHMA3, SurvivalData_b$ASTHMA4, useNA =
c("always"))

SurvivalData_b$ALCGRP <- 9
SurvivalData_b$ALCGRP[SurvivalData_b$ALCDAY5 < 200]<- 3
SurvivalData_b$ALCGRP[SurvivalData_b$ALCDAY5 >=200 &
SurvivalData_a$ALCDAY5 < 777] <- 2
SurvivalData_b$ALCGRP[SurvivalData_b$ALCDAY5 == 888] <- 1

table(SurvivalData_b$ALCDAY5, SurvivalData_b$ALCGRP, useNA =
c("always"))

SurvivalData_b$DRKMONTHLY <- 0
SurvivalData_b$DRKMONTHLY[SurvivalData_b$ALCGRP == 2] <- 1

table(SurvivalData_b$ALCGRP, SurvivalData_b$DRKMONTHLY, useNA =
c("always"))

SurvivalData_b$DRKWEEKLY <- 0
SurvivalData_b$DRKWEEKLY [SurvivalData_b$ALCGRP == 3] <- 1

table(SurvivalData_b$ALCGRP, SurvivalData_b$DRKWEEKLY, useNA =
c("always"))
```

```
SurvivalData_b$MALE <- 0
SurvivalData_b$MALE [SurvivalData_b$SEX == 1] <- 1

table(SurvivalData_b$MALE, SurvivalData_b$SEX, useNA =
c("always"))
```

Now is the time to start subsetting the dataset. We want to keep those with only valid `ASTHMA4` values (1 for yes and 0 for no), those with known veteran statuses (1 for yes and 2 for no), and those with a known `ALCGRP` (all except 9). To be able to monitor the number removed each time, in SAS, we want to increment the letter in the dataset for each data step so that we can rollback if there is a mistake. The resulting dataset should be tested with a `PROC FREQ` to ensure valid values.

```
data r.SurvivalData_c;
        set r.SurvivalData_b;
        if ASTHMA4 in (1,0);

data r.SurvivalData_d;
        set r.SurvivalData_c;
        if VETERAN3 in (1,2);

data r.SurvivalData_e;
        set r.SurvivalData_d;
        if ALCGRP ne 9;

run;

proc freq data=r.SurvivalData_e;
        table ASTHMA4 / list missing;
        table VETERAN3 / list missing;
        table ALCGRP / list missing;

run;
```

When we follow the same processes in R, we start with dataset `SurvivalData_b`, then increment it to `SurvivalData_c` by keeping only the valid values for `ASTHMA4`, and then checking results with a table command.

```
SurvivalData_c <- subset(SurvivalData_b, ASTHMA4 == 1 |
ASTHMA4 == 0)
table(SurvivalData_c$ASTHMA4)
```

We can now subset `SurvivalData_c` into `SurvivalData_d` based on the valid values of veteran status:

```
SurvivalData_d <- subset(SurvivalData_c, VETERAN3 == 1 |
VETERAN3 == 2)
table(SurvivalData_d$VETERAN3)
```

And finally, we subset SurvivalData_d into SurvivalData_e by known alcohol status.

```
SurvivalData_e <- subset(SurvivalData_d, ALCGRP != 9)
table(SurvivalData_e$ALCGRP)
```

In our next step, we need to remove records with ASTHMA4 = 1 but without a valid ASTHMAGE. To do this, a missing flag would be helpful to make, even though we realize those without asthma will be all missing for ASTHMAGE. Let us make the flag ASTHMAGE_MISS to help us figure out those who need to be removed because they have asthma, but their age of diagnosis is missing.

In SAS, we would pick up where we left off with SurvivalData_e, and with a data step, we would create SurvivalData_f which will include the ASTHMAGE_MISS flag. This will be set to 1 for the values 98 and 99 in ASTHMAGE (unknown), and also, when ASTHMAGE is missing, indicated by the period. This is followed by a check with PROC FREQ.

```
data r.SurvivalData_f;
        set r.SurvivalData_e;

        ASTHMAGE_MISS = 0;
        if ASTHMAGE in (98, 99,.)
               then ASTHMAGE_MISS = 1;

run;

proc freq data=r.SurvivalData_f;
        table ASTHMAGE * ASTHMAGE_MISS / list missing;

run;
```

Returning to R, we would do the same operation by adding ASTHMA_MISS as a variable to dataset SurvivalData_e. Instead of the period SAS uses for missing, we will use R's is.na function.

```
SurvivalData_e$ASTHMAGE_MISS <- 0
SurvivalData_e$ASTHMAGE_MISS[SurvivalData_e$ASTHMAGE == 98 |
      SurvivalData_e$ASTHMAGE == 99 | is.na(SurvivalData_
e$ASTHMAGE)] <- 1
table(SurvivalData_e$ASTHMAGE, SurvivalData_e$ASTHMAGE_MISS,
useNA = c("always")
```

Remember, having ASTHMAGE be missing is not a problem if ASTHMA4 = 0. It is only a problem when ASTHMA4 = 1, because it means that the respondent got the event, but we do not know when. For that reason, we cannot use that person's record in our survival analysis. Some analysts might choose to impute an ASTHMAGE for those individuals, but in this case, we will just remove them from the dataset because they are missing necessary information.

To do this, we will create a variable called NOASTHMAGE, which is set to 1 if the respondent reported having asthma, but ASTHMAGE_MISS = 1, and then remove the 1s from the dataset. In SAS, we do this by creating NOASTHMAGE in a data step that increments SurvivalData_f to SurvivalData_g. After checking the variable with PROC FREQ, we subset the dataset to SurvivalData_h by only keeping the records where NOASTHMAGE = 0.

```
data r.SurvivalData_g;
       set r.SurvivalData_f;

       NOASTHMAGE = 0;
       if (ASTHMA4 = 1 & ASTHMAGE_MISS = 1)
              then NOASTHMAGE = 1;

run;

proc freq data=r.SurvivalData_g;
       table ASTHMAGE_MISS * NOASTHMAGE / list missing;
       table ASTHMA4 * NOASTHMAGE / list missing;

run;

data r.SurvivalData_h;
       set r.SurvivalData_g;
       if NOASTHMAGE = 0;

run;
```

In R, we still use SurvivalData_e. We add NOASTHMAGE, check it with the table command, and then subset the dataset into SurvivalData_f.

```
SurvivalData_e$NOASTHMAGE <- 0
SurvivalData_e$NOASTHMAGE[SurvivalData_e$ASTHMA4 == 1 &
SurvivalData_e$ASTHMAGE_MISS == 1] <- 1

table(SurvivalData_e$ASTHMAGE_MISS, SurvivalData_e$NOASTHMAGE,
useNA = c("always"))
table(SurvivalData_e$ASTHMA4, SurvivalData_e$NOASTHMAGE, useNA =
c("always"))

SurvivalData_f <- subset(SurvivalData_e, NOASTHMAGE == 0)
```

Before we move on, it is important to check what proportion of asthmatics were removed because NOASTHMAGE = 1. Running a table command in R on the rollback dataset SurvivalData_e shows a disturbing reality.

Code:

```
table(SurvivalData_e$ASTHMA4, SurvivalData_e$NOASTHMAGE, useNA =
c("always"))
```

Output:

```
              0        1  <NA>
0        379081        0     0
1          1876    56644     0
<NA>          0        0     0
```

This represents the number of people reporting being diagnosed with asthma who did not have a valid ASTHMAGE and therefore are getting removed from the dataset. The 1,876 in the cell next to it represent the asthmatics with a valid ASHTMAGE. By removing 56,644 people, which represents 97% of the respondents reporting events in SurvivalData_e, we know our study will suffer from the selection bias. We cannot fix this; this is a result of problems with data collection or data preparation before this variable came to us. Imputing data in this case would not help us, since so much is missing, and we would end up making up 97% of the data. So we will continue to use this dataset for demonstration purposes only.

After removing those with NOASTHMAGE = 1, we need to clean up ASTHMAGE. Previously, it was stated that 97 was the code for "age 10 and under." For survival analysis, we could use the coding for ASTHMAGE except change 97 to 10, so we will do that in ASTHMAGE2. In SAS, we use a data step to increment SurvivalData_h to SurvivalData_i. We copy ASTHMAGE into ASTHMAGE2, then set ASTHMAGE2 to 10 if ASTHMAGE = 97, and check the variable with a PROC FREQ.

```
data r.SurvivalData_i;
        set r.SurvivalData_h;

        ASTHMAGE2 = ASTHMAGE;
        if ASTHMAGE = 97
                then ASTHMAGE2 = 10;

run;

proc freq data=r.SurvivalData_i;
        table ASTHMAGE * ASTHMAGE2 / list missing;

run;
```

In R, we add the ASTHMAGE2 variable and check it in a similar fashion, in SurvivalData_f.

```
SurvivalData_f$ASTHMAGE2 <- SurvivalData_f$ASTHMAGE
SurvivalData_f$ASTHMAGE2[SurvivalData_f$ASTHMAGE == 97] <- 10

table(SurvivalData_f$ASTHMAGE, SurvivalData_f$ASTHMAGE2, useNA =
c("always"))
```

Now that we have a valid event variable, ASTHMA4, and a valid time variable, ASTHMAGE2, we have to decide our window for survival analysis before we code our time and event variables, because we have to know what proportion of events will end up being censored, depending upon our choices. In SAS, we can run a PROC UNIVARIATE on ASHTMAGE2 to look at summary statistics, and add the normal plot options to look at a histogram and box plot.

```
proc univariate data=r.SurvivalData_i normal plot;
       var ASTHMAGE2;
run;
```

In R, we can use the describe command from the psych library to describe ASTHMAGE2, and we can visualize ASTHMAGE in a histogram and a box plot.

Code:

```
library(psych)
describe(SurvivalData_f$ASTHMAGE2)

#histogram

par(mfrow=c(1,2))

hist(SurvivalData_f$ASTHMAGE2,
       main = "Histogram of Age\n of Asthma Dx",
       xlab = "Class Age",
       ylab = "Frequency",
       xlim=c(0,100),
       ylim=c(0,800),
       border = "royalblue",
       col= "salmon",
       las = 1,
       breaks = 100)

#box plot

boxplot(SurvivalData_f$ASTHMAGE2,
       main = "Box Plot of Age\n of Asthma Dx",
       ylab = "Age at Dx",
```

```
        border = "maroon",
        col= "gold")
```

Output from the `describe` command:

```
  vars    n  mean    sd median trimmed   mad min max range skew kurtosis   se
1    1 1876 27.28 19.77     19   24.51 13.34  10  90    80 0.85    -0.56 0.46
```

In the inset, Figure 2.4 shows the histogram and the box plot. It is clear that the age of diagnosis is skewed low, and our median tells us that at least half of the events took place before age 19. As described earlier, ALCGRP is likely to be more accurate for older aged individuals. Therefore, we will select three potential time points: age 30, 50, and 80 as our period of study. Our survival analyses will examine the survival experience overall and in groups for the period birth to age 30, 50, and 80.

Assume that we start with the cutpoint of 30 years. We will need an event variable for having asthma at the age of 30 years or younger (ASTHMA30), and a time variable for how long it took to get diagnosed with asthma (with the maximum age possible as 30—we will call it TIME30). The actual value of TIME30 for those who got asthma at the age of 30 years or younger would be 10–30, and would be in ASTHMAGE2. The actual value of TIME30 for those who did not get asthma at the age of 30 years or younger (meaning they got it later or not at all), would be their age—but if their age is older than 30, it will be recoded to the end of the time period, which is 30.

In SAS, we would start by creating and checking the ASTHMA30 variable with a data step and a PROC FREQ.

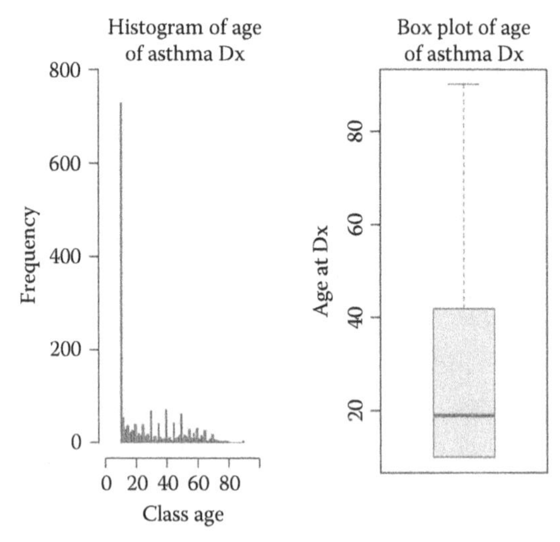

FIGURE 2.4
(See color insert.) Distribution of ASTHMAGE2.

```
data r.SurvivalData_j;
      set r.SurvivalData_i;

      ASTHMA30 = 0;
      if ASTHMA4 = 1 and ASTHMAGE2 le 30
            then ASTHMA30 = 1;

run;

proc freq data=r.SurvivalData_j;
      table ASTHMA30 * ASTHMAGE2 / list missing;
run;
```

In R, creating the ASTHMA30 variable is accomplished similarly and checked with the table command.

```
SurvivalData_g$ASTHMA30 <- 0
SurvivalData_g$ASTHMA30[SurvivalData_g$ASTHMA4 == 1 &
SurvivalData_g$ASTHMAGE2 <= 30] <- 1

table(SurvivalData_g$ASTHMA30, SurvivalData_g$ASTHMAGE2, useNA =
c("always"))
```

Next, we generate the TIME30 variable using SAS. We start by copying over the age variable into TIME30, and then updating that to ASTHMAGE2 if ASTHMA30 = 1. If the respondent is older than 30 and did not have asthma, this variable will be greater than 30, which is our time period in question. Therefore, if TIME30 is greater than 30, it is recoded to 30, and checked with PROC FREQ.

```
data r.SurvivalData_k;
      set r.SurvivalData_j;

      TIME30 = _AGE80;
      if ASTHMA30 = 1
            then TIME30 = ASTHMAGE2;
      if TIME30 >30
            then TIME30 = 30;

run;

proc freq data=r.SurvivalData_k;
      table TIME30 * ASTHMAGE2 / list missing;
run;
```

When we go to do this in R, we notice that for the first time, we need criteria on both sides of the equations when making variables. In the first line, which only applies to ASTHMA30 = 1, this criterion is placed on both sides of the equation to ensure that ASTHMAGE2 is only copied over for those with ASTHMA30 = 1. You will see in the second line, which applies only to ASTHMA30 not equal to 1 (meaning 0, since ASTHMA30 is binary), the criterion is again on both sides of the equation. Finally, the third line updates TIME30 to a maximum of 30, and a table command is used to check the recode.

```
SurvivalData_g$TIME30[SurvivalData_g$ASTHMA30 == 1] <-
        SurvivalData_g$ASTHMAGE2[SurvivalData_g$ASTHMA30 == 1]

SurvivalData_g$TIME30[SurvivalData_g$ASTHMA30 != 1] <-
        SurvivalData_g$X_AGE80[SurvivalData_g$ASTHMA30 != 1]

SurvivalData_g$TIME30[SurvivalData_g$TIME30 > 30] <- 30

table(SurvivalData_g$TIME30, SurvivalData_g$ASTHMAGE2, useNA =
c("always"))
```

Unlike in SAS, when continuous variables containing NAs are copied in R, R will throw up an error, because it does not want to copy the NAs. R only will count the populated rows in ASTHMAGE2 as the number of values for the variable, so when it goes to copy the variable into a new variable in the full dataset, it counts the dataset as having more rows than values of the variable and does not know what to do. In a data.frame, the rule is that each column has to apply to all the rows. So if the analyst removes the criterion from the right side of the first equation and run it, she will get this error:

```
Warning message:
In SurvivalData_g$TIME30[SurvivalData_g$ASTHMA30 == 1]
<- SurvivalData_g$ASTHMAGE2:
  number of items to replace is not a multiple of replacement
length
```

In order to demonstrate different time periods, we will make two more sets of time-to-event variables: ASTHMA50 and TIME50 for the period birth to age 50, and ASTHMA80 and TIME80 for birth to age 80. Here is how these variables would be created in SAS.

```
data r.SurvivalData_l;
       set r.SurvivalData_k;

       ASTHMA50 = 0;
       if ASTHMA4 = 1 and ASTHMAGE2 le 50
              then ASTHMA50 = 1;
       ASTHMA80 = 0;
       if ASTHMA4 = 1 and ASTHMAGE2 le 80
              then ASTHMA80 = 1;
```

```
        TIME50 = _AGE80;
        if ASTHMA50 = 1
                then TIME50 = ASTHMAGE2;
        if TIME50 > 50
                then TIME50 = 50;

        TIME80 = _AGE80;
        if ASTHMA80 = 1
                then TIME80 = ASTHMAGE2;
        if TIME80 > 80
                then TIME80 = 80;

run;

proc freq data=r.SurvivalData_1;
        table ASTHMA50 * ASTHMAGE2 / list missing;
        table ASTHMA80 * ASTHMAGE2 / list missing;
        table TIME50 * ASTHMAGE2 / list missing;
        table TIME80 * ASTHMAGE2 / list missing;
run;
```

Here if the same operation is done in R.

```
SurvivalData_g$ASTHMA50 <- 0
SurvivalData_g$ASTHMA50[SurvivalData_g$ASTHMA4 == 1 &
SurvivalData_g$ASTHMAGE2 <= 50] <- 1

table(SurvivalData_g$ASTHMA50, SurvivalData_g$ASTHMAGE2, useNA =
c("always"))

SurvivalData_g$TIME50[SurvivalData_g$ASTHMA50 == 1] <-
        SurvivalData_g$ASTHMAGE2[SurvivalData_g$ASTHMA50 == 1]

SurvivalData_g$TIME50[SurvivalData_g$ASTHMA50 != 1] <-
        SurvivalData_g$X_AGE80[SurvivalData_g$ASTHMA50 != 1]

SurvivalData_g$TIME50[SurvivalData_g$TIME50 > 50] <- 50

table(SurvivalData_g$TIME50, SurvivalData_g$ASTHMAGE2, useNA =
c("always"))

SurvivalData_g$ASTHMA80 <- 0
SurvivalData_g$ASTHMA80[SurvivalData_g$ASTHMA4 == 1 &
SurvivalData_g$ASTHMAGE2 <= 80] <- 1

table(SurvivalData_g$ASTHMA80, SurvivalData_g$ASTHMAGE2, useNA =
c("always"))

SurvivalData_g$TIME80[SurvivalData_g$ASTHMA80 == 1] <-
        SurvivalData_g$ASTHMAGE2[SurvivalData_g$ASTHMA80 == 1]
```

```
SurvivalData_g$TIME80[SurvivalData_g$ASTHMA80 != 1] <-
        SurvivalData_g$X_AGE80[SurvivalData_g$ASTHMA80 != 1]

SurvivalData_g$TIME80[SurvivalData_g$TIME80 > 80] <- 80

table(SurvivalData_g$TIME80, SurvivalData_g$ASTHMAGE2, useNA =
c("always"))
```

In SAS, we ended with `SurvivalData_1`, and in R, our last dataset was `SurvivalData_g`. Let us choose the name `SurvAnalytic` for this dataset to be used in analysis. In SAS, we could end our code by renaming the SAS dataset.

```
data r.SurvAnalytic;
        set r.SurvivalData_1;
run;
```

In R, we would write it out as a *.csv.

```
write.csv(SurvivalData_g, "SurvAnalytic.csv")
```

Dealing with Dates

Often in health-related datasets, there are a lot of dates, such as the date of visit or the date of having some outcome (such as a heart attack). These dates are often the items used when determining survival analysis windows and time-to-event for different time windows.

An exhaustive description of date handling in R is outside the scope of this book. This section will provide an overview of converting strings to date fields and calculating date windows. We will be manipulating date variables in the class "date," but the reader who needs to work extensively with dates in calculations should investigate the R classes `POSIXct` and `POSIXlt`, as these classes provide more extensive opportunities to work with dates and times. Also, Garrett Grolemund and colleagues have developed an excellent package called `lubridate` that makes date handling easier in R [55], and they have published a paper that carefully explains how to use their package [56].

See Table 2.9 for the example dataset that will be used for this demonstration, which is the list of hospitals in Rhode Island (excluding the Veterans Affairs hospital) and is available online from the American Hospital Directory (AHD.com) [57] The most recent Joint Commission accreditation date has been added to the dataset to provide an example date to work with.

This dataset has hospital names (`HospName`), cities (`HospCity`), number of staffed beds (`StBeds`), and most recent Joint Commission Accreditation Date (`AccredDate`). `AccredDate` will be used to demonstrate date manipulation.

This dataset was developed in Microsoft Excel and saved in the *.xlsx format. Excel can save spreadsheets with one tab in the comma separated values (CSV or *.csv) format, and can read *.csv files easily as well. This dataset was

TABLE 2.9
Rhode Island Hospital Dataset

HospName	HospCity	StBeds	AccredDate
Kent Hospital	Warwick	343	February 6, 2016
Landmark Medical Center	Woonsocket	141	August 17, 2013
Memorial Hospital of Rhode Island	Pawtucket	133	December 6, 2014
Newport Hospital	Newport	129	January 18, 2014
Our Lady of Fatima Hospital	North Providence	229	December 13, 2014
Rhode Island Hospital	Providence	686	November 22, 2014
Roger Williams Medical Center	Providence	160	September 13, 2014
South County Health	Wakefield	91	October 11, 2014
The Miriam Hospital	Providence	235	June 14, 2014
The Westerly Hospital	Westerly	89	August 7, 2015
Women & Infants Hospital	Providence	247	June 14, 2014

then subsequently saved in the *.csv format, and the R command `read.csv` was used to read it in.

```
RIHosp <- read.csv("C:/Users/Monika/Dropbox/R Stats Book/
Analytics/Data/RIHospitals.csv",
      header = TRUE, sep = ",")
RIHosp
```

Output:

```
                  HospName         HospCity StBeds AccredDate
1                Kent Hospital          Warwick    343   2/6/2016
2          Landmark Medical Center       Woonsocket    141  8/17/2013
3  Memorial Hospital of Rhode Island      Pawtucket    133  12/6/2014
4                Newport Hospital          Newport    129  1/18/2014
5      Our Lady of Fatima Hospital North Providence    229 12/13/2014
6            Rhode Island Hospital       Providence    686 11/22/2014
7    Roger Williams Medical Center       Providence    160  9/13/2014
8              South County Health        Wakefield     91 10/11/2014
9              The Miriam Hospital       Providence    235  6/14/2014
10           The Westerly Hospital         Westerly     89   8/7/2015
11        Women & Infants Hospital       Providence    247  6/14/2014
```

Note that in the `read.csv` command, `header = TRUE` was set because the first row contains headers (column names), and `sep = ","` designated that the fields were separated by commas (hence *.csv format). `AccredDate` may look like a date, but using the `class` command, we realize that it is a factor.

```
class(RIHosp$AccredDate)
```

Output:

```
[1] "factor"
```

In SAS, if we use the *.xlsx version of the dataset and read it in using the PROC IMPORT code, and then run a PROC CONTENTS command, we find a similar problem—AccredDate is read as a character of length 10.

```
PROC IMPORT OUT= R.RIHosp
            DATAFILE= "C:\Users\Monika\Dropbox\R Stats Book\
            Analytics\Data\RIHospitals.xlsx"
            DBMS=EXCEL REPLACE;
     RANGE="RIHospitals$";
     GETNAMES=YES;
     MIXED=NO;
     SCANTEXT=YES;
     USEDATE=YES;
     SCANTIME=YES;
RUN;

proc contents data=R.RIHosp;
      run;
```

In order to do date operations on this variable, it needs to be converted to a date format, not a character. In SAS, we could do this using a data step with format and input commands, followed by a PROC CONTENTS command to make sure we generated the correct variable. The following code creates AccredDate2, which is numeric and in the date format:

```
data R.RIHosp;
      set R.RIHosp;
      format AccredDate2 mmddyy10.;
      AccredDate2=input(trim(AccredDate),MMDDYY10.);
run;

proc contents data=R.RIHosp;
      run;
```

To do the same thing in R, we need to convert AccredDate to a date using the as.Date command; again, we will call the new field AccredDate2. In the as.Date command, we have to include the argument that explains how the date is formatted in the current factor class field.

```
RIHosp$AccredDate2 <- as.Date(RIHosp$AccredDate, "%m/%d/%Y")
RIHosp[, c('AccredDate', 'AccredDate2')]
```

Output:

```
   AccredDate AccredDate2
1    2/6/2016  2016-02-06
2   8/17/2013  2013-08-17
3   12/6/2014  2014-12-06
```

```
4    1/18/2014  2014-01-18
5   12/13/2014  2014-12-13
6   11/22/2014  2014-11-22
7    9/13/2014  2014-09-13
8   10/11/2014  2014-10-11
9    6/14/2014  2014-06-14
10    8/7/2015  2015-08-07
11  6/14/2014   2014-06-14
```

Please also notice that `AccredDate` as a factor is formatted month/day/year (using slashes). That is the meaning of the "`%m/%d/%Y`" argument in the `as.Date` command. `AccredDate2` may not look much different from `AccredDate`, but it is now in the date format as we can see by the class command.

```
class(RIHosp$AccredDate2)
```

Output:

```
[1] "Date"
```

Now that we have the date in the date format in `AccredDate2`, we can use that against other dates to make calculations. Imagine in our study, we decided to follow hospitals from accreditation date until a selected censoring date—let us imagine July 31, 2016. In SAS, we could create a column called `RefDate1` and put this date in that column. Then, we could use the `datdif` command to calculate the number of days in between the `RefDate1` and `AccredDate2`, with the difference being called `RefDate1Diff`.

```
data R.RIHosp;
      set R.RIHosp;
      RefDate1 = '31jul2016'D;
      RefDate1Diff = datdif(AccredDate2, RefDate1, 'act/act');
run;
```

In R, we would approach it slightly differently. We could start by creating `RefDate1` as an object:

```
RefDate1 <- as.Date(c("2016-07-31"))
```

Then, we could calculate the difference in days between `AccredDate2` and `RefDate1`, calculating `RefDate1Diff`.

```
RIHosp$RefDate1Diff <- RefDate1 - RIHosp$AccredDate2
RIHosp[, c('AccredDate2', 'RefDate1Diff')]
```

Output:

```
   AccredDate2  RefDate1Diff
1   2016-02-06      176 days
2   2013-08-17     1079 days
3   2014-12-06      603 days
4   2014-01-18      925 days
5   2014-12-13      596 days
6   2014-11-22      617 days
7   2014-09-13      687 days
8   2014-10-11      659 days
9   2014-06-14      778 days
10  2015-08-07      359 days
11  2014-06-14      778 days
```

Today's date can also be used as the reference date, as demonstrated with RefDate2:

```
RefDate2 <- Sys.Date()
```

Presumably, once these fields that count days exist, flagging events at different time points for survival analysis can be handled as we did with ASTHMAGE and incident asthma. However, sometimes, in survival analysis, we look into a window of a certain amount of days since a particular date (e.g., a window of 60 days since date of discharge), and not a calendar reference date. In that case, an extra step is required before calculating the days to an event.

Imagine we were studying a 60-day window after accreditation date. We would create a column for RefDate3, which would be a date 60 days after accreditation:

```
RIHosp$RefDate3 <- RIHosp$AccredDate2 + 60
RIHosp[, c('AccredDate2', 'RefDate3')]
```

Output:

```
   AccredDate2   RefDate3
1   2016-02-06 2016-04-06
2   2013-08-17 2013-10-16
3   2014-12-06 2015-02-04
4   2014-01-18 2014-03-19
5   2014-12-13 2015-02-11
6   2014-11-22 2015-01-21
7   2014-09-13 2014-11-12
8   2014-10-11 2014-12-10
9   2014-06-14 2014-08-13
10  2015-08-07 2015-10-06
11  2014-06-14 2014-08-13
```

There would need to be dates for subsequent events (such as reaccreditation), and those dates would then be compared to `RefDate3`. Records with events later than `RefDate3` would be excluded from the analysis (censored).

One of the main challenges in converting factor variables to dates is getting the incoming format correct. To give a quick overview, the dataset shown in Table 2.10 (called `DateExamples`) contains date strings of different formats. The following code successfully converts these dates.

TABLE 2.10

Formats for Example Dates Dataset (DateExamples)

AccredDateA	AccredDateB	AccredDateC	AccredDateD	AccredDateE
2016FEB 02	02-06-2016	February 2, 2016	Tuesday, 2/2/16	TUE FEB 02 16

```
DateExamples$AccredDateA2 <- as. Date(DateExamples$AccredDateA,
"%Y %b %d")
DateExamples$AccredDateB2 <- as. Date(DateExamples$AccredDateB,
"%m-%d-%Y")
DateExamples$AccredDateC2 <- as. Date(DateExamples$AccredDateC,
"%B %d, %Y")
DateExamples$AccredDateD2 <- as. Date(DateExamples$AccredDateD,
"%A, %m/%d/%y")
DateExamples$AccredDateE2 <- as. Date(DateExamples$AccredDateE,
"%a %b %d %y")
```

Table 2.11 is a summary of the terms used in the format of the date.

TABLE 2.11

Format Guide for Date Conversion

Format Code	Meaning	Example String	Example of Use in Format Code
`%d`	Day as number (0–31)	2016-02-02	`"%m-%d-%Y"`
`%a`	Abbreviated weekday	TUE FEB 02 16	`"%a %b %d %y"`
`%A`	Unabbreviated weekday	Tuesday, 2/2/16	`"%A, %m/%d/%y"`
`%m`	Month as a number (00–12)	2/6/2016	`"%m/%d/%Y"`
`%b`	Abbreviated month	2016FEB 02	`"%Y %b %d"`
`%B`	Unabbreviated month	February 2, 2016	`"%B %d, %Y"`
`%y`	2-digit year	TUE FEB 02 16	`"%a %b %d %y"`
`%Y`	4-digit year	2016-02-02	`"%m-%d-%Y"`

Recoding and Classifying Continuous Variables

A continuous independent variable does not need to be entered continuously into a model. For example, in our survival dataset, ASTHMAGE2 could be categorized. Viewing Figure 2.4 in the color inset as we did earlier when making time-to-event variables, we can see that there is a skewed distribution toward the younger years. Imagine that we want to create a grouping variable for ASTHMAGE2 called ASTHMAGEQUART that groups ASTHMAGE2 by quartiles.

In SAS, this is often handled by running PROC UNIVARIATE and using the ODS to output the results so that the quartile cutpoints can be referred to in the subsequent code. Then, those cutpoints are used as references to create a column with the quartiles classified as 1, 2, 3, and 4. Another approach in SAS is to use PROC RANK, as described in a white paper by Jonas V. Bilenas to create this classification variable [58]. Because this is such an involved operation that can be done many ways, the SAS code is not presented here.

Creating a quartile grouping variable is an example of a situation where the R code is easier to use than the SAS code. We can refer to our earlier use of the quantile command and first create a vector called ASTHMAGE2Quartiles from ASTHMAGE2:

```
ASTHMAGE2Quartiles <- quantile(SurvivalData_f$ASTHMAGE2,
na.rm=TRUE, prob = c(0.25, 0.50, 0.75))
```

Looking at this vector reveals the following:

```
ASTHMAGE2Quartiles
```

Output:

```
25% 50% 75%
 10  18  42
```

This vector is only three items, with 10 as the first item, 18 as the second item, and 42 as the third item. To refer to the first item, the following syntax is used: ASTHMAGE2Quartiles[1]. This is how we will refer to the quartiles in creating the new ASTHMAGEQUART variable.

```
SurvivalData_f$ASTHMAGEQUART <- NA
SurvivalData_f$ASTHMAGEQUART[SurvivalData_f$ASTHMAGE2 <=
ASTHMAGE2Quartiles[1]] <- 1
SurvivalData_f$ASTHMAGEQUART[(SurvivalData_f$ASTHMAGE2 >
ASTHMAGE2Quartiles[1]) &
      SurvivalData_f$ASTHMAGE2 <= ASTHMAGE2Quartiles[2]] <- 2
SurvivalData_f$ASTHMAGEQUART[(SurvivalData_f$ASTHMAGE2 >
ASTHMAGE2Quartiles[2]) &
      SurvivalData_f$ASTHMAGE2 <= ASTHMAGE2Quartiles[3]] <- 3
SurvivalData_f$ASTHMAGEQUART[SurvivalData_f$ASTHMAGE2 >
ASTHMAGE2Quartiles[3]] <- 4
```

The new variable begins with an NA, because all the people with no asthma in the dataset will have an NA for ASTHMAGE2. Next, this variable is populated with a 1 if ASTHMAGE2 is less than or equal to the first ASTHMAGE2 quartile, referred to as ASTHMAGE2Quartiles[1]. Notice how the other items in the list are referenced in the code. The table command confirms that the quartile grouping variable has been recoded properly.

```
table(SurvivalData_f$ASTHMAGE2, SurvivalData_f$ASTHMAGEQUART,
useNA = c("always"))
```

The output is long, but here is the beginning:
Output:

```
         1     2     3     4     <NA>
10     695     0     0     0        0
11       0    42     0     0        0
12       0    54     0     0        0
13       0    31     0     0        0
14       0    22     0     0        0
15       0    38     0     0        0
16       0    22     0     0        0
17       0    20     0     0        0
18       0    26     0     0        0
19       0     0    22     0        0
20       0     0    40     0        0
21       0     0    14     0        0
```

Recoding a Continuous Outcome Variable

As shown in Figure 2.4 and stated earlier, ASTHMAGE2 has a skewed distribution. If we were to use this as a continuous outcome variable in the linear regression, it would not meet the normality assumptions for the linear regression. Some data analysts address this issue by transforming the variable that does not follow a normal distribution. Log transformation is a popular approach. The following SAS code gives an example of using a data step to create a dataset called BRFSS_LogExample from BRFSS_a, and generates a logged version of ASTHMAGE called LOGASTHMAGE:

```
data r.BRFSS_LogExample;
      set r.BRFSS_a;
      LOGASTHMAGE = log(ASTHMAGE);
run;
```

We will demonstrate this log transformation in R by taking a subset of our data consisting only of people with a value for ASTHMAGE2, taking the log of ASTHMAGE2 (and placing this in the field LOGASTHMAGE), then visualizing it in a histogram.

```
AllAsthma <- subset(SurvivalData_f, !is.na(ASTHMAGE2))
AllAsthma$LOGASTHMAGE <- log(AllAsthma$ASTHMAGE2)
AllAsthma[, c('ASTHMAGE2', 'LOGASTHMAGE')]
```

Another approach is to take the square root of the variable:

```
AllAsthma$SQRTASTHMAGE <- sqrt(AllAsthma$ASTHMAGE2)
AllAsthma[, c('ASTHMAGE2', 'SQRTASTHMAGE')]
```

Now, we should look at the distribution of these two new variables, `LOGASTHMAGE` and `SQRTASTHMAGE`. We can plot a histogram and a box plot for each variable (4 plots) together in a matrix with this code:

```
layout(matrix(c(1,2,3,4),2,2)) # optional 4 graphs/page

hist(AllAsthma$LOGASTHMAGE,
       main = "Histogram of Log of Age\nof Asthma Dx",
       xlab = "Class Log Age",
       ylab = "Frequency",
       xlim=c(2,5),
       ylim=c(0,800),
       border = "mediumvioletred",
       col= "lightcoral",
       las = 1,
       breaks = 25)

boxplot(AllAsthma$LOGASTHMAGE,
       main = "Box Plot of Log of Age\nof Asthma Dx",
       ylab = "Log Age of Dx",
       border = "mediumvioletred",
       col= "lightcoral")

hist(AllAsthma$SQRTASTHMAGE,
       main = "Histogram of Square Root of Age of Asthma Dx",
       xlab = "Class Sqrt Age",
       ylab = "Frequency",
       xlim=c(2,10),
       ylim=c(0,800),
       border = "seagreen",
       col= "seagreen3",
       las = 1,
       breaks = 25)
```

```
boxplot(AllAsthma$SQRTASTHMAGE,
        main = "Box Plot of Square Root of Age of Asthma Dx",
        ylab = "Sqrt Age of Dx",
        border = "seagreen",
        col= "seagreen3")
```

Figure 2.5 in the inset shows this matrix of plots. By viewing Figure 2.5, the distribution of the LOGASTHMAGE and SQRTASTHMAG can be compared with Figure 2.4, the distribution of ASTHMAGE2, and we can see that applying the log function or the square root function did not fix the skewness of the variable. Notice in the two long titles, a **\n** breaks the line.

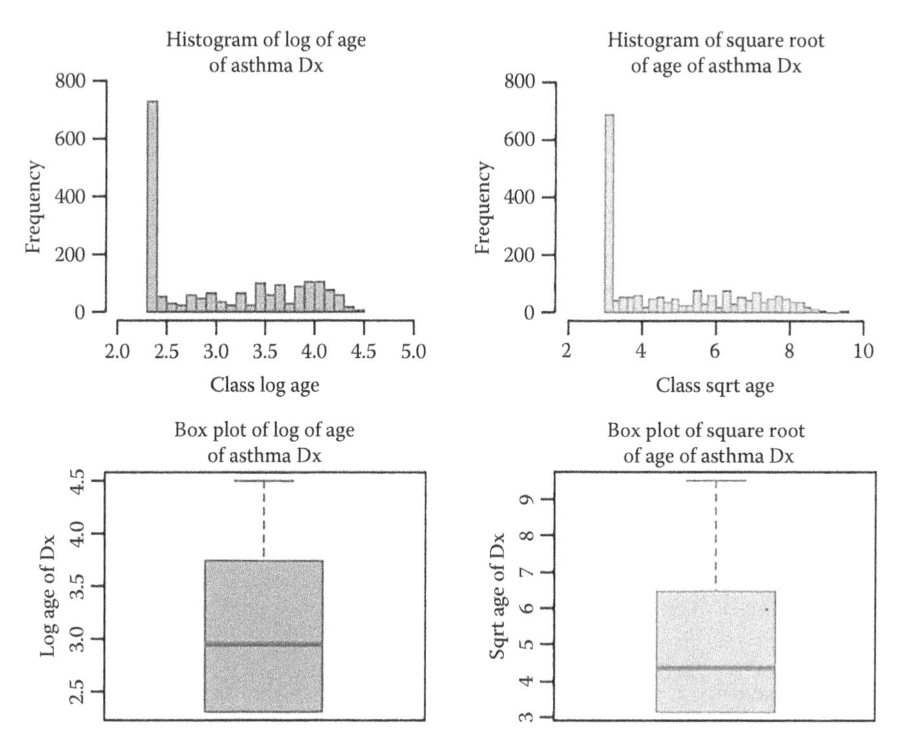

FIGURE 2.5
(See color insert.) Histogram and box plots of transformed ASTHMAGE2.

In addition to the natural log and square root, there are other operations that could be used, and these are summarized in Table 2.12.

TABLE 2.12

Examples of Transformation Operations

Function	Description	Code Example	X Value	Evaluated
`abs(x)`	Absolute value	`abs(-10)`	–10	10
`sqrt(x)`	Square root	`sqrt(25)`	25	5
`ceiling(x)`	Round up to next integer	`ceiling(5.25)`	5.25	6
`floor(x)`	Round down to last integer	`floor(5.25)`	5.25	5
`trunc(x)`	Truncate after integer	`trunc(47.23)`	47.23	47
`round(x, digits=n)`	Round to however many decimal places	`round(0.056239, digits = 4)`	0.05624	0.0562
`signif(x, digits=n)`	Round to however many significant digits	`signif(0.056239, digits = 4)`	0.05624	0.05624
`cos(x), sin(x), tan(x)`	Cosine, sine, and tangent. Other trigonometric functions also available in base R.	`cos(0.5)`	0.5	0.877583
`log(x)`	natural logarithm	`log(1)`	1	0
`log10(x)`	common logarithm	`log10(100)`	100	2
`exp(x)`	e^x	`exp(0)`	0	1

Code to demonstrate the examples in Table 2.12 is here:

```
abs(-10)
sqrt(25)
ceiling(5.25)
floor(5.25)
trunc(47.23)
round(0.056239, digits=4)
signif(0.056239, digits=4)
cos(0.5)
log(1)
log10(100)
exp(0)
```

The answers in the output are listed in the Evaluated column in Table 2.12.

Data Validation in R

Now that the dataset has been edited, it needs to be validated before it can be used in an analysis, as will be demonstrated in Chapters 3 and 4. This section will cover how to evaluate bivariate relationships between two continuous variables, a categorical and continuous variable, and two categorical variables. Next, power calculations will be covered, and finally, how to write the analytic file out to disk will be demonstrated.

Bivariate Relationships between Continuous Variables

Before doing linear regression modeling, it is helpful to examine bivariate relationships between the continuous dependent variable and potential independent variables. If some of those independent variables are also continuous, then it would be helpful to do correlations and make scatter plots to evaluate the relationship between the continuous independent variables and the continuous dependent variable.

In SAS, to make a scatter plot between age and sleep duration, we could use the GPLOT command:

```
TITLE 'Scatterplot - Age vs. Sleep Time';
PROC GPLOT DATA=r.BRFSS_a;
     PLOT _AGE80 * SLEPTIM1;
RUN;
```

In SAS, if we wanted to know the correlation between these variables, we could use different approaches, including PROC CORR:

```
proc corr data=r.BRFSS_a;
       var _AGE80 SLEPTIM1;
run;
```

To demonstrate these functions in R, we will create a dataset ScatterExample2 with three continuous variables (X_AGE80, SLEPTIM1, and ASTHMAGE) and SEX, a binary categorical variable. We will subset the dataset so that all values are not unknown or missing.

```
ScatterList <- c("X_AGE80", "SLEPTIM1", "ASTHMAGE", "SEX")
ScatterExample <- BRFSS_a[ScatterList]
ScatterExample2 <- subset(ScatterExample,
       !is.na(ScatterExample$SLEPTIM1)
       & ScatterExample$SLEPTIM1 != 77 &
ScatterExample$SLEPTIM1 != 99
       & !is.na(ScatterExample$ASTHMAGE) &
ScatterExample$ASTHMAGE <97)
```

Let us start by considering age (X_AGE80) and sleep duration (SLEPTIM1). The following code creates a scatter plot of these two variables:

```
plot(ScatterExample2$X_AGE80,ScatterExample2$SLEPTIM1,
       main = "Age vs. Sleep Duration in BRFSS 2014",
       xlab = "Age",
       ylab = "Avg Slp per Night",
       xlim=c(10,110),
       ylim=c(0,30),
       pch=2,
       cex =.8,
       col = "mediumorchid4")
```

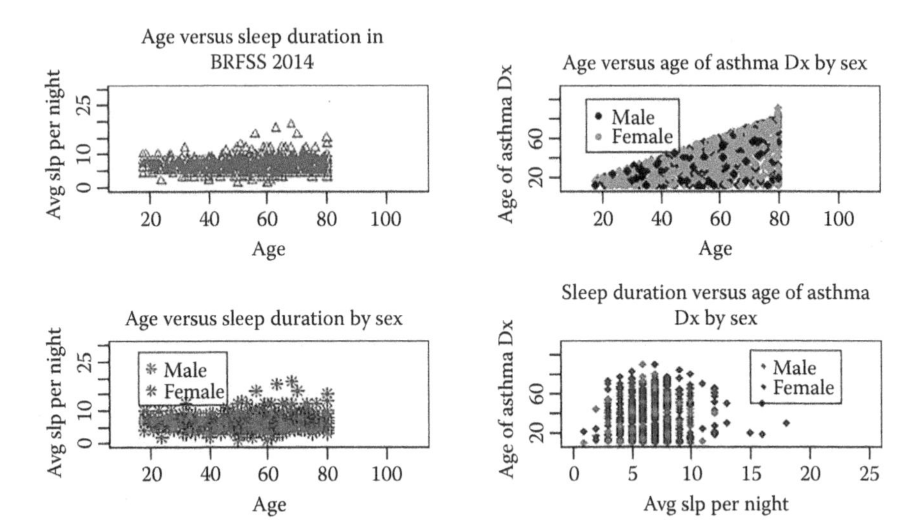

FIGURE 2.6
(See color insert.) Scatter plots.

This scatter plot is the upper-left plot in Figure 2.6. There appears to be a weak, positive correlation between the two variables. Notice the `pch` command; this designates the marker used in the scatter plot. There are many shapes of markers available; `pch = 2` is a triangle.

To calculate the correlation coefficient R, we can use the command `cor`:

```
cor(ScatterExample2$X_AGE80,ScatterExample2$SLEPTIM1,
use="all.obs", method="pearson")
```

This command will calculate the correlation coefficient using the two variables specified. The argument `all.obs` assumes no missing data; alternatives are `complete.obs` (listwise deletion) and `pairwise.complete.obs` (pairwise deletion). With our large dataset, we are using the method `pearson`, but alternatives are `spearman` and `kendall`.

Output:

```
[1] 0.1388027
```

This is the Pearson correlation coefficient for the correlation between age and sleep duration. Using only the dataset name in the `cor` command will produce a correlation matrix:

```
cor(ScatterExample2, use="all.obs", method="pearson")
```

Output:

```
               X_AGE80     SLEPTIM1    ASTHMAGE         SEX
X_AGE80   1.00000000 0.138802715 0.59242310 0.028145444
SLEPTIM1  0.13880271 1.000000000 0.11473477 0.004911634
ASTHMAGE  0.59242310 0.114734774 1.00000000 0.049571635
SEX       0.02814544 0.004911634 0.04957163 1.000000000
```

The main problem here is that *p*-values are not reported. These can be obtained using the `rcorr` command from the `Hmisc` library.

```
library(Hmisc)
res1<-rcorr(ScatterExample2$X_AGE80,ScatterExample2$SLEPTIM1,
type="pearson")
res1
```

Object `res1` is the correlation object produced by the `rcorr` command.

Output:

```
     x    y
x 1.00 0.14
y 0.14 1.00

n= 1176

P
  x y
x    0
y 0
```

The output is somewhat unintuitive. The correlation matrix at the top reports a correlation coefficient of 0.14 (as verified by the `cor` command run earlier), and the *p*-value is reported as 0 in the *p*-value matrix at the bottom. Running `rcorr` on the whole dataset makes the results easier to interpret, which we will do here and create correlation object `res2`.

```
res2<-rcorr(as.matrix(ScatterExample2, type="pearson"))
res2
```

Output:

```
          X_AGE80 SLEPTIM1 ASTHMAGE  SEX
X_AGE80      1.00     0.14     0.59 0.03
SLEPTIM1     0.14     1.00     0.11 0.00
ASTHMAGE     0.59     0.11     1.00 0.05
SEX          0.03     0.00     0.05 1.00

n= 1176
```

```
P
          X_AGE80  SLEPTIM1  ASTHMAGE  SEX
X_AGE80            0.0000    0.0000    0.3349
SLEPTIM1  0.0000             0.0000    0.8664
ASTHMAGE  0.0000   0.0000              0.0893
SEX       0.3349   0.8664    0.0893
```

This version reports correlation coefficients only out to two decimals, and the two tables are somewhat clumsy. A function has been written in R called `flattenCorrMatrix`:

```
flattenCorrMatrix <- function(cormat, pmat) {
  ut <- upper.tri(cormat)
  data.frame(
    row = rownames(cormat)[row(cormat)[ut]],
    column = rownames(cormat)[col(cormat)[ut]],
    cor =(cormat)[ut],
    p = pmat[ut]
    )
}
```

Functions are like macros in SAS, so running this code will create the function `flattenCorrMatrix`. This function can then be run on `res2` to produce an easier version to read:

```
flattenCorrMatrix(round(res2$r,4), round(res2$P, 4))
```

Output:

```
       row   column    cor      p
1  X_AGE80 SLEPTIM1 0.1388 0.0000
2  X_AGE80 ASTHMAGE 0.5924 0.0000
3 SLEPTIM1 ASTHMAGE 0.1147 0.0001
4  X_AGE80      SEX 0.0281 0.3349
5 SLEPTIM1      SEX 0.0049 0.8664
6 ASTHMAGE      SEX 0.0496 0.0893
```

Scatter plots are useful for each relationship, and in R, it is easy to arrange for images to be plotted in a 4 × 4 matrix. Also, it can be helpful to color code the points by sex to assess associations with this variable. The following code creates four scatter plots in a 4 × 4 matrix, with the last three plotting different colors by sex, and adding a legend.

```
layout(matrix(c(1,2,3,4),2,2)) # optional 4 graphs/page

plot(ScatterExample2$X_AGE80,ScatterExample2$SLEPTIM1,
       main = "Age vs. Sleep Duration in BRFSS 2014",
       xlab = "Age",
       ylab = "Avg Slp per Night",
       xlim=c(10,110),
       ylim=c(0,30),
```

```
        pch=2,
        cex =.8,
        col = "mediumorchid4")

plot(ScatterExample2$X_AGE80,ScatterExample2$SLEPTIM1,
        main = "Age vs. Sleep Duration by Sex",
        xlab = "Age",
        ylab = "Avg Slp per Night",
        xlim=c(10,110),
        ylim=c(0,30),
        pch=8,
        col = ifelse(ScatterExample2$SEX==1, "red", "blue"))

legend(20,28,
        pch=c(8,8),
        col=c("red", "blue"),
        c("Male", "Female"),
        bty="o",
        box.col="darkgreen",
        cex=.8)

plot(ScatterExample2$X_AGE80,ScatterExample2$ASTHMAGE,
        main = "Age vs. Age of Asthma\nDx by Sex",
        xlab = "Age",
        ylab = "Age of Asthma Dx",
        xlim=c(10,110),
        ylim=c(10,110),
        pch=16,
        col = ifelse(ScatterExample2$SEX==1, "gray25", "gray50"))

legend(20,100,
        pch=c(16,16),
        col=c("gray25", "gray50"),
        c("Male", "Female"),
        bty="o",
        box.col="darkgreen",
        cex=.8)

plot(ScatterExample2$SLEPTIM1,ScatterExample2$ASTHMAGE,
        main = "Sleep Duration vs. Age of Asthma\nDx by Sex",
        xlab = "Sleep Duration",
        ylab = "Age of Asthma Dx",
        xlim=c(0,25),
        ylim=c(10,110),
        pch=18,
        col = ifelse(ScatterExample2$SEX==1, "royalblue3",
        "palevioletred4"))

legend(15,105,
        pch=c(18,18),
        col=c("royalblue3", "palevioletred4"),
        c("Male", "Female"),
```

```
        bty="o",
        box.col="darkgreen",
        cex=.8)
```

Notice that the first two numbers in the legend command are the *x* and *y* coordinates of the upper-left corner of the legend. Also, notice that the pch command in the legend—this is how the legend knows what pch was used for the scatter plot. The argument bty = "o" indicates box type—it is either "o" (draw the box) or "n" (don't draw the box). Figure 2.6 in the inset provides the plots created from this code.

There are packages that provide excellent opportunities for data visualization of correlations. One is corrplot [59], which offers a heatmap-type display that can be configured in many ways, including changing the color palette, indicating a significant level on the plot, and showing confidence intervals on the plot. The following code creates the correlation object mcor and uses the corrplot command to produce Figure 2.7 in the inset.

```
ScatterExample3 <- ScatterExample2

colnames(ScatterExample3) <- c("Age", "Sleep","Age Asthma Dx",
"Sex")
library(corrplot)
mcor <- cor(ScatterExample3)
corrplot(mcor,
        type="upper",
        order="hclust",
        tl.col="black",
        tl.srt=45)
```

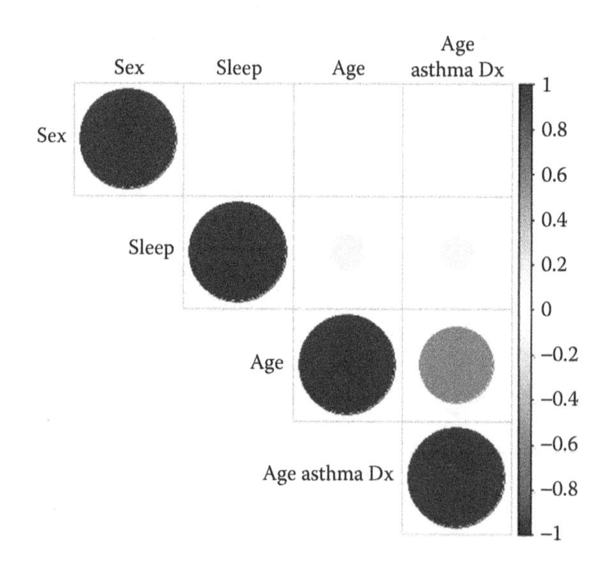

FIGURE 2.7
(See color insert.) Correlation plot.

`corrplot` does not offer an easy way to assign variable name labels, so we work around that by copying `ScatterExample2` to `ScatterExample3` and simply changing the column names to names we would normally see on a label with the `colnames` command. Note that in R, we can have column names with spaces, unlike in SAS. Next, we call up the library `corrplot`, then use the `cor` command on our dataset, `ScatterExample3`, to create the correlation object `mcor`. The `corrplot` command then creates the plot in Figure 2.7. In the `corrplot` code, upper specifies printing only the upper portion of the correlation matrix, `hclust` specifies to order the estimates by the correlation coefficient, `tl.col` specifies text label color, and `tl.srt` specifies a text label angle of 45°.

Bivariate Relationships between Categorical and Continuous Variables

In our linear regression demonstration in Chapter 4, we will use `SLEPTIM1`, or sleep duration as our dependent variable. When using a dependent continuous variable, it is helpful to first assess the relationships between categorical independent variables and this continuous variable before proceeding with regression modeling. Here, we will first examine the relationships between two two-level categorical variables, `ASTHMA4` (asthma status yes/no) and `SEX` (male/female), and `SLEPTIM1`. Next, we will examine the relationships between two multilevel categorical variables, `ALCGRP` (our alcohol grouping variable representing our hypothesized exposure) and `X_AGE_G` (age groups), and sleep duration.

Since both `ASTHMA4` and `SEX` have only two levels, to assess the relationship between these levels with `SLEPTIM1`, we could use an independent Student's *t*-test, as the SAS user would do using `PROC TTEST`. Note that in SAS, before doing a *t*-test comparing each level of `SEX`, the dataset would need to be sorted first by `SEX`.

```
proc sort data=r.BRFSS_a;
      by SEX;
proc ttest data=r.BRFSS_a;
      var SLEPTIM1;
      by SEX;
      run;
```

In R, there is no sorting required. The command we will use in R is called `t.test`, and it is followed by the argument for the dependent variable, a tilde, and the independent variable:

```
t.test(BRFSS_i$SLEPTIM1~BRFSS_i$ASTHMA4)
```

Output:

```
       Welch Two Sample t-test

data: BRFSS_i$SLEPTIM1 by BRFSS_i$ASTHMA4
t = 5.8738, df = 6060, p-value = 4.485e-09
alternative hypothesis: true difference in means is not equal
to 0
95 percent confidence interval:
 0.09852347 0.19722952
sample estimates:
mean in group 0 mean in group 1
       7.129348        6.981471
```

Although it is labeled Welch Two Sample *t*-test, this only refers to the fact that this *t*-test function calculates degrees of freedom using the formula of Welch–Satterthwaite [60]; it does not negate that this is indeed a Student *t*-test. Notice that the *t* value, df, and *p*-value are reported in the second line of the output, and the means are at the end. We can repeat this for sleep duration and sex:

```
t.test(BRFSS_i$SLEPTIM1~BRFSS_i$SEX)
```

Output:

```
       Welch Two Sample t-test

data: BRFSS_i$SLEPTIM1 by BRFSS_i$SEX
t = 12.658, df = 6146.6, p-value < 2.2e-16
alternative hypothesis: true difference in means is not equal
to 0
95 percent confidence interval:
 0.2342547 0.3201083
sample estimates:
mean in group 1 mean in group 2
       7.140360        6.863178
```

Again, there appear to be significant differences, so box plots can be helpful. Figure 2.8 shows box plots for sleep duration by asthma status and sleep duration by sex, side by side, made from this code:

```
par(mfrow=c(1,2))

boxplot(BRFSS_i$SLEPTIM1~BRFSS_i$ASTHMA4,
        main = "Sleep duration by Asthma status",
        ylab = "Avg Slp per Night",
        xlab = "Asthma Status",
        names = c("No asthma", "Has asthma"),
        border = "black",
        col=(c("deepskyblue3","darkgoldenrod")))
```

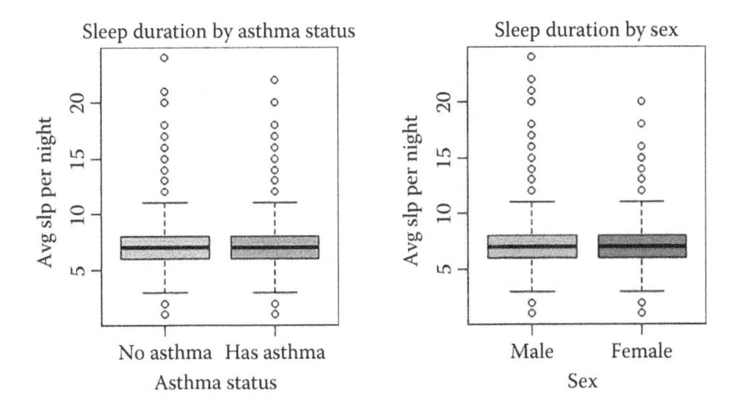

FIGURE 2.8
(See color insert.) Box plot of sleep duration by asthma status and sex.

```
boxplot(BRFSS_i$SLEPTIM1~BRFSS_i$SEX,
        main = "Sleep duration by Sex",
        ylab = "Avg Slp per Night",
        xlab = "Sex",
        names = c("Male", "Female"),
        border = "black",
        col=(c("darkorange","darkorchid")))
```

The visualizations are consistent with the estimates from the *t*-test. The following code compares sleep duration in terms of alcohol consumption status and age in a similar plot, which is the inset in Figure 2.9:

```
par(mfrow=c(1,2))

boxplot(BRFSS_i$SLEPTIM1~BRFSS_i$ALCGRP,
        main = "Sleep duration by Alcohol status",
        ylab = "Avg Slp per Night",
        xlab = "Alcohol Status",
        names = c("Nondrinker", "Monthly", "Weekly"),
        border = "black",
        col=(c("lightgoldenrod","lightpink","lightcoral")))

boxplot(BRFSS_i$SLEPTIM1~BRFSS_i$X_AGE_G,
        main = "Sleep duration by Age Group",
        ylab = "Avg Slp per Night",
        xlab = "Age Group",
        names = c("18-24", "25-34", "35-44", "45-54", "55-64",
        "65+"),
        border = "black",
        las = 2,
        col=(c("mediumslateblue","mediumpurple","mediumorchid1",
             "hotpink4", "indianred4", "indianred")))
```

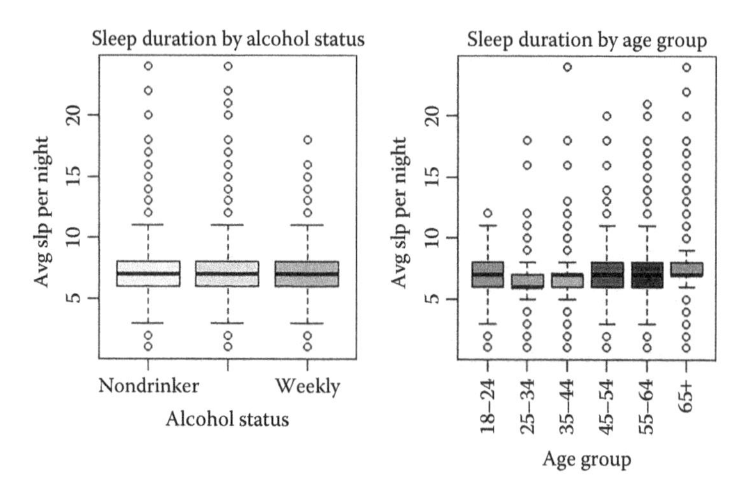

FIGURE 2.9
(See color insert.) Box plots of sleep duration by age and alcohol status.

The plots suggest that in bivariate modeling, age is more associated with sleep duration than alcohol status. Because age and alcohol group are multi-level categories, to assess their relationship with sleep duration, an analysis of variance, or ANOVA, should be used.

As a reminder, a one-way ANOVA asks for one independent variable, which can be continuous or ordinal, and a dependent variable that is continuous. In terms of alcohol consumption, because of how we coded this variable, we can use it as both continuous (with 1 being the lowest and 3 being the highest levels), or as an ordinal variable (with each level being in its own category).

In SAS, we could do a one-way ANOVA using `PROC GLM`, which is for "general linear modeling." Below are two examples—the first uses `ALCGRP` as a continuous independent variable, and the second includes the `CLASS` statement to model `ALCGRP` as an ordinal variable.

```
PROC GLM data=r.BRFSS_i
      model SLEPTIM1 = ALCGRP;
      run;

PRO CGLM data=r.BRFSS_i;
      class ALCGRP;
      model SLEPTIM1 = ALCGRP;
      run;
```

We will recreate these analyses in R. Notice that the following code creates a regression object named `AlcANOVA`, and the summary command displays the results. This code handles alcohol consumption as a continuous variable.

```
AlcANOVA <- lm(formula = SLEPTIM1 ~ ALCGRP,
        data = BRFSS_i)
summary(AlcANOVA)
```

Output:

```
Call:
lm(formula = SLEPTIM1 ~ ALCGRP, data = BRFSS_i)

Residuals:
    Min      1Q  Median      3Q     Max
-6.1173 -1.1149 -0.1149 0.8839 16.8851

Coefficients:
            Estimate Std. Error t value Pr(>|t|)
(Intercept) 7.113753   0.015596 456.129   <2e-16 ***
ALCGRP      0.001171   0.008396   0.139    0.889
---
Signif. codes: 0 '***' 0.001 '**' 0.01 '*' 0.05 '.' 0.1 ' ' 1

Residual standard error: 1.469 on 58129 degrees of freedom
Multiple R-squared: 3.347e-07, Adjusted R-squared: -1.687e-05
F-statistic: 0.01945 on 1 and 58129 DF, p-value: 0.8891
```

This code handles `ALCGRP` as an ordinal variable.

Code:

```
AlcANOVA2 <- lm(formula = SLEPTIM1 ~ as.factor(ALCGRP),
data = BRFSS_i)

summary(AlcANOVA2)
```

Output:

```
Call:
lm(formula = SLEPTIM1 ~ as.factor(ALCGRP), data = BRFSS_i)

Residuals:
    Min      1Q  Median      3Q     Max
-6.1487 -1.0903 -0.0903 0.8739 16.9097

Coefficients:
                    Estimate Std. Error t value Pr(>|t|)
(Intercept)         7.126103   0.009078 785.023  < 2e-16 ***
as.factor(ALCGRP)2 -0.035845   0.013328  -2.690  0.00716 **
as.factor(ALCGRP)3  0.022566   0.017716   1.274  0.20277
---
Signif. codes: 0 '***' 0.001 '**' 0.01 '*' 0.05 '.' 0.1 ' ' 1

Residual standard error: 1.468 on 58128 degrees of freedom
Multiple R-squared: 0.0002203, Adjusted R-squared: 0.0001859
F-statistic: 6.403 on 2 and 58128 DF, p-value: 0.001657
```

The `lm` command can be seen as similar to `PROC GLM` in SAS. As with the model statement in `PROC GLM`, the `formula` statement indicates the dependent variable followed by a tilde followed by the independent variable (or variables, in multiple linear regression). Instead of the CLASS statement used in SAS, the as.factor() function is used around ALCGRP to indicate that it should be handled as an ordinal variable as shown in the second example.

Note that simply viewing the objects AlcANOVA and AlcANOVA2 only reveals the intercepts and slopes for ALCGRP; the summary command must be run on each ANOVA object for the rest of the metrics to appear in the output.

As with PROG GLM, the summary statement produces linear regression estimates (which we will largely ignore for now) and ANOVA results (bottom of output). Please notice that the last line of the output contains the F-statistic, degrees of freedom, and *p*-value on the F-statistic. This output suggests that in bivariate analysis, ALCGRP is not associated with SLEPTIM1 when modeled continuously, but is statistically significantly associated with SLEPTIM1 when modeled ordinally.

We can also try age. We will use the ordinal age group variable X_AGE_G. First, we model it as a continuous independent variable:

```
AgeANOVA <- lm(formula = SLEPTIM1 ~ X_AGE_G,
        data = BRFSS_i)
summary(AgeANOVA)
```

Output:

```
Call:
lm(formula = SLEPTIM1 ~ X_AGE_G, data = BRFSS_i)

Residuals:
    Min       1Q   Median      3Q      Max
-6.3304  -0.8282  -0.0793 0.6696  17.4229

Coefficients:
             Estimate  Std. Error  t value  Pr(>|t|)
(Intercept)  5.823829    0.025087   232.15  <2e-16   ***
X_AGE_G      0.251102    0.004737    53.01  <2e-16   ***
---

Signif. codes: 0 '***' 0.001 '**' 0.01 '*' 0.05 '.' 0.1 ' ' 1

Residual standard error: 1.434 on 58129 degrees of freedom
Multiple R-squared: 0.04611, Adjusted R-squared: 0.0461
F-statistic: 2810 on 1 and 58129 DF, p-value: < 2.2e-16
```

Next, we model X_AGE_G as an ordinal variable.

Code:

```
AgeANOVA2 <- lm(formula = SLEPTIM1 ~ as.factor(X_AGE_G),
        data = BRFSS_i)
summary(AgeANOVA2)
```

Output:

```
Call:
lm(formula = SLEPTIM1 ~ as.factor(X_AGE_G), data = BRFSS_i)

Residuals:
    Min      1Q  Median      3Q     Max
-6.3859 -0.7033  0.0913  0.6141 17.4090

Coefficients:
                    Estimate Std. Error t value Pr(>|t|)
(Intercept)          6.52614    0.04769 136.840  < 2e-16 ***
as.factor(X_AGE_G)2 -0.07902    0.05517  -1.432 0.152089
as.factor(X_AGE_G)3  0.06483    0.05333   1.216 0.224122
as.factor(X_AGE_G)4  0.17721    0.05086   3.484 0.000494 ***
as.factor(X_AGE_G)5  0.38257    0.04965   7.705 1.33e-14 ***
as.factor(X_AGE_G)6  0.85976    0.04832  17.792  < 2e-16 ***
---
Signif. codes: 0 '***' 0.001 '**' 0.01 '*' 0.05 '.' 0.1 ' ' 1

Residual standard error: 1.43 on 58125 degrees of freedom
Multiple R-squared: 0.05202, Adjusted R-squared: 0.05194
F-statistic: 637.9 on 5 and 58125 DF, p-value: < 2.2e-16
```

This time, the F-statistic is significant in both analyses, as might have been predicted from Figure 2.10 below, which contains some plots run that we coded and ran earlier in the chapter. The second analysis suggests that in bivariate analysis, only older age groups are associated with sleep duration.

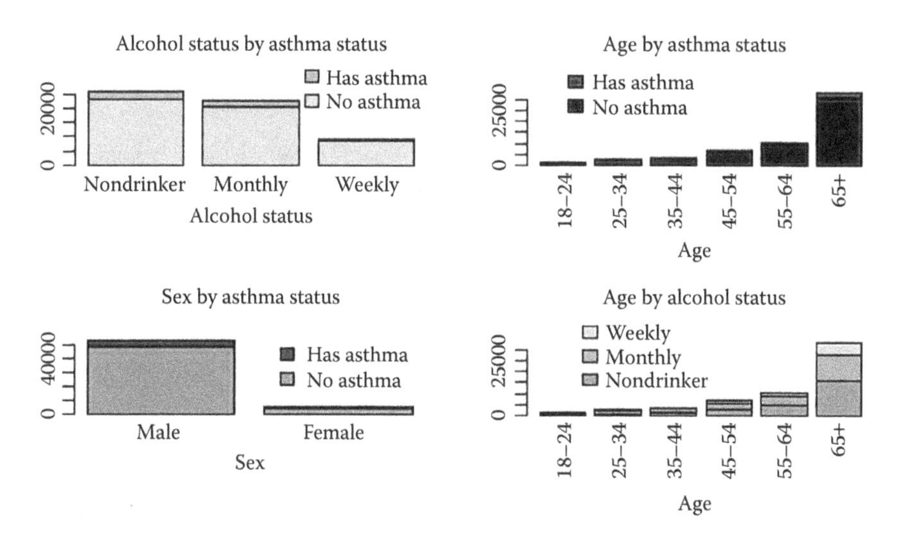

FIGURE 2.10
(See color insert.) Stacked bar chart example.

Bivariate Relationships between Categorical Variables

In the regression examples that will be provided in Chapter 4, logistic regression will be demonstrated by using the dependent variable ASTHMA4. It is helpful then to explore the bivariate relationships between independent categorical variables, such as SEX, X_AGE_G, and ALCGRP (our exposure), and ASTHMA4, our binary dependent variable.

As described earlier, a stacked barplot is helpful for visual comparisons. In SAS, a stacked bar chart could be made using PROC SGPLOT. The following SAS code is an example of using PROC SGPLOT to make a stacked bar chart of alcohol status by the asthma group.

```
proc sgplot data=r.BRFSS_h9;
  title 'Alcohol Status by Asthma Status';
  vbar ALCGRP / response=ALCGRP group=ASTHMA4 stat=sum;
  xaxis display=(nolabel);
  yaxis grid label='Frequency';
run;
```

R is quite extensible in making stacked bar plots. The following R code produces the inset in Figure 2.10.

```
#Make Labels

AsthmaLabels <- c("No Asthma","Has Asthma")
AlcLabels <- c("Nondrinker","Monthly","Weekly")
SexLabels <- c("Male","Female")
AgeLabels <- c("18-24", "25-34", "35-44", "45-54", "55-64",
"65+")

#Plots

layout(matrix(c(1,2,3,4),2,2)) # optional 4 graphs/page

AlcAsthmaFreq <- table(BRFSS_i$ASTHMA4, BRFSS_i$ALCGRP)

barplot(AlcAsthmaFreq,
        col= c("olivedrab3","rosybrown"),
        xlab="Alcohol Status",
        main="Alcohol Status by Asthma Status",
        names = AlcLabels,
        legend = AsthmaLabels,
        args.legend = list(
               x=4,
               y=20000,
               bty = "n"))

SexAsthmaFreq <- table(BRFSS_i$ASTHMA4, BRFSS_i$SEX)
```

```
barplot(SexAsthmaFreq,
       col=c("turquoise4","slateblue4"),
       xlab="Sex",
       main="Sex by Asthma Status",
       names = SexLabels,
       legend = AsthmaLabels,
       args.legend = list(
              x=2.5,
              y=30000,
              bty = "n"))

AgeAsthmaFreq <- table(BRFSS_i$ASTHMA4, BRFSS_i$X_AGE_G)

barplot(AgeAsthmaFreq,
       col=c("darkslategrey","firebrick"),
       xlab="Age",
       main="Age by Asthma Status",
       names = AgeLabels,
       legend = AsthmaLabels,
       las = 3,
       args.legend = list(
              x=4,
              y=25000,
              bty = "n"))

AgeAlcFreq <- table(BRFSS_i$ALCGRP, BRFSS_i$X_AGE_G)

barplot(AgeAlcFreq,
        col=c("lightblue4", "lightcoral", "lightgoldenrod3"),
        xlab="Age",
        main="Age by Alcohol Status",
        names = AgeLabels,
        legend = AlcLabels,
        las = 3,
        args.legend = list(
              x=4,
              y=25000,
              bty = "n"))
```

Notice the `args.legend` option in the `barplot` command that is used to position the legend on the plot. Also, `las=3` is used to reposition labels when crowding occurs. The stacked bar chart allows the analyst to consider overall distributions, as well as distributions within levels of a second categorical variable.

A mathematical assessment can be done using a chi-squared statistic or, if there are small cells, Fisher's exact test. In SAS, this is normally done as part of `PROC FREQ`, but it is a separate function in R. To run the chi-squared test, we will use the `chisq.test` function on the frequency table we made for alcohol and asthma:

```
chisq.test(AlcAsthmaFreq)
```

Output:

```
        Pearson's Chi-squared test

data: AlcAsthmaFreq
X-squared = 58.823, df = 2, p-value = 1.686e-13
```

Notice that the chi-square statistic, degrees of freedom, and *p*-value are reported. If a Fisher's exact test is needed, the analyst can use `fisher.test` as an alternative.

Power Calculations

Two power calculations that could be done here is one to estimate sample needed for the analysis of alcohol intake and sleep duration (continuous outcome), and one to estimate sample needed for the analysis of alcohol intake and asthma status (binary outcome). In both cases, we need an estimate of effect size. Cohen's *d* is a formula for estimating effect size that is commonly used in statistics. However, SAS does not have an easy way of calculating Cohen's *d*. Rajendra Kadel and Kevin Kip published a SAS white paper with a macro for calculating Cohen's *d* [61]. SAS users do not have a readily available `PROC` for calculating Cohen's *d*.

Calculating Cohen's *d* is considerably easier in R. The `lsr` package includes a command to calculate Cohen's *d* [62]. We can call up library `lsr`, and then calculate the variable `CohensDSleep` by using the `CohensD` command on our outcome, `SLEPTIM1`, and by a binary variable, `ASTHMA4`.

```
library(lsr)
CohensDSleep <- cohensD(BRFSS_i$SLEPTIM1, BRFSS_i$ASTHMA4)

CohensDSleep
```

Output:

```
[1] 6.636531
```

`CohensDSleep` has the value of 6.636531. Another way to think about effect size is to look at the raw differences in means. Here, we calculate variables `AsthmaMeanSleep` as the average sleep duration among respondents suffering from asthma, and `NoAsthmaMeanSleep` as the average sleep duration for those not suffering from asthma. We can make `DiffSleep` as the absolute difference between the two estimates.

```
AsthmaMeanSleep <- mean(BRFSS_i$SLEPTIM1[BRFSS_i$ASTHMA4 == 1])
NoAsthmaMeanSleep <- mean(BRFSS_i$SLEPTIM1[BRFSS_i$ASTHMA4 == 0])
DiffSleep <- abs(AsthmaMeanSleep - NoAsthmaMeanSleep)
```

The value of `DiffSleep` is 0.1478765. Imagine we wanted to calculate sample size for a study that would do a *t*-test between the two asthma groups, and used the effect size for `DiffSleep`. In SAS, `PROC POWER` is generally used. In `PROC POWER`, we could use the two sample means approach for this calculation, but we would have to put in an estimate of standard deviation. This is an example of `PROC POWER` that uses 1 as the standard deviation, the value of `DiffSleep` as the mean difference, restricts the power to 80%, and requests how many will be needed per group under those conditions.

```
proc power;
   twosamplemeans test=diff
   meandiff = .1478765
   stddev = 1
   power = .8
   npergroup = . ;
 run;
```

```
DiffSleep
```

Output:

```
[1] 0.1478765
```

In R, we could use the `pwr` package, which has several commands that can be used for power calculation [63]. All of the commands have the same structure; the function is stated, then all the arguments needed for a power calculation are designated except one, which is the one that is calculated.

For example, the *t*-test power calculation function, `pwr.t.test`, calls for *n* (sample size in one group), *d* (effect size), `sig.level` (significance level), and type ("two.sample," "one.sample" or "paired"). In the case where you have a fixed sample size, you can actually back-calculate effect size. Let us assume a fixed sample size of 50, a significance level of 0.05, and a power of 0.80.

```
library(pwr)
pwr.t.test(n= 50,
        sig.level = 0.05,
        power =.80,
        alternative ="two.sided")
```

Output:

```
     Two-sample t test power calculation

              n = 50
              d = 0.565858
```

```
     sig.level = 0.05
         power = 0.8
   alternative = two.sided

NOTE: n is number in *each* group
```

Notice that in the output, the effect size (d) is calculated to be 0.565858. Typically, we want to calculate n, so here is an example using the raw effect size (as a variable, `DiffSleep`) with the same significance, power, and type:

```
pwr.t.test(d = DiffSleep,
       sig.level = 0.05,
       power =.80,
       alternative ="two.sided")
```

Output:

```
     Two-sample t test power calculation

              n = 718.8192
              d = 0.1478765
      sig.level = 0.05
          power = 0.8
    alternative = two.sided

NOTE: n is number in *each* group
```

With this very small effect size, over 718 people would be needed in each group. We might want multiple effect sizes to be calculated. In that case, we can automate this somewhat with generating a sequence vector and using `lapply`. Let us start by creating a one-column data frame of a sequence of numbers between `DiffSleep` (low number) and `CohensDSleep` (high number) with steps of 0.25 in between. We will name the one column "`DiffLevel`."

```
SampleSize <- as.data.frame(seq(DiffSleep, CohensDSleep,0.25))
names(SampleSize) <- c("DiffLevel")
```

If you look at the `SampleSize` object, you will see 26 entries. The top looks like this:

```
  DiffLevel
1 0.1478765
2 0.3978765
3 0.6478765
4 0.8978765
5 1.1478765
```

Our next goal is to use the `lapply` function to make an object called `SampleResults`. This object will have the required sample at every level of `DiffLevel`. However, trying to use `lapply` on `SampleSize` would not work, because there are `DiffLevels` that are too high for which to calculate results. Therefore, it is important that we remove the `DiffLevels` that are too high first, before we run the `lapply`. We make `SampleSize2` as a subset of `SampleSize` where the `DiffLevel` is less than 5.

```
SampleSize2 <- subset(SampleSize, DiffLevel < 5)
```

Using the `SampleSize2` object, we can automate the development of the object `SampleResults` using the `lapply` function and specifying our one-column dataset:

```
SampleResults <- lapply(SampleSize2[, c('DiffLevel')],
function(x)
       {pwr.t.test(d = x[1],
       sig.level = 0.05,
       power =.80,
       alternative = "two.sided")
       })
```

Viewing the object `SampleResults` will provide calculations of sample needed for the various effect sizes from the raw value of `DiffSleep` up to the highest value less than 5 in our dataset.

This last demonstration was for a *t*-test power calculation, but the `pwr` package offers several options for other types of power calculations.

The regressions demonstrated in Chapter 4 include linear regression (hypothesized exposure = alcohol consumption, outcome = sleep duration) and logistic regression (same exposure, with outcome = asthma status). Here, the commands from the `pwr` package will be used to calculate sample size needed for both these regressions.

Many analysts use the *t*-test formula when calculating sample size for an ultimate regression. This is fine because power calculation is not an exact science. However, if the analyst really wants to power her study for a linear regression analysis, she can use `pwr.f2.test` (see Table 2.13). This function requires numerator degrees of freedom (u) as an argument in order to produce v, denominator degrees of freedom, which will lead us to a sample size estimate. The u variable refers to the degrees of freedom in the ANOVA table for the regression. Assuming a simple regression with `ALCGRP` as the only independent variable, u would be two degrees of freedom. The argument `f2` is the effect size; we will use `lapply` and our `SampleSize2` object for this, but first, let us estimate effect size using our sample.

With `ALCGRP`, we have three levels: No drinking, monthly drinking, and weekly drinking. We can generate Cohens's d for this variable, and call it `CohensDAlc`:

TABLE 2.13

Commands in the pwr Package

Function	Description	Arguments	Code Example	n, n2, N, or v
pwr.2p.test	Two proportions (equal n)	h =, n =, sig.level =, power =	pwr.2p.test(h = 0.15, sig.level = 0.05,power = 0.80)	697.68
pwr.2p2n.test	Two proportions (unequal n)	h =, n1 =, n2 =, sig.level =, power =	pwr.2p2n.test(h = .15,n1 = 1000,sig.level = 0.05, power = 0.80)	535.72
pwr.anova.test	Balanced one way ANOVA	k =, n =, f =, sig.level =, power =	pwr.anova.test (k = 5, f = 0.15,sig.level = 0.05, power = 0.80)	107.04
pwr.chisq.test	Chi-square test	w =, N =, df =, sig.level =, power =	pwr.chisq.test (w = 0.15, df = 3, sig.level = 0.05, power = 0.80)	484.56
pwr.f2.test	General linear model	u =, v =, f2 =, sig.level =, power =	pwr.f2.test (u = 2,f2 = 0.15,sig.level = 0.05, power = 0.80)	64.32
pwr.p.test	Proportion (one sample)	h =, n =, sig.level = power =	pwr.p.test(h = 0.15, sig.level = 0.05, power = 0.80)	348.84
pwr.r.test	Correlation	n =, r =, sig.level =, power =	pwr.r.test(r = 0.15, sig.level = 0.05, power = 0.80)	345.70
pwr.t.test	*t*-tests (one-sample, two-sample, paired)	n =, d =, sig.level =, power =, type = c("two.sample," "one.sample," "paired")	pwr.t.test(d = 0.15,sig.level = 0.05,power = 0.80,alternative ="two.sided")	698.64
pwr.t2n.test	*t*-test (two samples with unequal n)	n1 =, n2=, d =, sig.level =, power =	pwr.t2n.test(n1 = 1000, d = 0.15, sig.level = 0.05, power = 0.80)	536.75

Key: n = number in each group, n1 = number in first group, n2 = number in second group, h = proportion of n (or n1), k = number of groups, f = value of f statistic, w =effect size in chi-square, N = total sample size, u = numerator degrees of freedom, v = denominator degrees of freedom, f2 = effect size in linear models, r = value of r statstic, d = effect size in *t*-test.

```
CohensDAlc<- cohensD(BRFSS_i$SLEPTIM1, BRFSS_i$ALCGRP)
```

```
CohensDAlc
```

Output:

```
[1] 4.667021
```

Cohen's D is large again; it is 4.667021. It is, however, less than 5, so we can use it as our upper boundary of effect size levels in our sequence. For the lower boundary, we can compare the mean sleep duration in each alcohol group. We will generate means for each alcohol level as objects here named `NoDrinkMeanSleep`, `MonthlyMeanSleep`, and `WeeklyMeanSleep`:

```
NoDrinkMeanSleep <- mean(BRFSS_i$SLEPTIM1[BRFSS_i$ALCGRP == 1])
MonthlyMeanSleep <- mean(BRFSS_i$SLEPTIM1[BRFSS_i$ALCGRP == 2])
WeeklyMeanSleep <- mean(BRFSS_i$SLEPTIM1[BRFSS_i$ALCGRP == 3])
```

Next, we can use those variables to calculate the three raw differences between the three variables as `Diff1`, `Diff2`, and `Diff3`:

```
Diff1 <- abs(NoDrinkMeanSleep - MonthlyMeanSleep)
Diff2 <- abs(NoDrinkMeanSleep - WeeklyMeanSleep)
Diff3 <- abs(MonthlyMeanSleep - WeeklyMeanSleep)
```

Finally, we can take the lower boundary of our sequence by taking the minimum raw difference and calling it `DiffSleep`:

```
DiffSleep <- min(Diff1, Diff2, Diff3)
```

Using our new `DiffSleep` and `CohensDAlc`, we can generate a new sequence of effect size levels:

```
SampleSize <- as.data.frame(seq(DiffSleep, CohensDAlc,0.25))
names(SampleSize) <- c("DiffLevel")
```

Finally, using the `lapply` command, we can get estimates of v for all the different effect size levels in our sequence which is placed in the object `LMResults`:

```
LMResults <- lapply(SampleSize[, c('DiffLevel')], function(x)
        {pwr.f2.test (u = 2,
        f2 = x[1],
        sig.level = 0.05,
        power = 0.80)
        })
```

In the first set of results in `LMResults` (output not shown), where `f2` = 0.02256555, v is calculated to be 426.9744, meaning 428 people would be required under those parameters. The v estimate drops drastically at the next effect size of 0.2725656, where $v = 35.50796$, suggesting 36 people would be required under those parameters.

Finally, to estimate the logistic regression sample, we turn again to a function in the `pwr` package and estimates from our data. The function we will be using is `pwr.2p2n.test`, which is a two-proportion test (unequal n), because we are limited by the number of people we have in our dataset who have asthma, so we have to set that at `n1` in the set of arguments. Notice how we calculate objects holding the values of total sample (`TotalVets`), total rows with asthma (`YesAsthma`), total rows without asthma (`NoAsthma`), and the proportions of each of these asthma groups in drinking monthly and weekly (`AsthmaMonthlyProp`, `AsthmaWeeklyProp`, `NoAsthmaMonthlyProp`, and `NoAsthmaWeeklyProp`).

```
TotalVets <- nrow(BRFSS_i)
YesAsthma <- nrow(BRFSS_i[BRFSS_i$ASTHMA4 == 1,])
NoAsthma <- nrow(BRFSS_i[BRFSS_i$ASTHMA4 == 0,])

AsthmaMonthlyProp <- nrow(BRFSS_i[BRFSS_i$ASTHMA4 == 1 &
        BRFSS_i$DRKMONTHLY == 1,])/YesAsthma
AsthmaWeeklyProp <- nrow(BRFSS_i[BRFSS_i$ASTHMA4 == 1 &
        BRFSS_i$DRKWEEKLY == 1,])/YesAsthma

NoAsthmaMonthlyProp <- nrow(BRFSS_i[BRFSS_i$ASTHMA4 == 0 &
        BRFSS_i$DRKMONTHLY == 1,])/NoAsthma
NoAsthmaWeeklyProp <- nrow(BRFSS_i[BRFSS_i$ASTHMA4 == 0 &
        BRFSS_i$DRKWEEKLY == 1,])/NoAsthma
```

We know that `n1` in our code will be set to `YesAsthma`, but we need to calculate `f2`, or effect size. We can look at the differences in proportions of alcohol groups by asthma status in a similar way as to how we looked at them with respect to sleep duration—by calculating absolute differences, and taking the minimum and maximum of these differences as a sequence:

```
Diff1 <- abs(AsthmaMonthlyProp - NoAsthmaMonthlyProp)
Diff2 <- abs(AsthmaMonthlyProp - NoAsthmaWeeklyProp)
Diff3 <- abs(AsthmaWeeklyProp - NoAsthmaMonthlyProp)
Diff4 <- abs(AsthmaWeeklyProp - NoAsthmaWeeklyProp)

MinDiff <- min(Diff1, Diff2, Diff3, Diff4)
MaxDiff <- max(Diff1, Diff2, Diff3, Diff4)

SampleSize <- as.data.frame(seq(MinDiff, MaxDiff, 0.02))
names(SampleSize) <- c("DiffLevel")
SampleSize2 <- subset(SampleSize, DiffLevel > 0.05)
```

You will notice that we subsetted SampleSize into SampleSize2, again because effect sizes less than 0.05 were too small to be handled by the calculation. Again, lapply can be used to create a series of calculations for different effect sizes represented in our DiffLevels:

```
PropResults <- lapply(SampleSize2[, c('DiffLevel')], function(x)
       {pwr.2p2n.test(h = x[1],
       n1 = YesAsthma,
       sig.level = 0.05,
       power = 0.80)
       })
```

Please notice that the first entry in PropResults (output not shown) estimates n2 at 4,481.484, while the next estimate drops to 1,775.222. Nevertheless, we can convince ourselves that our analytic dataset has enough sample in each asthma group to be powerful enough to test very small differences in the prevalence of exposure in each group.

Write Out Analytic File

The last step after developing and validating an analytic dataset is to write it out to a *.csv using a particular name (in this case, analytic.csv). That way, if the dataset needs to be regenerated due to changes in editing in earlier files in the "movie," the name of the analytic file will not need to be changed in the analysis code. Also, having the analysis code start with reading in the current analytic.csv dataset is a way to ensure that one is using the most up-to-date version of the analytic dataset.

In SAS, writing out a dataset as a *.csv would be handled with a PROC EXPORT command:

```
PROC EXPORT DATA= R.BRFSS_i
            OUTFILE= "C:\Users\Monika\Dropbox\R Stats Book\
            Analytics\Data\Analytic.csv"
            DBMS=CSV REPLACE;
     PUTNAMES=YES;
RUN;
```

We will do the same in R. Using the write.csv code, the dataset in memory BRFSS_i is written out to the directory pointed to earlier using the Change Dir command from the menu. Notice that the rest of the descriptive analysis and the linear and logistic regression discussed in Chapters 3 and 4 will use the dataset "analytic" for demonstration.

```
write.csv(BRFSS_i, file = "analytic.csv")
```

Theoretically, it would have been possible to write out each iteration of the BRFSS file we were editing (`BRFSS_a`, `BRFSS_b`, etc.). This was not necessary because there was only one programmer involved. However, in a group programming effort, writing out each of these steps as a *.csv might be helpful because other programmers could read in those iterations and thus the work of editing variables could be split up among a programming team.

Now that our analytic dataset is developed, we can move on to conducting a descriptive analysis of it in Chapter 3.

Optional Exercises

Section "Reading Data into R"

Questions

1. What package in R can be used to read in data in many different formats?
2. What command in R can be used to get all the variable names in a data frame?
3. What command is used to identify data type of the variable in R?
4. In the chapter, a table of Rhode Island hospitals was provided, along with code to read it into R. Read this table in. Using R, calculate how many rows are in the file.
5. Using R, print out the column names of the Rhode Island hospital table.
6. Using R, find the class of the variable `StBeds`.
7. Using R, find the maximum length of the variable `StBeds`.

Answers

1. The `foreign` package.
2. The `colnames` command.
3. Data types in R are referred to as "classes." The `class` command is used for this.
4. Answer:

   Code:

   ```
   nrow(RIHosp)
   ```

   Output:

   ```
   [1] 11
   ```

5. Answer

   Code:

   ```
   colnames(RIHosp)
   ```

   Output:

   ```
   [1] "HospName" "HospCity" "StBeds" "AccredDate"
   ```

6. Answer:

   Code:

   ```
   class(RIHosp$StBeds)
   ```

   Output:

   ```
   [1] "integer"
   ```

7. Answer:

   Code:

   ```
   max(nchar(as.character(RIHosp$StBeds)))
   ```

   Output:

   ```
   [1] 3
   ```

Section "Checking Data in R"

Questions

1. Use the `summary` command in R on the Rhode Island hospital dataset to generate summary statistics of `StBeds`.
2. Using the `quantiles` command in R, generate the same `quantiles` for `StBeds` as would be calculated in `PROC UNIVARIATE` in SAS.
3. Install the `psych` package in R, and use the `describe` function to create summary statistics of `StBeds`.
4. Create a histogram of the `StBeds` variable using R. Manipulate the `xlim`, `ylim`, and `breaks` options to improve readability. Optionally, change the colors from what was demonstrated.
5. Create a box plot of the `StBeds` variable using R. Optionally, change the colors from what was demonstrated.
6. Create a QQ plot of the `StBeds` variable using R. Optionally, change the colors from what was demonstrated.
7. Create a frequency table in R of the `HospCity` variable using the `table` command and also, using the `freq` command from the `summarytools` package. Include the missings in the counts.
8. Create a pie chart in R of the distribution of hospitals by `HospCity`. Optionally, change the palette from what was demonstrated.

9. Create a bar chart in R of the distribution of hospitals by `HospCity`. Optionally, change the palette from what was demonstrated.
10. Using the BRFSS dataset, run a crosstab between the variables `VETERAN3` and `SEX` using the table command in R, and the `CrossTable` command from the `gmodels` package.
11. Using the BRFSS dataset, use the table command in R to create an object of the `VETERAN3` and `SEX` crosstab. Run `prop.table` on this object to produce row percents.
12. Using R, create a stacked barplot using the table created in Question 11. Optionally, change the palette from what was demonstrated.

Answers

1. Answer:

   Code:

   ```
   summary(RIHosp$StBeds)
   ```

   Output:

   ```
   Min. 1st Qu. Median  Mean 3rd Qu.  Max.
   89.0  131.0   160.0 225.7   241.0 686.0
   ```

2. Answer:

   Code:

   ```
   quantile(RIHosp$StBeds, na.rm=TRUE, prob = c(0.00,
   0.01, 0.05, 0.10, 0.25, 0.50, 0.75, 0.90, 0.95,
   0.99, 1.00))
   ```

   Output:

   ```
     0%   1%   5%  10%   25%   50%   75%   90%   95%   99%  100%
   89.0 89.2 90.0 91.0 131.0 160.0 241.0 343.0 514.5 651.7 686.0
   ```

3. Answer:

   Code:

   ```
   library(psych)
   describe(RIHosp$StBeds)
   ```

   Output:

   ```
   vars n mean sd median trimmed mad min max range skew
   kurtosis se
   1 1 11 225.73 171.01 160 189.78 102.3 89 686 597 1.66
   1.89 51.56
   ```

4. Possible answer:

   Code:

```
hist(RIHosp$StBeds,
        main = "Histogram of Staffed Beds",
        xlab = "Class Staffed Beds",
        ylab = "Frequency",
        xlim=c(0,800),
        ylim=c(0,6),
        border = "cornsilk4",
        col= "cornflowerblue",
        las = 1,
        breaks = 8)
```

   Output not shown.

5. Possible answer:

   Code:

```
boxplot(RIHosp$StBeds,
        main = "Box Plot of Staffed Beds",
        ylab = "Staffed Beds",
        border = "cornsilk4",
        col= "cornflowerblue")
```

   Output not shown.

6. Possible answer:

```
qqnorm(RIHosp$StBeds,
        main = "Q-Q Plot of Staffed Beds",
        col= "cornflowerblue")
qqline(RIHosp$StBeds,
        col = "cornsilk4")
```

   Output not shown.

7. Answer:

   Code:

```
table(RIHosp$HospCity, useNA = c("always"))
library(summarytools)
freq(RIHosp$HospCity)
```

   Output:

```
      Newport  North Providence  Pawtucket Providence
            1                 1          1          4
    Wakefield           Warwick   Westerly Woonsocket
            1                 1          1          1
         <NA>
            0
```

```
Frequencies

Dataframe name: RIHosp
Variable name: HospCity

                     N   %Valid    %Cum.    %Total    %Cum.
                                   Valid              Total
-----------------------------------------------------------
          Newport    1     9.09     9.09      9.09     9.09
North Providence     1     9.09    18.18      9.09    18.18
        Pawtucket    1     9.09    27.27      9.09    27.27
       Providence    4    36.36    63.64     36.36    63.64
        Wakefield    1     9.09    72.73      9.09    72.73
          Warwick    1     9.09    81.82      9.09    81.82
         Westerly    1     9.09    90.91      9.09    90.91
       Woonsocket    1     9.09      100      9.09      100
             <NA>    0       NA       NA         0      100
            Total   11      100      100       100      100
```

8. Possible answer:

```
HospCityFreq <- table(RIHosp$HospCity, useNA =
c("always"))
pie(HospCityFreq,
      col = cm.colors(8),
      main = "Pie Chart of HospCity")
```

Output not shown.

9. Possible answer:

Code:

```
barplot(HospCityFreq,
      col = cm.colors(8),
      xlab = "Distribution of HospCity",
      las = 2,
      main = "Bar Chart of HospCity")
```

Output not shown.

10. Answer:

Code:

```
table(BRFSS_a$VETERAN3, BRFSS_a$SEX, useNA =
c("always"))
library(gmodels)
CrossTable(BRFSS_a$VETERAN3, BRFSS_a$SEX)
```

Output:

```
              1        2      <NA>
  1       56596     5524         0
  2      135840   265721         0
  7          68       32         0
  9         213       81         0
  <NA>      253      336         0
     Cell Contents
  |----------------------------|
  |                          N |
  |    Chi-square contribution |
  |              N / Row Total |
  |              N / Col Total |
  |            N / Table Total |
  |----------------------------|

Total Observations in Table: 464075

               | BRFSS_a$SEX

BRFSS_a$VETERAN3 |          1 |           2 | Row Total |
-----------------|------------|-------------|-----------|
               1 |      56596 |        5524 |     62120 |
                 |  36772.218 |   26115.432 |           |
                 |      0.911 |       0.089 |     0.134 |
                 |      0.294 |       0.020 |           |
                 |      0.122 |       0.012 |           |
-----------------|------------|-------------|-----------|
               2 |     135840 |      265721 |    401561 |
                 |   5731.969 |    4070.814 |           |
                 |      0.338 |       0.662 |     0.865 |
                 |      0.705 |       0.979 |           |
                 |      0.293 |       0.573 |           |
-----------------|------------|-------------|-----------|
               7 |         68 |          32 |       100 |
                 |     16.876 |      11.985 |           |
                 |      0.680 |       0.320 |     0.000 |
                 |      0.000 |       0.000 |           |
                 |      0.000 |       0.000 |           |
-----------------|------------|-------------|-----------|
               9 |        213 |          81 |       294 |
                 |     67.693 |      48.076 |           |
                 |      0.724 |       0.276 |     0.001 |
                 |      0.001 |       0.000 |           |
                 |      0.000 |       0.000 |           |
```

```
-----------------|-----------|-----------|----------|
Column Total     |    192717 |    271358 |   464075 |
                 |     0.415 |     0.585 |          |
-----------------|-----------|-----------|----------|
```

11. Possible answer:

    Code:

```
VetSexFreq <- table(BRFSS_a$VETERAN3, BRFSS_a$SEX,
useNA = c("always"))
prop.table(VetSexFreq, 1)
```

    Output:

```
                 1          2       <NA>
1       0.91107534 0.08892466 0.00000000
2       0.33827986 0.66172014 0.00000000
7       0.68000000 0.32000000 0.00000000
9       0.72448980 0.27551020 0.00000000
<NA>    0.42954160 0.57045840 0.00000000
```

12. Possible answer:

    Code:

```
SexLabels <- c("Male", "Female", "Missing")
VetLabels <- c("Yes","No","Don't Know", "Refused",
"Missing")


barplot(VetSexFreq,
        col=cm.colors(5),
        xlab="Sex",
        main="Sex by Veteran Status",
        names = SexLabels,
        legend = VetLabels)
```

    Output not shown.

Section "Editing Data in R"

Questions

1. Using R, copy dataset `BRFSS_a` into `BRFSS_example1` keeping only the variables `SMOKE100`, `EDUCA`, `INCOME2`, and `EXERANY2`.
2. Using R, subset dataset `BRFSS_a` into men only (`SEX=1`) and women only (`SEX=2`).

3. Using R, count the number of rows in each of the datasets you made in Question 2. Verify that all the rows in the dataset are accounted for.
4. Create a table to guide yourself in developing the grouping variable for income (`INCOME2`) called `INCOME_EXP` which has four categories: 1=Up to $34,999, 2=$35,000–74,999, 3=$75,000 or more, 9=don't know, refused, missing or unknown. Check to make sure the variable is recoded correctly.
5. Using R, copy the dataset `BRFSS_a` into `BRFSS_example2`. In the new dataset, using R, create the grouping variable `INCOME_EXP` you designed in Question 4 using the `in` statement. Check to make sure the variable is recoded correctly.
6. Using the same dataset as in Question 5, in R, create an indicator variable called `INCOME_UNK` which is set to 1 where `INCOME_EXP` is unknown and 0 in all other cases. Check to make sure the variable is recoded correctly.
7. Imagine you wanted to use `INCOME_EXP` in a regression, so you plan to make a set of indicator variables. What levels would you put in your comparison group (code = 0 on all indicator variables), and why?
8. Using the dataset `BRFSS_example2`, in R, create an indicator flag called `SMOKE100_MISS` for those missing a value in `SMOKE100`. Check to make sure the variable was coded properly.
9. Starting with `BRFSS_a`, using R, recreate the survival dataset demonstrated by rerunning the code up to `SurvivalData_g`. Create `ASTHMA70` and `TIME70` time-to-event variables to facilitate an analysis with a time period from birth to age 70.
10. Using the Rhode Island hospital dataset, using R, create a fourth reference date of March 15, 2016, and create a variable with the difference between the accreditation date and this fourth reference date. Check to make sure the variable was coded properly.
11. Using the dataset `BRFSS_example2`, in R, create the grouping variable `AGEQUART` that classifies quartiles of age (`X_AGE80`) and contains a 1 for the first quartile, 2 for the second quartile, 3 for the third quartile, and 4 for the fourth quartile. Check to make sure the variable was coded properly.
12. Using the dataset `BRFSS_example2`, in R, create a log-transformed version of the variable for age (`X_AGE80`) called `LOGX_AGE80`, and check its distribution. Create a histogram and box plot of `LOGX_AGE80`. Manipulate the `xlim`, `ylim`, and `breaks` options to improve readability. Optionally, change the colors from what was demonstrated.

Answers

1. Possible answer:

```
BRFSSVarListExample1 <- c("SMOKE100", "EDUCA",
"INCOME2", "EXERANY2")
BRFSS_example1 <- BRFSS_a[BRFSSVarListExample1]
```

2. Possible answer:

```
MenOnly <- subset(BRFSS_a, SEX==1)
WomenOnly <- subset(BRFSS_a, SEX==2)
```

3. Answer:

Code:

```
nrow(MenOnly)
nrow(WomenOnly)
identical(nrow(BRFSS_a), nrow(MenOnly) +
nrow(WomenOnly))
```

Output:

```
[1] 192970
[1] 271694
[1] TRUE
```

4. Possible answer:

INCOME2	Description	INCOME_EXP
1	<$10,000	1
2	$10,000–14,999	1
3	$15,000–19,999	1
4	$20,000–24,999	1
5	$25,000–34,999	1
6	$35,000–49,999	2
7	$50,000–74,999	2
8	$75,000 or more	3
	Missing	9

5. Possible answer:

Code:

```
BRFSS_example2 <- BRFSS_a
BRFSS_example2$INCOME_EXP <- 9
BRFSS_example2$INCOME_EXP[BRFSS_example2$INCOME2 %in%
1:5] <- 1
BRFSS_example2$INCOME_EXP[BRFSS_example2$INCOME2 %in%
6:7] <- 2
```

```
BRFSS_example2$INCOME_EXP[BRFSS_example2$INCOME2 == 8]
<- 3
table(BRFSS_example2$INCOME_EXP, BRFSS_
example2$INCOME2, useNA = c("always"))
```

Output:

```
          1     2     3     4     5     6     7      8    77    99  <NA>
1     21199 22943 30511 37531 44315     0     0      0     0     0     0
2         0     0     0     0     0 57418 62175      0     0     0     0
3         0     0     0     0     0     0     0 117176     0     0     0
9         0     0     0     0     0     0     0      0 31622 35553  4221
<NA>      0     0     0     0     0     0     0      0     0     0     0
```

6. Answer:

   Code:

```
BRFSS_example2$INCOME_UNK <- 0
BRFSS_example2$INCOME_UNK[BRFSS_example2$INCOME_EXP
==9] <- 1
table(BRFSS_example2$INCOME_UNK,
BRFSS_example2$INCOME_EXP)
```

   Output:

```
       1      2      3     9
0 156499 119593 117176     0
1      0      0      0 71396
```

7. Possible answer: I would choose levels 3 (the highest income group) and 9 (unknown) as the reference group for all indicator variables. That is because I suspect this group has the lowest risk of the outcome.

8. Possible answer:

   Code:

```
BRFSS_example2$SMOKE100_MISS <- 0
BRFSS_example2$SMOKE100_MISS[is.na(BRFSS_
example2$SMOKE100)] <- 1
table(BRFSS_example2$SMOKE100, BRFSS_example2$SMOKE100_
MISS, useNA = c("always"))
```

   Output:

```
            0      1  <NA>
1      195411      0     0
2      248500      0     0
7        1815      0     0
9        1044      0     0
<NA>        0  17894     0
```

9. Possible answer:

```
SurvivalData_g$ASTHMA70 <- 0
SurvivalData_g$ASTHMA70[SurvivalData_g$ASTHMA4 == 1 &
SurvivalData_g$ASTHMAGE2 <= 80] <- 1

table(SurvivalData_g$ASTHMA70, SurvivalData_g$ASTHMAGE2,
useNA = c("always"))

SurvivalData_g$TIME70[SurvivalData_g$ASTHMA70 == 1]
<- SurvivalData_g$ASTHMAGE2[SurvivalData_g$ASTHMA70 == 1]
      SurvivalData_g$TIME70[SurvivalData_g$ASTHMA70 != 1]
      <- SurvivalData_g$X_AGE80[SurvivalData_g$ASTHMA70
      != 1]
SurvivalData_g$TIME70[SurvivalData_g$TIME70 > 70] <- 70

table(SurvivalData_g$TIME70, SurvivalData_g$ASTHMAGE2,
useNA = c("always"))
```

Output not shown.

10. Answer:

Code:

```
RefDate4 <- as. Date(c("2016-03-15"))
RIHosp$RefDate4Diff <- RefDate4 - RIHosp$AccredDate2
RIHosp[, c('AccredDate2', 'RefDate4Diff')]
```

Output:

```
     AccredDate2   RefDate4Diff
1     2016-02-06        38 days
2     2013-08-17       941 days
3     2014-12-06       465 days
4     2014-01-18       787 days
5     2014-12-13       458 days
6     2014-11-22       479 days
7     2014-09-13       549 days
8     2014-10-11       521 days
9     2014-06-14       640 days
10    2015-08-07       221 days
11    2014-06-14       640 days
```

11. Possible answer:

Code:

```
AGEQuartiles <- quantile(BRFSS_example2$X_AGE80,
na.rm=TRUE, prob = c(0.25, 0.50, 0.75))

BRFSS_example2$AGEQUART <- NA
BRFSS_example2$AGEQUART[BRFSS_example2$X_AGE80 <=
AGEQuartiles[1]] <- 1
BRFSS_example2$AGEQUART[(BRFSS_example2$X_AGE80 >
AGEQuartiles[1]) &
```

```
    BRFSS_example2$X_AGE80 <= AGEQuartiles[2]] <- 2
BRFSS_example2$AGEQUART[(BRFSS_example2$X_AGE80 >
AGEQuartiles[2]) &
    BRFSS_example2$X_AGE80 <= AGEQuartiles[3]] <- 3
BRFSS_example2$AGEQUART[BRFSS_example2$X_AGE80 >
AGEQuartiles[3]] <- 4

table(BRFSS_example2$X_AGE80, BRFSS_example2$AGEQUART,
useNA = c("always"))
```

Output not shown.

12. Possible answer:

```
BRFSS_example2$LOGX_AGE80 <- log(BRFSS_example2$X_AGE80)

hist(BRFSS_example2$LOGX_AGE80,
      main = "Histogram of Log of Age",
      xlab = "Class Log Age",
      ylab = "Log of Age",
      xlim=c(2,5),
      ylim=c(0,50000),
      border = "cornsilk4",
      col= "cornflowerblue",
      las = 1,
      breaks = 25)

boxplot(BRFSS_example2$LOGX_AGE80,
      main = "Box Plot of Log of Age",
      ylab = "Log of Age",
      border = "cornsilk4",
      col= "cornflowerblue")
```

Plots not shown.

Section "Data Validation in R"

Questions

1. Using the Rhode Island hospital dataset, in R, create a scatter plot between staffed beds (`StBeds`) and `RefDate4Diff` (created in Section 3, Question 10). Manipulate the `xlim`, `ylim`, and `breaks` options to improve readability. Optionally, change the colors from what was demonstrated.
2. Using the `BRFSS_example2` dataset (used in Section 3 questions), in R, run a correlation between the log of age variable you made in Section 3 questions (`LOGX_AGE80`) and `SLEPTIM1`. Obtain *p*-values.

3. Using the BRFSS_example2 dataset (used in Section 3 questions), in R, create a scatter plot between LOGX_AGE80 and SLEPTIM1, color-coded for SEX. Manipulate the options to improve readability. Optionally, change the colors from what was demonstrated.
4. Using the BRFSS_example2 dataset, conduct a *t*-test in R of LOGX_AGE80 between SEX=1 and SEX=2.
5. Using the BRFSS_example2 dataset, make side by side box plots of LOGX_AGE80 for SEX=1 and SEX=2. Manipulate the options to improve readability. Optionally, change the colors from what was demonstrated.
6. Using the BRFSS_example2 dataset, in R, create an ANOVA object with the dependent variable LOGX_AGE80 and the independent variable NUMADULT. Use NUMADULT as a continuous variable in one ANOVA, and an ordinal variable in the subsequent ANOVA.
7. Using the BRFSS_example2 dataset, in R, create a stacked bar chart for VETERAN3 by X_AGE_G (age group). Manipulate the options to improve readability. Optionally, change the colors from what was demonstrated.
8. Using R, conduct a chi-square test on the frequency table you made for Question 7.
9. Using R and the pwr package, calculate how many people would be needed per group for an effect size of 0.5678 with a two-sided significance level of 0.05, and a power of 80%.
10. Using R, subset BRFSS_example2 by VETERAN3 = 1 and create a new dataset called BRFSS_example 3. Using the write.csv command in R, write out dataset BRFSS_example3 as a *.csv named "Example3.csv".

Answers

1. Possible answer:

```
plot(RIHosp$StBeds, RIHosp$RefDate4Diff,
        main = "Staffed Beds vs. Days from Reference\n
        Date in RI Hospitals",
        xlab = "Staffed Beds",
        ylab = "Days from Ref",
        xlim=c(0,700),
        ylim=c(0,1000),
        pch=2,
        cex =.8,
        col = "cornflowerblue")
```

Plot not shown.

2. Answer:

   Code:

```
library(Hmisc)
res1<-rcorr(BRFSS_example2$LOGX_AGE80,
BRFSS_example2$SLEPTIM1, type="pearson")
res1
```

   Output:

```
       x y
x 1.00 0.06
y 0.06 1.00

n= 464664

P
  x  y
x     0
y  0
```

3. Possible answer:

```
plot(BRFSS_example2$LOGX_AGE80,BRFSS_example2$SLEPTIM1,
       main = "Log Age vs. Sleep Duration by Sex",
       xlab = "Log Age",
       ylab = "Sleep Duration",
       xlim=c(2.5,5),
       ylim=c(0,30),
       pch=15,
       col = ifelse(BRFSS_example2$SEX==1,
       "darkorange4", "darkorange"))
legend(4.5,28,
       pch=c(15,15),
       col=c("darkorange4", "darkorange"),
       c("Male", "Female"),
       bty="o",
       box.col="black",
       cex=.8)
```

   Plot not shown.

4. Answer:

```
t.test(BRFSS_example2$LOGX_AGE80~BRFSS_example2$SEX)
```

5. Possible answer:

```
boxplot(BRFSS_example2$LOGX_AGE80~BRFSS_example2$SEX,
       main = "Log of Age by Sex",
```

```
          ylab = "Log of Age",
          xlab = "Sex",
          names = c("Male", "Female"),
          border = "black",
          col=(c("darkorange4","darkorange")))
```

Plot not shown.

6. Possible answer:

   Code:

```
AdultANOVA <- lm(formula = LOGX_AGE80 ~ NUMADULT,
       data = BRFSS_example2)
summary(AdultANOVA)
```

   Output:

```
  Call:
  lm(formula = LOGX_AGE80 ~ NUMADULT, data =
  BRFSS_example2)

Residuals:
       Min        1Q   Median       3Q      Max
  -1.26287 -0.12638 0.06773 0.20535 1.86158

Coefficients:
              Estimate Std. Error t value Pr(>|t|)
  (Intercept) 4.263339 0.001253 3403.3 <2e-16 ***
  NUMADULT   -0.110099 0.000636 -173.1 <2e-16 ***
  ---

Signif. codes: 0 '***' 0.001 '**' 0.01 '*' 0.05 '.' 0.1 ' ' 1

Residual standard error: 0.2768 on 298553 degrees of
freedom
(166109 observations deleted due to missingness)
Multiple R-squared: 0.09122, Adjusted R-squared: 0.09121
F-statistic: 2.997e+04 on 1 and 298553 DF, p-value: <
2.2e-16
```

Code:

```
AdultANOVA2 <- lm(formula = LOGX_AGE80 ~
as.factor(NUMADULT),
       data = BRFSS_example2)
summary(AdultANOVA2)
```

Output:

```
  Call:
  lm(formula = LOGX_AGE80 ~ as.factor(NUMADULT), data =
  BRFSS_example2)
```

```
Residuals:
     Min       1Q   Median       3Q      Max
-1.26885 -0.11617 0.07002 0.20764 0.63432

Coefficients:
Estimate Std. Error t value Pr(>|t|)
(Intercept)             4.1592250 0.0008311 5004.660   < 2e-16 ***
as.factor(NUMADULT)2   -0.1183745 0.0010935 -108.251   < 2e-16 ***
as.factor(NUMADULT)3   -0.2497764 0.0018975 -131.637   < 2e-16 ***
as.factor(NUMADULT)4   -0.3352193 0.0031587 -106.124   < 2e-16 ***
as.factor(NUMADULT)5   -0.3716768 0.0064390  -57.723   < 2e-16 ***
as.factor(NUMADULT)6   -0.3722786 0.0130065  -28.623   < 2e-16 ***
as.factor(NUMADULT)7   -0.4078708 0.0273666  -14.904   < 2e-16 ***
as.factor(NUMADULT)8   -0.3702135 0.0460511   -8.039  9.08e-16 ***
as.factor(NUMADULT)9   -0.5030879 0.0690705   -7.284  3.26e-13 ***
as.factor(NUMADULT)10  -0.3003177 0.0651209   -4.612  4.00e-06 ***
as.factor(NUMADULT)11  -0.3548842 0.1381334   -2.569  0.010196 *
as.factor(NUMADULT)12  -0.5237840 0.1595020   -3.284  0.001024 **
as.factor(NUMADULT)14   0.0892702 0.2762631    0.323  0.746593
as.factor(NUMADULT)15  -0.9403492 0.2762631   -3.404  0.000665 ***
as.factor(NUMADULT)17  -0.3488725 0.1953484   -1.786  0.074117 .
as.factor(NUMADULT)18  -0.0160903 0.2762631   -0.058  0.953555
---
Signif. codes: 0 '***' 0.001 '**' 0.01 '*' 0.05 '.' 0.1 ' ' 1

Residual standard error: 0.2763 on 298539 degrees of
  freedom
(166109 observations deleted due to missingness)
Multiple R-squared: 0.09451, Adjusted R-squared: 0.09447
F-statistic: 2077 on 15 and 298539 DF, p-value: < 2.2e-16
```

7. Possible answer:

```
VetLabels <- c("Yes","No","Don't Know", "Refused",
"Missing")
AgeLabels <- c("18-24", "25-34", "35-44", "45-54",
"55-64", "65+")

VetAgeGrpFreq <- table(BRFSS_example2$VETERAN3,
BRFSS_example2$X_AGE_G)

barplot(VetAgeGrpFreq,
col=c("cornsilk", "cornsilk3", "cornsilk4",
"cornflowerblue", "darkblue"),
xlab="Age",
main="Age by Veteran Status",
names = AgeLabels,
legend = VetLabels,
las = 3,
args.legend = list(
```

```
         x=4,
         y=125000,
         bty = "n"))
```

Plot not shown.

8. Possible answer:

   Code:

   ```
   chisq.test(VetAgeGrpFreq)
   ```

   Output:

   ```
   Pearson's Chi-squared test

   data: VetAgeGrpFreq
   X-squared = 19147, df = 15, p-value < 2.2e-16
   ```

9. Answer:

   Code:

   ```
   library(pwr)
   pwr.t.test(d =.5678,
         sig.level = 0.05,
         power =.80,
         alternative ="two.sided")
   ```

   Output:

   ```
   Two-sample t test power calculation

               n = 49.66954
               d = 0.5678
       sig.level = 0.05
           power = 0.8
     alternative = two.sided

   NOTE: n is number in *each* group
   ```

10. Possible answer:

    ```
    BRFSS_example3 <- subset(BRFSS_example2, VETERAN3 == 1)
    write.csv(BRFSS_example3, file = "Example3.csv")
    ```

3

Basic Descriptive Analysis

Once the analytic dataset is developed and written out to *.csv format, as we did in Chapter 2, we are ready to begin the first step of our analysis, which is a descriptive analysis. This means making the archetypal "Table 1," which is the deliverable that documents the results of our descriptive analysis. The structure of Table 1 can differ from publication to publication depending upon the analyst's preferred style, and also, depending upon whether the dependent variable is categorical or continuous.

This chapter will present ways to use R to make Table 1 using a style that most journals find appropriate because it includes both summary statistics and bivariate statistical tests that can help the reader understand the nature of the sample in the analytic dataset. Although there are other ways to conduct and present descriptive analyses [64], this book will recommend a particular structure for Table 1s.

The first section of this chapter will start with a review of how SAS is used to make categorical Table 1s, and will then demonstrate how to use R to make Table 1 for our example hypothesis with a categorical dependent variable or outcome. After that, the second section will give an example of how to develop Table 1 using R for our example hypothesis with a continuous dependent variable or outcome. Finally, the third section will present some descriptive analyses that can be done in R in preparation for survival analysis.

Making "Table 1"—Categorical Outcome

This section will describe the steps for making a Table 1 for the categorical outcome asthma (yes/no), or `ASTHMA4`. It will begin with a discussion of the end goal—a table structured appropriately for a journal article. Next, SAS approaches to developing this type of Table 1 will be reviewed. After that, the `table` command in R will be discussed. Finally, approaches to developing categorical Table 1 in R that parallel approaches used in SAS will be presented.

Structure of Categorical Table 1

Let us revisit our hypothesis with the categorical outcome variable: Among veterans, alcohol consumption is associated with asthma. Therefore, what becomes important in our descriptive analysis is how the potential confounders are distributed by the outcome of asthma. The prevalence of the asthma outcome in each level of each potential confounder should definitely be a component of Table 1. Frequencies are helpful as well, and bivariate statistical test results can be added. Table 3.1 is an example of a Table 1 structure for our categorical outcome, asthma versus no asthma.

Please note some features of this table. First, the columns report the prevalence of the candidate confounder in the entire analytic dataset as well as in each category (asthma/no asthma), and also include the frequencies. Next, results at all of the levels of the grouping variables are reported for the potential confounders, including "not reported." The potential confounders are

TABLE 3.1

Example of Completed Table 3.1: Binary Dependent Variable

Category	Level	Total n, (%)	Has Asthma n, (%)	No Asthma n, (%)	Chi-Squared p-Value
	All	58,131, 100%	5,343, 9%	52,788, 91%	NA
Alcohol status	Nondrinker	26,169, 45%	2,671, 50%	23,498, 45%	<0.0001
	Monthly drinker	22,646, 39%	1,897, 36%	20,749, 39%	
	Weekly drinker	9,316, 16%	775, 15%	8541, 16%	
Age	Age 18–24	899, 2%	90, 2%	809, 2%	<0.0001
	Age 25–34	2,657, 5%	264, 5%	2,393, 5%	
	Age 35–44	3,589, 6%	325, 6%	3,264, 6%	
	Age 45–54	6,543, 11%	637, 12%	5,906, 11%	
	Age 55–64	10,724, 18%	1,153, 22%	9,571, 18%	
	Age 65 or older	33,719, 58%	2,874, 54%	30,845, 58%	
Sex	Male	52,971, 91%	4,555, 85%	48,416, 92%	<0.0001
	Female	5,160, 9%	788, 15%	4,372, 8%	
Ethnicity	Hispanic	2,262, 4%	236, 4%	2,026, 4%	0.0930
	Non-Hispanic	55,262, 95%	5,056, 95%	50,206, 95%	
	Not reported	607, 1%	51, 1%	556, 1%	
Race	White	49,394, 85%	4,362, 82%	45,032, 85%	<0.0001
	Black/African American	3,939, 7%	411, 8%	3,528, 7%	
	Asian	930, 2%	153, 3%	777, 1%	
	American Indian/ Alaskan Native	557, 1%	51, 1%	506, 1%	
	Native Hawaiian/ Pacific Islander	261, 0%	20, 0%	241, 0%	
	Other race/ Multi-racial	2,056, 4%	252, 5%	1,804, 3%	
	Not reported	994, 2%	94, 2%	900, 2%	

(Continued)

TABLE 3.1 (*Continued*)

Example of Completed Table 3.1: Binary Dependent Variable

Category	Level	Total *n*, (%)	Has Asthma *n*, (%)	No Asthma *n*, (%)	Chi-Squared *p*-Value
Marital status	Currently married	40,551, 70%	3,530, 66%	37,021, 70%	<0.0001
	Divorced, widowed, separated	15,588, 27%	1,577, 30%	14,011, 27%	
	Never married	982, 2%	134, 3%	848, 2%	
	Not reported	1,010, 2%	102, 2%	908, 2%	
Highest education level	Less than high school	2,483, 4%	318, 6%	2165, 4%	<0.0001
	High school graduate	16,241, 28%	1,430, 27%	14,811, 28%	
	Some college/ technical	17,559, 30%	1,720, 32%	15,839, 30%	
	Four or more years of college	21,742, 37%	1,868, 35%	19,874, 38%	
	Not reported	106, 0%	7, 0%	99, 0%	
Annual household income	<$10k	1,165, 2%	187, 3%	978, 2%	<0.0001
	$10k to <$15k	2,111, 4%	305, 6%	1,806, 3%	
	$15k to <$20k	3,148, 5%	418, 8%	2,730, 5%	
	$20k to <$25k	4,774, 8%	509, 10%	4265, 8%	
	$25k to <$35k	6,491, 11%	609, 11%	5,882, 11%	
	$35k to <$50k	9,305, 16%	765, 14%	8,540, 16%	
	$50k to <$75k	9,636, 17%	825, 15%	8,811, 17%	
	$75k or more	15,230, 26%	1,167, 22%	14,063, 27%	
	Not reported	6,271, 11%	558, 10%	5,713, 11%	
Obesity status	Underweight	478, 1%	61, 1%	417, 1%	<0.0001
	Normal	14,340, 25%	1,171, 22%	13,169, 25%	
	Overweight	25,572, 44%	2,098, 39%	23,474, 44%	
	Obese	16,871, 29%	1,909, 36%	14,962, 28%	
	Not reported	870, 1%	104, 2%	766, 1%	
Smoking status	Smoker	8,571, 15%	931, 17%	7,640, 14%	<0.0001
	Non-smoker	26,639, 46%	4,389, 82%	44,872, 85%	
	Not reported	22,921, 39%	23, 0%	276, 1%	
Exercise status	Exercised in the last month	8,571, 15%	3,759, 70%	40,598, 77%	<0.0001
	Did not exercise in the last month	49,261, 85%	1,572, 29%	12,069, 23%	
	Not reported	299, 1%	12, 0%	121, 0%	
Health plan	Has a health plan	55,795, 96%	5,095, 95%	50,700, 96%	0.0418
	No health plan	2,203, 4%	236, 4%	1,967, 4%	
	Not reported	133, 0%	12, 0%	121, 0%	

(*Continued*)

TABLE 3.1 (*Continued*)

Example of Completed Table 3.1: Binary Dependent Variable

Category	Level	Total *n*, (%)	Has Asthma *n*, (%)	No Asthma *n*, (%)	Chi-Squared *p*-Value
General health	Excellent	9,016, 16%	465, 9%	8,551, 16%	<0.0001
	Very good	18,111, 31%	1,253, 23%	16,858, 32%	
	Good	18,797, 32%	1,741, 33%	17,056, 32%	
	Fair	8,436, 15%	1,187, 22%	7,249, 14%	
	Poor	3,569, 6%	673, 13%	2,896, 5%	
	Not reported	202, 0%	24, 0%	178, 0%	

ordered starting with the hypothesized exposure (alcohol consumption categories), followed by demographic categories, socioeconomic categories, and comorbidity categories. Finally, on the right, the results of chi-squared tests are reported.

This table represents the deliverable that would be printed in a journal for Table 1 for the asthma analysis. Regardless of whether SAS, SPSS, or R is used for the analysis, there is a variety of strategies for producing this deliverable. Several strategies used in SAS will be reviewed first. This will be followed by a review of similar strategies in R, and one particular strategy to produce Table 3.1 in R will be demonstrated.

SAS Approaches to Categorical Table 1 Structure

As pointed out earlier, Table 1 contains frequencies. In SAS, the famous `PROC FREQ` is typically used for calculating the frequencies in categorical Table 1. Using `PROC FREQ` without any options set will produce a very dense table. An example is given below that produces a crosstab between the exposure grouping variable, `ALCGRP`, and the outcome variable, `ASTHMA4` (Table 3.2).

Code:

```
proc freq data=r.analytic;
        tables ALCGRP*ASTHMA4;
run;
```

Although `PROC FREQ` outputs much useful information, including frequencies and percentages, there is an overwhelming amount of information in the table, so analysts usually suppress some of it [65]. One approach is to use the `/list option` (Table 3.3).

TABLE 3.2

Example of `PROC FREQ` Output

Frequency

Percent

Row Pct

Col Pct

Table of `ALCGRP` by `ASTHMA4`

	ASTHMA4		
ALCGRP	**0**	**1**	**Total**
1	23498 40.42 89.79 44.51	2671 4.59 10.21 49.99	26169 45.02
2	20749 35.69 91.62 39.31	1897 3.26 8.38 35.50	22646 38.96
3	8541 14.69 91.68 16.18	775 1.33 8.32 14.50	9316 16.03
Total	52788 90.81	5343 9.19	58131 100.00

Code:

```
proc freq data=r.analytic;
        tables ALCGRP*ASTHMA4 /list;
run;
```

Although this produces the information we want, it is not in the structure that we want. Although it is possible to use the ODS to output a `PROC FREQ`

TABLE 3.3

Example of `PROC FREQ` Output with List Option

ALCGRP	ASTHMA4	Frequency	Percent	Cumulative Frequency	Cumulative Percent
1	0	23498	40.42	23498	40.42
1	1	2671	4.59	26169	45.02
2	0	20749	35.69	46918	80.71
2	1	1897	3.26	48815	83.97
3	0	8541	14.69	57356	98.67
3	1	775	1.33	58131	100.00

table in either structure (with or without the `list` option) to a *.csv file [66], this is generally not helpful unless the table can be structured in SAS so it has the columns and the rows as shown in Table 3.1. For example, consider the following SAS code that creates our crosstab of `ALCGRP` and `ASTHMA4`, but outputs it as a dataset using the ODS, which is then exported as a *.csv:

Code:

```
ods output CrossTabFreqs = AlcFreq;
ods trace on;
proc freq data=r.analytic;
      tables ALCGRP*ASTHMA4;
run;
ods output close;
PROC EXPORT DATA= WORK.ALCFREQ
           OUTFILE= "C:\Users\Monika\Dropbox\R Stats
           Book\Analytics\Data\AlcFreq_sas.csv"
           DBMS=CSV REPLACE;
     PUTNAMES=YES;
RUN
```

The resulting *.csv looks like Table 3.4.

Because of this challenge, SAS developed a few `PROC`s aimed at making "journal-style" or "journal-ready" tables, a particularly famous one being `PROC TABULATE`. A white paper from the SAS Global Forum 2008 by Janet Grubber and colleagues is titled "Creating Journal-Style Tables in an Easy Way (with `PROC TABULATE`, `PROC TEMPLATE`, `PROC FORMAT` and `ODS RTF`)," which is an excellent overview of using these approaches [67]. A feature of these approaches, which is both an advantage and a limitation, is that the tables are output in HTML. This is an advantage because of the professional graphical quality of the HTML image, but a limitation because, unlike in Excel, these images are not easy to edit. For example, in Excel, borders can be easily darkened or suppressed using point-and-click procedures, whereas in `PROC TABULATE`, this must be done with code [67].

Although these `PROC`s in SAS for making journal-ready tables are usable and produce amazing results, they are very complicated to program. In fact, the white paper's title is somewhat ironic because after declaring this can be done "in an easy way," the paper contains 14 pages, with much of that code. Briefly, these authors recommend using `PROC FORMAT` to label the levels of the categorical variables, using `PROC TEMPLATE` to design a style sheet, using `label` commands to label the covariates, then building the HTML table using `PROC TABULATE` code [67]. Within that code are instructions as to how to apply formats (such as making a number appear as a percent) as well as instructions on how to actually run the calculations (as in `PROC FREQ`) [67].

Without going into too much detail, here is an example of a snippet of `PROC TABULATE` code that could be used to build upon to eventually achieve a

TABLE 3.4

Example of PROC FREQ Output Using ODS

Table	ALCGRP	ASTHMA4	_TYPE_	_TABLE_	Frequency	Percent	RowPercent	ColPercent	Missing
Table ALCGRP * ASTHMA4	1	0	11	1	23498	40.42249402	89.79326684	44.51390468	
Table ALCGRP * ASTHMA4	1	1	11	1	2671	4.594794516	10.20673316	49.99064196	
Table ALCGRP * ASTHMA4	1		10	1	26169	45.01728854			
Table ALCGRP * ASTHMA4	2	0	11	1	20749	35.69351981	91.62324472	39.30628173	
Table ALCGRP * ASTHMA4	2	1	11	1	1897	3.263319055	8.376755277	35.50439828	
Table ALCGRP * ASTHMA4	2		10	1	22646	38.95683886			
Table ALCGRP * ASTHMA4	3	0	11	1	8541	14.69267689	91.68097896	16.17981359	
Table ALCGRP * ASTHMA4	3	1	11	1	775	1.333195713	8.319021039	14.50495976	
Table ALCGRP * ASTHMA4	3		10	1	9316	16.0258726			
Table ALCGRP * ASTHMA4		0	1	1	52788	90.80869072			
Table ALCGRP * ASTHMA4		1	1	1	5343	9.191309284			
Table ALCGRP * ASTHMA4			0	1	58131	100			0

categorical Table 1 in the format desired. First, the analytic table is copied into a table called "example." This is because SAS formats and labels will be applied for PROC TABULATE, and these are not needed in the analytic dataset. During the copying of the dataset, labels are applied to the ASTHMA4 and ALCGRP variables, as these will be used in the example. Next, formats are set up for ASTHMA4 and ALCGRP levels using PROC FORMAT. Finally, PROC TABULATE code is used, which applies the formats.

Code:

```
data r.example;
       set r.analytic;
       label ASTHMA4 = "Asthma Status";
       label ALCGRP = "Alcohol Consumption";
run;

/*set up formats*/

proc format;
        value asthma_f
        0 = "No Asthma"
        1 = "Has Asthma";
        value alcohol_f
        1 = "Nondrinker"
        2 = "Monthly Drinker"
        3 = "Weekly Drinker"
        ;
run;

/*apply formats in proc tabulate*/

proc tabulate data=r.example;
        format ALCGRP alcohol_f.
               ASTHMA4 asthma_f.;
        class ALCGRP ASTHMA4;
        table (ALCGRP ALL),
               ASTHMA4 * N;
run;
```

Output is shown in Table 3.5.

This code could provide the basic building blocks for a table that could be built out in PROC TABULATE. Total frequencies and percentages could be added, and the output formatted to display commas after thousands, percent signs, and other features.

Another SAS PROC that is used to develop Table 1 is PROC REPORT. Similar to PROC TABULATE, PROC REPORT is used to develop journal-ready tables as reports that can be output in SAS's HTML window and optionally printed as a PDF—not written out as a data file that could be transferred to Excel. Ben

TABLE 3.5

Example of PROC TABULATE Output—Categorical Outcome

	Asthma Status	
	No Asthma	Has Asthma
	N	N
Alcohol consumption	23498	2671
Nondrinker		
Monthly drinker	20749	1897
Weekly drinker	8541	775
All	52788	5343

Cochran wrote an excellent white paper on using PROC REPORT [68]. Like with PROC TABULATE, there are many options that can be set both within the PROC and on the ODS portion of the code that outputs the report, thus making the procedure ultimately customizable, but also complicated [68].

SAS includes a macro language; users who are familiar with this language can adapt published macros built in SAS for the purpose of developing a structured Table 1, or build their own macros that they reuse from project to project. Zbigniew Kaziola wrote an instructive white paper with an easy-to-use table-formatting macro in SAS [69]. Although Kaziola makes the steps very clear and is very neat in the white paper's presentation, the annotated code is still quite complex [69].

Because SAS has existed a long time, many different approaches have been developed for structuring the descriptive statistics reported in Table 1, and a few of these approaches were reviewed here. It is unknown how often these SAS approaches are used in practice, however. Tables appearing in reports and submitted to journals are often ultimately formatted in Excel, not in HTML. The next part of this section will describe how SAS users leverage Excel combined with SAS to present journal-ready tables in Excel.

SAS Approaches to Table Presentation Using Excel

SAS users may opt to present their results as journal-ready tables in Excel* rather than using SAS to develop using approaches like PROC TABULATE and PROC REPORT [70,71]. Using Excel as a supplemental tool to SAS in the development of descriptive tables can be accomplished using one of two basic approaches: (1) creating blank tables in Excel and copying and pasting information manually from SAS output into Excel and (2) using SAS features (such as the ODS and data steps) to format results in SAS that can be

* Manuscripts are generally in Microsoft Word, so the tables may be formatted in Excel and copied and pasted into Word.

exported out as a file that can be read by Excel (such as *.csv). In the second approach, only a small amount of editing is required to prepare the exported Excel file for presentation, and this editing is easily done.

From the standpoint of accuracy, the second approach is preferred because it reduces the likelihood of transcription errors [70,71]. But from the standpoint of efficiency, the programming to produce and export properly formatted tables using SAS can be extensive. A particularly elegant approach to quick formatting of tables and exporting them using SAS's `PROC SQL` for post-processing in Excel is demonstrated in Ralph Winter's humorously titled white paper, "Excellent Ways of Exporting SAS Data to Excel" [72]. But part of the simplicity of this approach is that it avoids the SAS data step, using instead `PROC SQL` code, which may be too inefficient to run on large datasets [72].

In summary, if the analyst chooses to conduct the analysis in SAS and present the tables in Excel, the optimal approach is to develop code to export a formatted table from SAS into a file that can be read by Excel. However, this may require a considerable amount of expertise with SAS programming. The next part of this section reviews how SAS is used in producing the bivariate statistical tests that are presented in categorical Table 1.

SAS Bivariate Categorical Tests

In addition to producing frequencies, `PROC FREQ` has another feature that is used in developing categorical Table 1, which is performing bivariate statistical tests. The following code includes the `chisq` option:

Code:

```
proc freq data=r.analytic;
        tables ALCGRP*ASTHMA4 /chisq;
run;
```

This produces the same tabular results as the basic `PROC FREQ` table shown earlier, but adds an extra table shown in Table 3.6.

TABLE 3.6

Example of `PROC FREQ` Output with `CHISQ` Option

Statistic	DF	Value	Prob
Chi-square	2	58.8228	<0.0001
Likelihood ratio chi-square	2	58.5632	<0.0001
Mantel–Haenszel chi-square	1	47.1422	<0.0001
Phi coefficient		0.0318	
Contingency coefficient		0.0318	
Cramer's V		0.0318	

The statistics normally needed from this table are in the first row—the F-statistic and degrees of freedom, as well as the associated *p*-value. When working with small cells, a Fisher's Exact Test is used, in which case, the "`fisher`" instead of "`chisq`" option would be used.

So far, this section has reviewed approaches used in SAS to develop journal-ready tables. It started by describing how `PROC FREQ` is a mainstay for SAS users for calculating frequencies and percentages needed for categorical Table 1. It also reviewed using SAS `PROC`s to make journal-ready tables by way of HTML output, as well as using Excel as a supplemental tool along with SAS in developing journal-ready descriptive tables. Conducting bivariate tests in SAS whose results can be reported in Table 1 was also reviewed.

The next part of this section will review the `table` command in R, which has many of the same uses as SAS's `PROC FREQ`.

The Table Command in R

R's equivalent of `PROC FREQ` is roughly the "`table`" command, but unlike `PROC FREQ`, the default output is very sparse. Like with `PROC FREQ`, the `table` command can be used with one field as an argument, and that will produce one-way frequencies. For example, to see frequencies of asthma (yes/no) in the analytic dataset, we can run the `table` command on the `ASTHMA4` field:

Code:

```
table(analytic$ASTHMA4)
```

Output:

```
    0      1
52788   5343
```

The columns are labeled with the value of the level. Unlike with `PROC FREQ`, there are no proportions output. However, this can be easily arranged if the frequency table is saved as a table object. This code saves the results of the table command in a table object called `AsthmaFreq`.

Code:

```
AsthmaFreq <- table(analytic$ASTHMA4)
```

Now that this table is saved as an object called `AsthmaFreq`, we revisit the `prop.table` command. We can run the `prop.table` command on `AsthmaFreq`, and the results will be the cell proportions.

Code:

```
prop.table(AsthmaFreq)
```

Output:

```
         0           1
0.90808691  0.09191309
```

For a crosstab, another field can be added to the table argument. We will add `ALCGRP` for a crosstab of asthma status by alcohol status:

Code:

```
table(analytic$ASTHMA4, analytic$ALCGRP)
```

Output:

```
       1      2     3
0  23498  20749  8541
1   2671   1897   775
```

Again, proportions may be of interest. As we did before, let us save this first crosstab table as a table object called `AsthmaAlcFreq`.

Code:

```
AsthmaAlcFreq <- table(analytic$ASTHMA4, analytic$ALCGRP)
```

Now that the table is saved as an object, we can use `prop.table` again on the saved table object. This time, we will add the 1 option, and this will give us row proportions.

Code:

```
prop.table(AsthmaAlcFreq, 1)
```

Output:

```
             1          2          3
0    0.4451390  0.3930628  0.1617981
1    0.4999064  0.3550440  0.1450496
```

If we instead add the 2 option, we will get the column proportions.

Code:

```
prop.table(AsthmaAlcFreq, 2)
```

Output:

```
              1           2           3
0    0.89793267  0.91623245  0.91680979
1    0.10206733  0.08376755  0.08319021
```

The `table` command provides the information, but if the ultimate goal is a table structured like Table 3.1, then this output would need to be edited, because none of the `table commands` run so far produce a table in our desired structure for Table 1. This is the same challenge seen with SAS. In addition, because `ALCGRP` is a three-level variable and `ASTHMA4` contains only two levels, it is easy to tell variable is on which axis in the output. However, for presentation, this part of the table would need editing for clarity as well.

As with SAS, variety of approaches exist to constructing the formatted Table 1. As described with SAS, one way is to format tables in R as deliverables directly from R (that are output in HTML or other format that produces the table as an image). A second way is to involve Excel in the development of the journal-ready table.

The next part of the section will describe R approaches that are similar to `PROC TABULATE` and `PROC REPORT`, that result in tables in HTML output. In R, these approaches are more readily used for online presentation of data rather than journal manuscripts; Excel is often preferred to be used during the development of manuscript drafts because of the relative simplicity of manually editing Excel files to make minor revisions. Therefore, this part will be followed by a more extensive explanation of one strategy to develop a fully formatted Table 1 using R, and output it as a *.csv that can be converted to an *.xlsx and edited in Excel.

R Approaches to Categorical Table 1

In SAS, the "best" approach to developing Table 1 depends on the expertise of the analyst. If an analyst is proficient at `PROC TABULATE`, or has built a particularly efficient macro she reuses, then those would be the most efficient for her. Because R lends itself to easy editing of tables, a particularly efficient way to approach this problem in R is to structure the Table 1 in R, and then export it as a *.csv which can be converted to an *.xlsx in Excel, with final editing done.

Although like with SAS, the "best" R approach for the analyst depends on the analyst's expertise, using Excel as part of developing Table 1 is probably more often the "best" approach in R. This is because the SAS approach to exporting tabular results for Excel to read requires ODS language, thus adding to its complexity, whereas R can do a similar operation with code that is more uniform, so it may be easier to grasp. The R approach of developing a table that is in our desired output format and exporting it to be post-processed in Excel is parallel to the SAS approaches described in Winter's white paper discussed earlier, where SAS was used to format tables that were output into Excel-readable files [70,71].

Although involving Excel in developing Table 1 in R is probably more often the "best" approach, R indeed has capabilities for outputting a fully formatted table as an image the way `PROC TABULATE` or `PROC REPORT` can, but these are generally calibrated for online presentation. For example, both the `stargazer` [73] and `tables` [74] packages produce high-quality tables that appear as if they were printed in a journal. However, they both require other components besides R, such as Latex, which is an environment that manages graphical output not unlike SAS's ODS [75]. In fact, Duncan Murdoch, the author of the `tables` package, admits he was "inspired by my 20-year-old memories of SAS `PROC TABULATE`" to develop the package [74].

But when developing a manuscript to be submitted to a journal, which will likely undergo multiple revisions, unless the analyst is well-versed in Latex or other graphical output programming, it is probably easier to use Excel for table presentation. As described before with SAS, if going the Excel route, there are two main approaches to creating a presentation-ready Table 1: (1) copying and pasting results from R output into Excel manually or (2) formatting the table in R and exporting it as a file that can be read by Excel. As mentioned earlier, compared with SAS, R is more adept for restructuring and outputting data in *.csv format, which can be read by Excel, mainly because it does not require the use of a separate ODS. Also, as mentioned before, the second approach is preferred (regardless of software used) because it reduces the possibility of transcription errors. Should the analyst choose second approach for developing Table 1 in R, it must also be decided how much editing of the table should be done in R, and how much should be left to post-processing in Excel. Like with SAS, the analyst's familiarity with various R packages and adeptness with R versus Excel will guide these decisions.

In making these decisions, one consideration is that Excel can easily calculate and display percentages. Therefore, outputting frequencies into a *.csv using R might be the most efficient way of developing a finished table with both frequencies and percentages in Excel because Excel would provide the percentages. If this choice is made, a simple approach would be to output each frequency table as its own *.csv and copy and paste the results into an Excel presentation spreadsheet. For example, to produce the asthma frequencies we did earlier, the following code could be used:

Code:

```
AsthmaFreq <- table(analytic$ASTHMA4)
write.csv(AsthmaFreq, file = "AsthmaFreq.csv")
```

This code creates the table object `AsthmaFreq`, then writes this out as a *.csv to the directory set as default. Opening the *.csv in Excel shows the Table 3.7. From this point, the frequencies could be copied and pasted into the Excel table shell quite easily. Notice that Table 3.7 is naturally formatted similarly to the desired format of Table 1 in terms of rows and columns.

A person more adept at R programming might want to push further, and do more to build the table in R before outputting it as a *.csv. This would

TABLE 3.7
Asthma Frequency Table

	Var1	Freq
1	0	52788
2	1	5343

be parallel to a person working hard to learn PROC TABULATE code, but the advantage of this approach is the output is a *.csv that is easy to edit by hand, whereas PROC TABULATE code produces HTML output that typically would be modified using graphic editing software.

Here is an example in R that parallels what was demonstrated earlier, in PROC TABULATE. It involves using tables as data.frame objects. A data.frame object has properties that are slightly different from a table object, which will become evident in this example. The goal of this example is to use R to prepare a data.frame object that is close to the desired table structure shown earlier, and then write this out as a *.csv to make the final editing in Excel very minimal.

To do this, first, a blank table should be created that is a data.frame object. Subsequent programming will be aimed at adding the numbers to this object so that it can be completed and written out as a *.csv. The code to create the blank table follows.

Code:

```
Table1Cat <- data.frame(Category=character(),
             Level=character(),
             TotalN=integer(),
             TotalProp=numeric(),
             HasAsthmaN=integer(),
             HasAsthmaProp=numeric(),
             NoAsthmaN=integer(),
             NoAsthmaProp=numeric())
```

The code generates a blank data.frame called Table1Cat by using the data.frame command and then labeling and creating the fields desired in our final table, and specifying the field type. Category and Level refer to the labels along the *y*-axis of the table and are designated as character fields. TotalN and TotalProp refer to the total number in the dataset and proportion of total dataset. HasAsthmaN is the frequency in the category and level having asthma (ASTHMA4=1), and NoAsthmaN is the frequency in the category and level of not having asthma (ASTHMA4=0). HasAsthmaProp is the category and level's proportion of the total who have asthma, and NoAsthmaProp is the proportion among those who do not have asthma. These are column proportions. Note that `numeric()` is necessary for fields that will contain decimals.

To fill in the table, the first step is to complete the first row, which contains all respondents in the sample. It shows the total frequency and proportion in each asthma group. We will create this row, and bind it to the blank `Table1Cat`. The next step will be to create frequency tables for each of the bivariate comparisons, meaning the exposure and each potential confounder crosstabbed by asthma status, in the exactly the same structure as this table, and bind them to `Table1Cat` in the correct order. We will create each of these sets of rows as smaller tables, and then bind them to `Table1Cat`.

But before we start the procedure of building out `Table1Cat`, let us look at the differences between a table object and a `data.frame` object. In the following code, we will create the table `AsthmaFreq` as a `data.frame` using the `as.data.frame` command, and not just as a table. After creating these objects, we will run `nrow` and `ncol` on them to see the numbers of rows and columns in them.

Code:

```
#as a table
AsthmaFreq <- table(analytic$ASTHMA4)
nrow(AsthmaFreq)
ncol(AsthmaFreq)

#as a data frame
AsthmaFreq <- as.data.frame(table(analytic$ASTHMA4))
nrow(AsthmaFreq)
ncol(AsthmaFreq)
```

Output:

```
> AsthmaFreq <- table(analytic$ASTHMA4)
> nrow(AsthmaFreq)
[1] 2
> ncol(AsthmaFreq)
[1] NA
> AsthmaFreq <- as.data.frame(table(analytic$ASTHMA4))
> nrow(AsthmaFreq)
[1] 2
> ncol(AsthmaFreq)
[1] 2
```

Notice how the table `AsthmaFreq` has 2 rows and 0 columns, while the `data.frame` `AsthmaFreq` has 2 rows and 2 columns, allowing us to refer to the columns in subsequent code. `AsthmaFreq` as a `data.frame` appears this way:

Code:

```
AsthmaFreq
```

Output:

```
     Var1     Freq
1       0    52788
2       1     5343
```

The output is similar in structure to when `PROC FREQ` is used with the list option. This `data.frame` will be used to populate the main `data.frame` we are building, which is `Table1Cat`.

At this point, defining some variables would be helpful. `TotalObs` will be total observations, and is the number of rows in our analytic dataset.

Code:

```
TotalObs <- nrow(analytic)
```

The variables `TotalAsthma` (number of respondents with asthma) and `TotalNoAsthma` (number of respondents with no asthma) are also helpful, as they will be the denominators of the column proportions we calculate in the code. We create these variables by selecting the correct numbers out of `AsthmaFreq` and copying them into the variable name. Looking at the output of `AsthmaFreq`, we see that the total frequency of those who have asthma is 5343, which is in the second row and the second column. We also see the total frequency of those who do not have asthma is 52,788, which is located in the first row and the second column. This code picks out these exact numbers by defining the row and column of the table where the numbers are located and places these numbers in the variable names.

Code:

```
TotalAsthma <- AsthmaFreq[2,2]
TotalNoAsthma <- AsthmaFreq[1,2]
```

Now that we have these variables set and our blank data.frame generated as `Table1Cat`, we can start building out the table. First, we will generate the top row of the table, which reports overall frequencies and proportions in the dataset. To make that first entry (`Entry1`), we will have to build it as a `data.frame` and append—called "row bind" in R—the `Entry1 data.frame` with the `Table1Cat data.frame`. Here is the code to make the `Entry1 data.frame`.

Code:

```
Entry1 <- data.frame(Category="All",
                     Level="All",
                     TotalN=TotalObs,
                     TotalProp=TotalObs/TotalObs,
                     HasAsthmaN=TotalAsthma,
                     HasAsthmaProp=TotalAsthma/TotalObs,
                     NoAsthmaN=TotalNoAsthma,
                     NoAsthmaProp=TotalNoAsthma/TotalObs)
```

Notice that this code specifies all the columns we contemplated earlier. Because we are working on only the first entry to the table, we enter "All" into both `Category` and `Level`. We enter the value of the variable `TotalObs` for `TotalN` (because this is the frequency in the entire dataset) and `TotalObs/TotalObs` for `TotalProp` (because this is the proportion in the entire dataset). Next, we repeat the process using the `TotalAsthma` and `TotalNoAsthma` values as frequencies and numerators in proportions, with the denominator being `TotalObs`. After running the above, `Entry1` looks like this:

Output:

```
  Category Level TotalN TotalProp HasAsthmaN HasAsthmaProp NoAsthmaN NoAsthmaProp
1      All   All  58131         1       5343    0.09191309     52788    0.9080869
```

Now, we will "row bind," or `rbind`, this `Entry1` to `Table1Cat` and call the results `Table1Cat`.

Code:

```
Table1Cat <- rbind(Table1Cat, Entry1)
```

`Table1Cat` now looks like this:

Output:

```
  Category Level TotalN TotalProp HasAsthmaN HasAsthmaProp NoAsthmaN NoAsthmaProp
1      All   All  58131         1       5343    0.09191309     52788    0.9080869
```

It looks identical to `Entry1`, but making the blank version first and binding `Entry1` to it was a way to force the data fields to have a particular structure (e.g., `numeric()` versus `decimal()`).

Making entries to row bind to finish the table will take a different approach because crosstabs need to be used. An example for the first grouping variable, `ALCGRP`, will be given here. This process can be repeated with all the grouping variables.

Like with the first entry, this process starts by making a crosstab table called `AlcFreq` from `ALCGRP`, the grouping variable, and `ASTHMA4`, the outcome.

Code:

```
AlcFreq <- table(analytic$ALCGRP, analytic$ASTHMA4)
nrow(AlcFreq)
ncol(AlcFreq)
```

Output:

```
nrow(AlcFreq)
[1]    3
ncol(AlcFreq)
[1]    2
```

The `AlcFreq` table looks like this:

Output:

```
      0     1
1 23498  2671
2 20749  1897
3  8541   775
```

As can be seen, this is a table with two columns (for each `ASTHMA4` level) and three rows (for each `ALCGRP` level). From our metadata, we know 0=no asthma and 1=asthma for the outcome, and for alcohol consumption, 1=nondrinker, 2=monthly drinker, and 3=weekly drinker. So, as an example, the frequency of weekly drinkers with asthma is 775, and that is in row 3 and column 2.

Now that these frequencies are available to us in a table, we need to build the next entry in `Table1Cat`, which will have the alcohol group levels on the *y*-axis, and the frequencies and proportions going across the *x*-axis. This entry will have three rows, one for each alcohol level, and as many columns as in the original `Table1Cat`.

To build the next entry, we will start by building each column separately. Next, we will "column bind" (`cbind`) them together to turn the separate columns into a table. We will simultaneously turn the table into a data.frame that then can be appended with `rbind` to `Table1Cat`, which we continue to build. We will build each column in the second entry as a vector of three values (because there are three alcohol categories) and name the vector after the column we are building.

Code:

```
Category <- c("Alcohol Status", "", "")
Level <- c("Nondrinker", "Monthly Drinker", "Weekly Drinker")
TotalN <- c("","","")
TotalProp <- c("","","")
HasAsthmaN <- AlcFreq[,2]
HasAsthmaProp <- c("","","")
NoAsthmaN <- AlcFreq[,1]
NoAsthmaProp <- c("","","")
```

Referencing our desired final table structure, the Category values for this part of the table have "Alcohol Status" in the first cell, with the lower cells blank. This is specified by `""` in the coding to make the `Category` vector. Next, for the `Level` vector, the levels are specified in the order top to bottom. Notice that for `TotalN`, `TotalProp`, `HasAsthmaProp`, and `NoAsthmaProp`, all of the values are left blank. That is because we will calculate them later using values we are actually entering into the table in this step.

Of particular interest is `HasAsthmaN` and `NoAsthmaN`. The use of brackets specifies the columns and rows. For example, looking at `AlcFreq`, if we wanted to specify the 775 frequency of those who are weekly drinkers with asthma, we would specify `AlcFreq[3,2]`. If we wanted to specify the entire row of weekly drinkers (with no asthma and asthma frequencies), we would just specify the first entry and leave the column blank: `AlcFreq[3,]`. Likewise, if we wanted the column of asthma frequencies for each level, we would specify the column only, after the comma: `AlcFreq[,2]`. This explains why in our code, we insert `AlcFreq[2]` into `HasAsthmaN` and `AlcFreq[,1]` into `NoAsthmaN`.

Now that we have essentially created all the columns in our table that will make up `Entry2`, we will column bind, or `cbind`, them together. We will use the `as.data.frame` command to output the resulting table as a `data.frame`, and we will name it `AlcTbl`.

Code:

```
AlcTbl <- as.data.frame(cbind(Category, Level, TotalN, TotalProp,
       HasAsthmaN, HasAsthmaProp, NoAsthmaN, NoAsthmaProp))
```

Now that `AlcTbl` is a `data.frame`, we can populate the metrics that were originally set to blank.

```
AlcTbl$TotalN <- HasAsthmaN + NoAsthmaN
AlcTbl$TotalProp <- AlcTbl$TotalN/TotalObs
AlcTbl$HasAsthmaProp <- AlcFreq[,2]/TotalAsthma
AlcTbl$NoAsthmaProp <- AlcFreq[,1]/TotalNoAsthma
```

The `TotalN`, or row total, is updated by adding the frequencies `HasAsthmaN` and `NoAsthmaN` together, and the `TotalProp` is calculated by dividing the `TotalN` by the variable, `TotalObs`. To calculate the other proportions, the numerator is expressed as we expressed it earlier: `AlcFreq[,2]` for the asthma frequencies and `AlcFreq[,1]` for the no asthma frequencies. The denominators are the variables `TotalAsthma` and `TotalNoAsthma`, respectively. The resulting `AlcTbl` looks like this:

Output:

```
       Category             Level TotalN TotalProp HasAsthmaN HasAsthmaProp
1  Alcohol Status        Nondrinker  26169 0.4501729       2671     0.4999064
2                 Monthly Drinker  22646 0.3895684       1897     0.3550440
3                  Weekly Drinker   9316 0.1602587        775     0.1450496
  NoAsthmaN NoAsthmaProp
1     23498    0.4451390
2     20749    0.3930628
3      8541    0.1617981
```

The next step is to `rbind AlcTbl` to `Table1Cat`, which already has our overall summary statistics in it.

Code:

```
Table1Cat <- rbind(Table1Cat, AlcTbl)
```

The resulting `Table1Cat` looks like this:

```
        Category          Level TotalN TotalProp HasAsthmaN HasAsthmaProp NoAsthmaN
1            All            All  58131 1.0000000       5343    0.09191309     52788
11 Alcohol Status    Nondrinker  26169 0.4501729       2671    0.49990642     23498
2             Monthly Drinker  22646 0.3895684       1897    0.35504398     20749
3              Weekly Drinker   9316 0.1602587        775    0.14504960      8541
   NoAsthmaProp
1     0.9080869
11    0.4451390
2     0.3930628
3     0.1617981
```

Notice that the table now includes the alcohol statistics. Using the approach of making a separate table for each candidate confounding variable and row binding it to `Table1Cat` could be done for each variable in the order of presentation of Table 1. The final result could be written out as a *.csv and easily edited in Excel for final presentation in the journal. Code to write out the *.csv is as follows.

Code:

```
write.csv(Table1Cat, file = "Table1Cat.csv")
```

Approaches to Automating Table Generation in R

As described earlier, SAS users can approach automating table generation through using macros in SAS macro language. R does not have a direct parallel to SAS macro language because it is built differently. In SAS, new `PROCS` that are developed can start as macros; therefore, macro language in SAS becomes the main building block for automation in SAS. R, on the other hand, has many different types of building blocks for automation. An extensive explanation of these is outside the scope of this book, but the curious reader can explore using user-defined functions in R [76], the "`apply`" family of functions in R [77], and the "`defmacro`" command in the `gtools` package for making SAS-like macros in R [78]. Also, one brief example will be given here and annotated.

Imagine we wanted to automate creating crosstabs of a list of particular variables by `ASTHMA4`, and then writing each table out as uniquely named *.csv files. First, we could start by making a vector with the list of variables we want to include. For this short example, we will only include three variables–`ALCGRP`, `X_AGE_G`, and `SEX`–but we could include as many as we wanted. We will name the vector `GrpVars`.

```
GrpVars <- c("ALCGRP", "X_AGE_G", "SEX")
```

When automating updating data in R, we have found it is easier to refer to columns by their column number rather than their field name. Since we will be referring to the `ASTHMA4` column over and over, we can find out its column number and store that in a variable called ASTHMA4cn (for column number) using the which command.

```
ASTHMA4cn <- which(colnames(analytic)=="ASTHMA4")
```

In the code, the which command queries the analytic file for the number of the column named "ASTHMA4," and this value is placed in the ASTHMA4cn variable.

Next, using a loop, we will create three tables that are written out as *.csv files: ALCGRPfreq.csv, X_AGE_Gfreq.csv, and SEXfreq.csv.

```
for (i in 1:length(GrpVars)){
        GrpVarcn <- which(colnames(analytic)==GrpVars[i])
        Tbl <- table(analytic[,GrpVarcn], analytic[,ASTHMA4cn])
        write.csv(Tbl, paste(GrpVars[i],"freq.csv",sep=""))
}
```

Although this is a small amount of code, it is quite complicated. Notice that it starts with a for loop. The syntax starts with the word for, followed by a parenthesis and the variable i, which will be set as the number of the current iteration in the code loop when it runs. The number of the iterations is specified by "in," and because we want it to go from the first entry in GrpVars to the last entry, instead of saying 1:3 because we have three variables now, we can set it to 1:length(GrpVars), which will set the maximum number of iterations to the number of variables in the vector GrpVars. That way, if we add more variables to GrpVars, the loop will run through all of them.

After that, a { is placed, and then the next lines will be what happens in each iteration of the loop. After those lines, there will be a solitary } on the last line to finish the code and say where the loop ends.

The first line of the code in the loop sets the variable GrpVarcn (for column number) to the column number of the current GrpVar, which is designated as GrpVar[i], meaning the group variable from GrpVar which is the subject of the current iteration. This is similar to the code above that was used to set ASTHMA4cn, only GrpVarcn will only be set for the current iteration, and then reset the next time the loop iterates. GrpVarcn can now be used to designate the grouping column in analytic that we want to do a crosstab for in the current iteration.

On the next line, a table is created named Tbl using the table command, listing the current iteration GrpVars as the first argument, and then ASTHMA4 as the second argument, but referring to them using the variables for their column names. Notice we are using the syntax construction of referring to columns by filling in only the y of analytic[x,y].

At this point in the code, Tbl is the crosstab between the grouping variable in the current iteration and the ASTHMA4 variable. Therefore, the last thing to do in this iteration is to write out Tbl because it will be replaced in the next iteration by the new frequency table with the next grouping variable. However, when we write it out, we want to make sure we remember which of the grouping variables was used in the table. For this reason, we need to come up with a unique name each time for the table that is exported that is based on the `GroupVar[i]` value.

To do that, we use the `paste` command, which creates strings. The `paste` command takes in both numeric and character string arguments. The `sep=""` option removes any spaces between the arguments in the result (which appear by default in the `paste` command unless specifically handled using the `sep=` option). By using `GrpVars[i]` in the `paste` command followed by "`freq.csv`" and adding the `sep=""` option, the table that is exported to *.csv will be named whatever the current `GrpVar` value is followed by `freq.csv`. As described before, the results of the code presented are separate frequency tables written out to *.csv into the designated data directory named `ALCGRPfreq.csv`, `X_AGE_Gfreq.csv`, and `SEXfreq.csv`.

This book will not use automation approaches because they are difficult to grasp for a beginning R user. Once the reader masters techniques in this book, the reader is encouraged to advance to learning automation techniques in R such as those mentioned in this part.

R Bivariate Statistical Tests

The last part of Table 1 categorical that needs to be addressed is statistical tests. As you will recall, in SAS, chi-square and Fisher's exact tests are options in `PROC FREQ`. In R, these tests are achieved by running code on the frequency table object that is the subject of the test. In R, the command `chisq.test` is used for the chi-square test, and `fisher.test` used for Fisher's exact test. The argument in the command is the crosstab table object developed by the `table` command as was demonstrated earlier, with `AlcFreq`. The code follows:

Code:

```
chisq.test(AlcFreq)
```

Output:

```
        Pearson's Chi-squared test

data: AlcFreq
X-squared = 58.823, df = 2, p-value = 1.686e-13
```

Note that the output includes the chi-squared statistic (`X-squared`), degrees of freedom (`df`), and the p-value on the chi-squared statistic in scientific notation. In Table 1, extremely small p-values will be notated < 0.0001. These results can be easily manually added to Table 1.

This section began with a description of various SAS approaches to developing categorical Table 1 and covered using graphical output approaches, involving Excel in processing, and conducting bivariate categorical tests. Next, the section gave an overview of using similar processes in R and demonstrated with an example that builds a categorical Table 1 in R that is outputted as a *.csv, which can be read into Excel for post-processing. Also, conducting bivariate categorical statistical tests in R was reviewed.

The next section describes how to develop a Table 1 for a continuous outcome variable. As with this section, first SAS approaches will be reviewed, then an R approach will be demonstrated.

Making "Table 1"—Continuous Outcome

This section will provide an example of making Table 1 for a continuous outcome, sleep duration, or `SLEPTIM2`. First, a structure of continuous Table 1 will be proposed. Next, an explanation of how SAS is typically used as a tool to populate Table 1 continuous will be provided, along with how bivariate statistical tests are computed in SAS. After that, an approach to populating Table 1 using R will be presented, which will parallel the process in SAS. The section will end with an explanation of how to do bivariate statistical tests on the continuous variable in R that can be included in continuous Table 1.

Structure of Continuous Table 1

The previous section covered how to make a Table 1 for a binary categorical outcome variable, which was `ASTHMA4`. This section will explain how to make a Table 1 for a continuous outcome variable, which is sleep duration (`SLEPTIME2`). As with categorical Table 1, there is a variety of ways to present this information in the literature. Table 3.8 provides a structure we will use. Like with Table 1 categorical, this table lists the covariate categories and levels along the *y*-axis. There is a column that includes the frequency and column percentage for each level, a column that reports the mean and standard deviation of sleep duration for each level, and a final column for statistical tests.

First, this section will look at how an analyst might construct this table using SAS, and next, alternative approaches in R will be presented.

SAS Approaches to Continuous Table 1

As with categorical outcomes, SAS does not have an easy way to output calculations as *.csv that are in the format of Table 3.8. Therefore, as described in the Making "Table 1"—Categorical Outcome section regarding developing journal-ready categorical Table 1s, SAS users may use HTML approaches like

TABLE 3.8

Example of Completed Table 1: Continuous Dependent Variable

Category	Level	*n*, (%)	Sleep Duration (hours) m, sd	*t*-Test or ANOVA *p*-Value
	All	58,131, 100%	7.1, 1.5	NA
Alcohol status	Nondrinker	26,169, 45%	7.1, 1.6	0.00167
	Monthly drinker	22,646, 39%	7.1, 1.4	
	Weekly drinker	9,316, 16%	7.1, 1.3	
Asthma status	Has asthma	5,343, 9%	7.0, 1.8	<0.0001
	No asthma	52,788, 91%	7.1, 1.4	
Age	Age 18–24	899, 2%	6.5, 1.5	<0.0001
	Age 25–34	2,657, 5%	6.4, 1.4	
	Age 35–44	3,589, 6%	6.6, 1.4	
	Age 45–54	6,543, 11%	6.7, 1.4	
	Age 55–64	10,724, 18%	6.9, 1.5	
	Age 65 or older	33,719, 58%	7.4, 1.4	
Sex	Male	52,971, 91%	7.1, 1.5	<0.0001
	Female	5,160, 9%	6.9, 1.5	
Ethnicity	Hispanic	2,262, 4%	6.8, 1.5	<0.0001
	Non-Hispanic	55,262, 95%	7.1, 1.5	
	Not reported	607, 1%	7.1, 1.9	
Race	White	49,394, 85%	7.2, 1.4	<0.0001
	Black/African American	3,939, 7%	6.7, 1.8	
	Asian	930, 2%	6.9, 1.9	
	American Indian/ Alaskan Native	557, 1%	6.7, 1.5	
	Native Hawaiian/Pacific Islander	261, 0%	6.4, 1.6	
	Other Race/Multiracial	2056, 4%	6.8, 1.7	
	Not reported	994, 2%	7.0, 1.7	
Marital status	Currently married	40,551, 70%	7.1, 1.4	<0.0001
	Divorced, widowed, separated	15,588, 27%	7.1, 1.6	
	Never married	982, 2%	6.6, 1.8	
	Not reported	1,010, 2%	6.9, 1.6	
Highest education level	Less than high school	2,483, 4%	7.2, 2	<0.0001
	High school graduate	16,241, 28%	7.1, 1.6	
	Some college/technical	17,559, 30%	7, 1.5	
	Four or more years of college	21,742, 37%	7.2, 1.3	
	Not reported	106, 0%	7.2, 1.4	

(Continued)

TABLE 3.8 (*Continued*)

Example of Completed Table 1: Continuous Dependent Variable

Category	Level	*n*, (%)	Sleep Duration (hours) m, sd	*t*-Test or ANOVA *p*-Value
Annual household income	<$10k	1,165, 2%	6.8, 2.3	<0.0001
	$10k to <$15k	2,111, 4%	6.9, 2.0	
	$15k to <$20k	3,148, 5%	7.1, 1.8	
	$20k to <$25k	4,774, 8%	7.1, 1.7	
	$25k to <$35k	6,491, 11%	7.2, 1.5	
	$35k to <$50k	9,305, 16%	7.1, 1.4	
	$50k to <$75k	9,636, 17%	7.1, 1.3	
	$75k or more	15,230, 26%	7.1, 1.2	
	Not reported	6,271, 11%	7.2, 1.5	
Obesity status	Underweight	478, 1%	7.1, 2.1	<0.0001
	Normal	14,340, 25%	7.2, 1.5	
	Overweight	25,572, 44%	7.1, 1.4	
	Obese	16,871, 29%	7.0, 1.5	
	Not reported	870, 1%	7.0, 1.7	
Smoking status	Smoker	8,571, 15%	6.8, 1.7	<0.0001
	Nonsmoker	26,639, 46%	7.2, 1.4	
	Not reported	22,921, 39%	7.2, 1.4	
Exercise status	Exercised in the last month	8,571, 15%	7.1, 1.4	0.2281
	Did not exercise in the last month	49,261, 85%	7.1, 1.8	
	Not reported	299, 1%	7.3, 1.7	
Health plan	Has a health plan	55,795, 96%	7.1, 1.5	<0.0001
	No health plan	2,203, 4%	6.8, 1.7	
	Not reported	133, 0%	7.2, 1.5	
General health	Excellent	9,016, 16%	7.2, 1.3	<0.0001
	Very good	18,111, 31%	7.2, 1.2	
	Good	18,797, 32%	7.1, 1.4	
	Fair	8,436, 15%	7.0, 1.8	
	Poor	3,569, 6%	7.0, 2.3	
	Not reported	202, 0%	7.4, 2.2	

`PROC TABULATE` and `PROC REPORT`, or may use approaches that involve Excel in the development of the final table.

To calculate the numbers that will appear in Table 1 continuous using SAS, `PROC FREQ` is used for frequencies and percentages (as described in the last section), and means and standard deviations can be obtained from using PROC UNIVARIATE.* Here is PROC UNIVARIATE code for sleep duration to produce summary statistics for the entire dataset. Only the top of the output—the moments—are shown.

Code:

```
proc univariate data=r.analytic;
      var SLEPTIM2;
run;
```

Table 3.9 shows the output.

TABLE 3.9

PROC UNIVARIATE Output for SLEPTIM2

Moments			
N	58131	Sum weights	58131
Mean	7.11575579	Sum observations	413646
Std deviation	1.46860065	Variance	2.15678788
Skewness	0.51824615	Kurtosis	5.48634619
Uncorrected SS	3068778	Corrected SS	125374.079
Coeff variation	20.6387163	Std error mean	0.00609116

To generate summary statistics by a grouping variable, such as ALCGRP, the BY argument can be used in PROC UNIVARIATE, but please understand the code must be preceded by a SORT command that sorts by the BY variable. Otherwise, SAS will give an error worded similarly to this: "ERROR: Data set R.ANALYTIC is not sorted in ascending sequence. The current BY group has ALCGRP = 2 and the next BY group has ALCGRP = 1." This error shows up because SAS requires this presort for its indexing function.

The output is shown in Table 3.10. Please also note that the output provides the moments separated by ALCGRP, and preceded by a title indicating which group is the subject of the statistics.

Code:

```
proc sort data=r.analytic;
      by ALCGRP;

proc univariate data=r.analytic;
      var SLEPTIM2;
      by ALCGRP;
run;
```

* One may observe that PROC UNIVARIATE also produces n's, but PROC FREQ would still be needed for the proportions, as those are not available in PROC UNVARIATE.

TABLE 3.10

PROC UNIVARIATE Output for SLEPTIM2 by ALCGRP

ALCGRP=1 Moments			
N	26169	Sum weights	26169
Mean	7.1261034	Sum observations	186483
Std deviation	1.59387128	Variance	2.54042566
Skewness	0.54109281	Kurtosis	4.8451737
Uncorrected SS	1395375	Corrected SS	66477.8588
Coeff variation	22.3666595	Std error mean	0.0098528

While PROC UNIVARIATE provides the results of calculations, it does not provide them in an easy way to export as a *.csv in the format desired. Again, we can use the ODS to output the results, but the output is not structured in an easy way for us to use for our table display.

To illustrate this, in the following code, the ODS is turned on, and we request the moments table from the PROC UNIVARIATE results be placed as a SAS dataset in the directory mapped to LIBNAME "r." Then, we run the PROC UNIVARIATE code for summary statistics by ALCGRP level, and turn off the ODS.

Code:

```
ods trace on /listing;
ods output Moments=r.AlcMoments;
proc univariate data=r.analytic;
        var SLEPTIM2;
        by ALCGRP;
run;
ods listing close;
ods trace off;
```

This SAS dataset can be exported to *.csv using the export wizard, which writes the following code:

Code:

```
PROC EXPORT DATA= r.AlcMoments
            OUTFILE= "C:\Users\Monika\Dropbox\R Stats Book\
            Analytics\Data\AlcMoments.csv"
            DBMS=CSV REPLACE;
     PUTNAMES=YES;
RUN;
```

TABLE 3.11

ALCMOMENTS Dataset

ALCGRP	VarName	Label1	cValue1	nValue1	Label2	cValue2	nValue2
1	SLEPTIM2	N	26169	26169	Sum weights	26169	26169
1	SLEPTIM2	Mean	7.126103	7.126103	Sum observations	186483	186483
1	SLEPTIM2	Std deviation	1.593871	1.593871	Variance	2.540426	2.540426
1	SLEPTIM2	Skewness	0.541093	0.541093	Kurtosis	4.845174	4.845174
1	SLEPTIM2	Uncorrected SS	1395375	1395375	Corrected SS	66477.86	66478
1	SLEPTIM2	Coeff variation	22.36666	22.36666	Std error mean	0.009853	0.009853
2	SLEPTIM2	N	22646	22646	Sum weights	22646	22646
2	SLEPTIM2	Mean	7.090259	7.090259	Sum observations	160566	160566
2	SLEPTIM2	Std deviation	1.375262	1.375262	Variance	1.891345	1.891345
2	SLEPTIM2	Skewness	0.560816	0.560816	Kurtosis	6.490695	6.490695
2	SLEPTIM2	Uncorrected SS	1181284	1181284	Corrected SS	42829.51	42830
2	SLEPTIM2	Coeff variation	19.3965	19.3965	Std error mean	0.009139	0.009139
3	SLEPTIM2	N	9316	9316	Sum weights	9316	9316
3	SLEPTIM2	Mean	7.148669	7.148669	Sum observations	66597	66597
3	SLEPTIM2	Std deviation	1.312195	1.312195	Variance	1.721857	1.721857
3	SLEPTIM2	Skewness	0.222834	0.222834	Kurtosis	4.293913	4.293913
3	SLEPTIM2	Uncorrected SS	492119	492119	Corrected SS	16039.09	16039
3	SLEPTIM2	Coeff variation	18.3558	18.3558	Std error mean	0.013595	0.013595

But as with `PROC FREQ`, the output, although containing all the needed information, is not in a desirable format (Table 3.8). The moments table that is output is shown in Table 3.11.*

Code or manual manipulation could be used to extract these metrics from this table and place them in an Excel table for presentation. As reviewed earlier, this is one of the approaches that can be used for presenting Table 1 that involves Excel.

`PROC TABULATE` in SAS can be used also for continuous outcomes, but as shown in the last section, the coding is hairy and output hard to manipulate without a full grasp of `PROC TABULATE` syntax. The following is the code that will produce part of the desired Table 1 continuous is `PROC TABULATE`:

Code:

```
/*copy dataset and add labels*/

data r.example;
        set r.analytic;
        label SLEPTIM2 = "Sleep Duration";
        label ALCGRP = "Alcohol Consumption"
        label ASTHMA4 = "Asthma Status";
run;
```

* It is acknowledged that it is also possible to use `PROC MEANS` with the `out=` option in SAS to export means by groups, but this table also would need to be formatted further.

```
/*set up formats*/

proc format;
        value asthma_f
        0 = "No Asthma"
        1 = "Has Asthma";
        value alcohol_f
        1 = "Nondrinker"
        2 = "Monthly Drinker"
        3 = "Weekly Drinker"
        ;
run;

/*apply formats in proc tabulate*/

proc tabulate data=r.example;
        title "Continuous Variable Table 1";
        format ALCGRP alcohol_f.
               ASTHMA4 asthma_f.;
        class ALCGRP ASTHMA4;
        var SLEPTIM2;
        TABLE ALCGRP ASTHMA4,
               SLEPTIM1 * (N Mean STD);
run;
```

The output is shown in Table 3.12. As can be seen, much more work would need to be done in `PROC TABULATE` to have the output reflect our desired Table 1 continuous format.

Another approach that can be used to develop continuous Table 1 is the one described by Winters, which was discussed earlier, where a table is structured inside SAS and then exported to *.csv [72]. As mentioned earlier, this is a viable approach but does require some advanced knowledge of SAS coding, as it involves the ODS.

TABLE 3.12

Example of `PROC TABULATE` Output—Continuous Outcome

	Sleep Duration		
	N	**Mean**	**Std**
Alcohol consumption label	26169	7.13	1.59
Nondrinker			
Monthly drinker	22646	7.09	1.38
Weekly drinker	9316	7.15	1.31
Asthma status	52788	7.13	1.43
No asthma			
Has asthma	5343	6.98	1.78

In summary, the approaches used in SAS to develop continuous Table 1 are basically the same approaches used in SAS to develop categorical Table 1, with only minor differences (such as the use of PROC UNIVARIATE instead of PROC FREQ). A SAS analyst may choose a graphical output approach such as PROC TABULATE or PROC REPORT. Alternatively, the analyst can build and reuse (or adapt) a macro in SAS macro language. Or, the analyst may involve Excel at various levels in developing the final presentation table.

The next part of this section reviews using SAS to develop bivariate continuous tests to add to continuous Table 1.

Continuous Bivariate Statistical Tests in SAS

The final touch to add to Table 1 continuous is comprised of results from statistical tests. If the dependent variable, SLEPTIM2, is assumed to be normally distributed (as well as meeting other assumptions), a *t*-test is used to compare means in binary groups (e.g., Male vs. Female), and an ANOVA is used to compare means in groups with three or more levels (e.g., ALCGRP). If linearity cannot be assumed, then nonparametric tests are used. In lieu of the parametric *t*-test, the Mann–Whitney *U*-test* may be used, and in lieu of the ANOVA, a Kruskal–Wallis test may be used.

SAS development started in 1966 [79], and over the years, many PROCs have been programmed to produce *t*-test results. This example will use PROC TTEST to *t*-test the mean of sleep duration between independent groups, MALE = 0 (females) and MALE = 1 (males). Please note that because we are using MALE in the "by" option of PROC TTEST, we must precede the PROC TTEST code with PROC SORT by the MALE variable. The output shown is just the results from the *t*-test, and not the other output that is provided with PROC TTEST†.

Code:

```
proc sort data=r.analytic;
        by MALE;
proc ttest data=r.analytic;
        var SLEPTIM2;
        by MALE;
run;
```

The output is shown in Table 3.13.

* This test is also called the Mann-Whitney-Wilcoxon, Wilcoxon rank-sum test, and Wilcoxon-Mann-Whitney test.

† Using the class option in PROC TTEST would prevent needing to sort by MALE before conducting the test.

TABLE 3.13

Output from PROC TTEST for Sleep Duration by Sex

DF	*t* Value	Pr > |*t*|
5159	327.52	<.0001

The output provides the *t*-value, degrees of freedom, and *p*-value on the *t*-statistic. For a Mann–Whitney *U*-test, `PROC NPAR1WAY` could be used with the `wilcoxon` option.

Code:

```
proc npar1way data = r.analytic wilcoxon;
  class MALE;
  var SLEPTIM2;
run;
```

The relevant output from `PROC NPAR1WAY` is presented in Table 3.14.

Next, for categorical variables with three or more levels, an ANOVA could be used. Because `ALCGRP` is an ordinal variable, we will use the `CLASS` statement and run a `PROC GLM` one-way ANOVA between `ALCGRP` and `SLEPTIM2`.

Code:

```
PROC GLM data=r.analytic;
        class ALCGRP;
        model SLEPTIM2 = ALCGRP;
run;
```

The resulting ANOVA table is provided in Table 3.15.

TABLE 3.14

Output from PROC NPAR1WAY for Sleep Duration by Sex

Wilcoxon Two-Sample Test	
Statistic	134689720.5000
Normal approximation	
Z	–13.7149
One-sided Pr < Z	<.0001
Two-sided Pr > |Z|	<.0001
t Approximation	
One-sided Pr < Z	<.0001
Two-sided Pr > |Z|	<.0001
Z includes a continuity correction of 0.5.	

TABLE 3.15

Output from `PROC GLM` for Sleep Duration by Alcohol Consumption Group

Source	DF	Sum of Squares	Mean Square	F Value	Pr > F
Model	2	27.6159	13.8080	6.40	0.0017
Error	58,128	125346.4633	2.1564		
Corrected total	58,130	125374.0793			

TABLE 3.16

Output from `PROC NPAR1WAY` for Sleep Duration by Alcohol Consumption Group

Kruskal–Wallis Test	
Chi-square	22.8400
DF	2
Pr > Chi-square	<0.0001

The output includes a Kruskal–Wallis Test table, which is presented in Table 3.16.

These results could be manually added to the table structure shown in Table 3.8. The first part of this section gave an overview of SAS approaches to developing continuous Table 1, which are roughly the same as the SAS approaches to developing categorical Table 1, with some minor differences in the `PROC`s used. The next part of this section discusses parallel approaches in R and provides a demonstration of one approach, where R is used to build a continuous Table 1 that is exported as a *.csv and post-processed in Excel.

R Approaches to Continuous Table 1

Although there are graphical alternatives, as demonstrated in the first section, it is not difficult in R to build a table as a `data.frame` and then export it as a *.csv to generate a base file that can be post-processed in Excel that is close in format to Table 3.8, our desired format. Therefore, we will use this Excel-supplemented approach with R in building continuous Table 1 as we did building categorical Table 1.

R does not have a perfect parallel to `PROC UNIVARIATE`, which produces a full list of moments. As demonstrated in earlier chapters, the `summary` command in R produces calculations that could be of interest, including the mean. The following code runs the `summary` command on our dependent variable, `SLEPTIM2`.

Code:

```
summary(analytic$SLEPTIM2)
```

Output:

```
Min.   1st Qu.  Median    Mean  3rd Qu.    Max.
1.000    6.000    7.000   7.116    8.000   24.000
```

The mean SLEPTIM2 for the entire dataset is 7.116 hours, as shown above. However, for means for each ALCGRP, we will use the aggregate command in R.

Code:

```
aggregate(analytic$SLEPTIM2, list(analytic$ALCGRP), mean)
```

Output:

```
   Group.1          x
1        1   7.126103
2        2   7.090259
3        3   7.148669
```

The first argument of the aggregate command is the variable that will be used in the operation, which is SLEPTIM2. The next argument says to list the results of the operation by the levels of a grouping variable, which for us, is ALCGRP. Finally, the "mean" option determines the function behind the calculation. The Quick-R blog provides a quick list of functions that could be used here, which include median and range [80].

These are calculations of means, but for Table 3.8, we still need a calculation of variance. The standard deviation of SLEPTIM2 in the entire dataset can be easily calculated with the sd command:

Code:

```
sd(analytic$SLEPTIM2)
```

Output:

```
[1]  1.468601
```

Note that the above code can only run if there are no missing values ("NA"s) in the field analytic$SLEPTIM2. We insured that there were no NAs in this field because we removed them as part of building the analytic dataset. However, if there were any NAs in analytic$SLEPTIM2, R would register an error. To get around that error, the na.rm ("remove NAs") option could be specified. The default is na.rm=FALSE, meaning that NAs are not removed. This was not a problem for our situation because we did not have any NAs in our field. But if we had, we would need to set na.rm=TRUE, telling R to remove the NAs from analytic$SLEPTIM2 and then calculate the standard deviation from the populated values. The code would be formulated like this:

Code:

```
sd(analytic$SLEPTIM2, na.rm=TRUE)
```

Because there were already no NAs in the field we were analyzing, the output from this code is the same as for the previous code.

The calculated sd of 1.468601 refers to the entire dataset, but we also need sd calculated for each ALCGRP level. Just as we used aggregate to calculate the means in each alcohol group, now we will use it again to calculate standard deviations. Notice the code is identical to the earlier code, except the function we are requesting is sd, not mean.

Code:

```
aggregate(analytic$SLEPTIM2, list(analytic$ALCGRP), sd)
```

Output:

```
   Group.1          x
1        1   1.593871
2        2   1.375262
3        3   1.312195
```

As we saw with SAS, this default output from the aggregate command in R is not in the desired format, which is shown in the structure of Table 3.8. Therefore, our next approach is to use R to construct a table closer in structure to Table 3.8 and export that as a *.csv, so we minimize the amount of retyping we will need to do to make the table journal-ready.

As with categorical Table 1, continuous Table 1 starts with code to construct the table, called Table1Cont:

Code:

```
Table1Cont <- data.frame(Category=character(),
                 Level=character(),
                 TotalN=integer(),
                 TotalProp=numeric(),
                 SleepMean=numeric(),
                 SleepSD=numeric())
```

Notice that this table is similar in format to Table 3.8. Like with Table 1 categorical, it starts out with Category and Level as labels for the variables on the *y*-axis. The TotalN and TotalProp are similar to the ones used in Table 1 categorical. New in this table are SleepMean, which will be the mean of SLEPTIM2 at that category and level, and SleepSD, which will be the standard deviation of SLEPTIM2 at that category and level.

As with Table 1 categorical, our strategy will be to make separate entries in the same format as the table, and then row bind these entries onto the table.

Also, as with Table 1 categorical, the first row is for the overall dataset. Therefore, we will need to set up variables for the number of observations (as we did before—`TotalObs`), the mean for `SLEPTIM2` in the entire dataset (`TotalMean`), and the standard deviation for `SLEPTIM2` in the entire dataset (`TotalSD`). We will be able to calculate proportions and fill them in using `TotalObs` as the denominator.

Code:

```
TotalObs <- nrow(analytic)
TotalMean <- mean(analytic$SLEPTIM2)
TotalSD <- sd(analytic$SLEPTIM2)
```

Using these variables, we can now construct the first entry in `Table1Cont`, which we will name `Entry1`.

Code:

```
Entry1 <- data.frame(Category="All",
               Level="All",
               TotalN=TotalObs,
               TotalProp=TotalObs/TotalObs,
               SleepMean=TotalMean,
               SleepSD=TotalSD)
```

Notice how Category and Level are set to `"All,"` and `TotalN` is set to `TotalObs`, and `TotalProp` is set to the ratio of `TotalObs` to `TotalObs` (which will be 1.0). `Entry1` looks like this:

Output:

```
  Category Level TotalN TotalProp SleepMean  SleepSD
1      All   All  58131         1  7.115756 1.468601
```

The next step is to row bind this to the blank `Table1Cont`.

Code:

```
Table1Cont <- rbind(Table1Cont, Entry1)
```

The resulting `Table1Cont` looks like this:

Output:

```
  Category Level TotalN TotalProp SleepMean  SleepSD
1      All   All  58131         1  7.115756 1.468601
```

Like with `Table1Cat`, it looks identical to `Entry1`, but this step enforces that we have the data types specified in `Table1Cont`. It is not possible to row bind together tables with different structures to achieve the results for which we are striving.

As with `Table1Cat`, the next step is to develop tables for each of the covariates—alcohol consumption group, sex, age group, and the others—and row bind them to `Table1Cont`. These tables need to be in the same format and contain the appropriate metrics for each `Category` and `Level`. Like we did with `Table1Cat`, let us do this for the alcohol groups in `Table1Cont`.

To facilitate this, we will first make three `data.frames` that we can use to help populate the entry for alcohol group in `Table1Cont`. The first is `AlcFreq`, which will contain the frequencies of `AlcGroup` (which is the same step we did under `Table1Cat` for this). Next, we will make the `data.frame` `AlcMeans` out of using the `aggregate` command for alcohol group means (as demonstrated earlier). Finally, we will make the `data.frame` `AlcSDs` using the `aggregate` code for standard deviations for groups shown earlier.

Code:

```
AlcFreq <- as.data.frame(table(analytic$ALCGRP))
AlcMeans <- as.data.frame(aggregate(analytic$SLEPTIM2,
   by=list(analytic$ALCGRP), mean))
AlcSDs <- as.data.frame(aggregate(analytic$SLEPTIM2,
   by=list(analytic$ALCGRP), sd))
```

The `data.frame` `AlcFreq` looks the same as the earlier demonstration. `AlcMeans` and `AlcSDs` are shown here.

Output:

```
> AlcMeans
  Group.1          x
1       1   7.126103
2       2   7.090259
3       3   7.148669
> AlcSDs
  Group.1          x
1       1   1.593871
2       2   1.375262
3       3   1.312195
```

Next, just like we did with `Table1Cat`, we will construct columns that we will column bind together to make the alcohol entry. We will perform this task by referring to these tables.

Code:

```
Category <- c("Alcohol Status", "", "")
Level <- c("Nondrinker", "Monthly Drinker", "Weekly Drinker")
TotalN <- AlcFreq[,2]
TotalProp <- AlcFreq[,2]/TotalObs
SleepMean <- AlcMeans[,2]
SleepSD <- AlcSDs[,2]
```

Note that `Category` and `Level` are filled in the way we did them with `Table1Cat`. `TotalN` uses the second column of `AlcFreq`, which has the frequencies for each level. `TotalProp` uses the frequencies of `AlcFreq` as the numerator, and the variable `TotalObs` as the denominator, to calculate the proportion of that category and level in the dataset. `SleepMean` copies in the second column from `AlcMeans`, and `SleepSD` copies in the second column of `AlcSDs`. The next step is to column bind these columns together to produce a `data.frame` called `AlcTbl` that represents the `Table1Cont` entry for alcohol group.

Code:

```
AlcTbl <- as.data.frame(cbind(Category, Level, TotalN, TotalProp,
        SleepMean, SleepSD))
```

At this point, `AlcTbl` looks like this:

Output:

```
        Category            Level TotalN        TotalProp        SleepMean
1 Alcohol Status      Nondrinker  26169 0.450172885379574 7.12610340479193
2              Monthly Drinker  22646 0.389568388639452 7.09025876534487
3               Weekly Drinker   9316 0.160258725980974 7.14866895663375
           SleepSD
1 1.59387128199415
2 1.37526185039389
3 1.31219530604596
```

It is in the correct structure and populated, so we will then row bind it onto the `Table1Cont` we are building.

Code:

```
Table1Cont <- rbind(Table1Cont, AlcTbl)
```

Now, `Table1Cont` looks like this:

Output:

```
        Category            Level TotalN        TotalProp        SleepMean
1            All              All  58131                 1  7.1157557929504
2 Alcohol Status      Nondrinker  26169 0.450172885379574 7.12610340479193
3              Monthly Drinker  22646 0.389568388639452 7.09025876534487
4               Weekly Drinker   9316 0.160258725980974 7.14866895663375
           SleepSD
1 1.46860065254059
2 1.59387128199415
3 1.37526185039389
4 1.31219530604596
```

Notice that, as with `Table1Cat`, we can continue using this approach to build entry tables for the other covariates and then row bind them to `Table1Cont` until it is complete. Once it is complete, like with `Table1Cat`, it can be written out as a *.csv.

Code:

```
write.csv(Table1Cont, file = "Table1Cont.csv")
```

This *.csv is closer to the format of Table 3.8, our desired format, than the `PROC UNIVARIATE` output was from SAS. Therefore, constructing a continuous journal-ready Table 1 could be more efficient in R because the numbers will not need to be manually entered.

The next part of this section covers conducting the statistical tests in R that can be added to continuous Table 1.

Continuous Bivariate Statistical Tests in R

Bivariate tests between two groups would be a *t*-test of means, which is a parametric test, or a Mann–Whitney *U*-test, which is non-parametric. In SAS, we went over `PROC TTEST` for the *t*-test, and `PROC NPAR1WAY` with the Wilcoxon option for the Mann–Whitney *U*-test. In R, the commands for *t*-test and Mann–Whitney *U*-test are `t.test` and `wilcox.test`, respectively.

The `t.test` command in R has several options that can be set. An important consideration is whether or not the variances are equal or homogenous. If we were to conduct an independent *t*-test between males and females for `SLEPTIM2`, we would need to know if we thought the variances were equal or homogenous or not in order to use the *t*-test command properly. To make this decision, one could simply eyeball the results for standard deviation and decide on the basis of that. To do that, we could use our aggregate code. We will use `MALE` (1=Male, 0=Female) as our sex covariate.

Code:

```
aggregate(analytic$SLEPTIM2, list(analytic$MALE), sd)
```

Output:

```
  Group.1        x
1       0 1.505267
2       1 1.462665
```

A rule of thumb that can be used is if one standard deviation is not at least twice the other, then the variances can be said to be homogenous. However, there are a few tests that can be used that are more scientific. Bartlett's Test for Homogeneity of Variances [80] is one such test and is available in R outside of a package. We will use Bartlett's test to see if variances in `SLEPTIM2` are equal or unequal between the two sexes in our dataset.

Code:

```
bartlett.test(SLEPTIM2 ~ MALE, data=analytic)
```

Output:

```
        Bartlett test of homogeneity of variances

data: SLEPTIM2 by MALE
Bartlett's K-squared = 7.8725, df = 1, p-value = 0.005019
```

Bartlett's test renders a p-value of 0.005019. This small p-value suggests that the variances are indeed unequal between the two groups, which contradicts our instinct that both standard deviations looked similar. If we are not sure which is the best choice, we can start by trying the t-test both ways—one specifying equal variance and the other specifying unequal variance—and see if the results differ.

Below is the t-test code. The default option is to set the variances as unequal*, so to choose equal variance, we must set the option `var.equal` to `TRUE`. The first code will run the *t*.test assuming equal variances.

Here is an example of using `t.test` to test the mean `SLEPTIM2` between males and females using the `SEX` variable as the grouping variable.

Code:

```
t.test(analytic$SLEPTIM2 ~ analytic$MALE, var.equal=TRUE)
```

Output:

```
        Two Sample t-test

data: analytic$SLEPTIM2 by analytic$MALE
t = -12.961, df = 58129, p-value < 2.2e-16
alternative hypothesis: true difference in means is not equal
to 0
95 percent confidence interval:
-0.3190993 -0.2352638
sample estimates:
mean in group 0 mean in group 1
       6.863178        7.140360
```

The output is a little cluttered, but the first line clearly lists the t-statistic, the degrees of freedom, and the p-value on the t-test. The 95% confidence interval for the difference is listed, as well as the means in each group.

It is possible to extract particular statistics from the t-test output. To do that, let us start by creating an object called `MaleTTest` from the results of our t-test.

* The analyst can either specify `var.equal=FALSE` or simply not specify `var.equal`, and the t-test code will assume unequal variances.

Code:

```
MaleTTest <- t.test(analytic$SLEPTIM2 ~ analytic$MALE,
var.equal=TRUE)
```

Now, we can use the `str()` command, known as the "structure" command, to see the structure of this object.

Code:

```
str(MaleTTest)
```

Output:

```
List of 9
 $ statistic  : Named num -13
  ..- attr(*, "names")= chr "t"
 $ parameter  : Named num 58129
  ..- attr(*, "names")= chr "df"
 $ p.value    : num 2.31e-38
 $ conf.int   : atomic [1:2] -0.319 -0.235
  ..- attr(*, "conf.level")= num 0.95
 $ estimate   : Named num [1:2] 6.86 7.14
  ..- attr(*, "names")= chr [1:2] "mean in group 0" "mean in
      group 1"
 $ null.value : Named num 0
  ..- attr(*, "names")= chr "difference in means"
 $ alternative: chr "two.sided"
 $ method     : chr " Two Sample t-test"
 $ data.name  : chr "analytic$SLEPTIM2 by analytic$MALE"
 - attr(*, "class")= chr "htest"
```

The output is a little confusing, but a take-home message is that within this `MaleTTest` object, `$statistic` would extract the *t*- value from the test, and `$p.value` would extract the *p*-value of the test. See the following code:

Code:

```
t.test(analytic$SLEPTIM2 ~ analytic$MALE, var.equal=TRUE)$statistic
t.test(analytic$SLEPTIM2 ~ analytic$MALE, var.equal=TRUE)$p.value
```

Output:

```
        t
-12.96055
[1] 2.314708e-38
```

By using the <-, these exact values could be saved as variables.

As far as interpretation is concerned, the results from our *t*-test with equal variances is a very small *p*-value. Let us see what happens when we set the variance to unequal (which we will do by simply leaving off the `var.equal` option, because the default is `var.equal=FALSE`).

Code:

```
t.test(analytic$SLEPTIM2 ~ analytic$MALE)
```

Output:

```
        Welch Two Sample t-test

data: analytic$SLEPTIM2 by analytic$MALE
t = -12.658, df = 6146.6, p-value < 2.2e-16
alternative hypothesis: true difference in means is not equal
        to 0
95 percent confidence interval:
 -0.3201083 -0.2342547
sample estimates:
mean in group 0 mean in group 1
        6.863178        7.140360
```

As we can see, the `unequal` option gives us an unequal variances *t*-test, also known as a Welch `t-test`. The results are the same—a very small *p*-value—so we could choose equal or unequal variances in this case, and we would get the same answer.

Imagine we viewed `SLEPTIM2` as skewed and wanted to do a nonparametric Mann–Whitney *U*-test. We use the same arguments as we did in `t.test`, only this time, we will use `wilcox.test`.

Code:

```
wilcox.test(analytic$SLEPTIM2 ~ analytic$MALE)
```

Output:

```
        Wilcoxon rank sum test with continuity correction

data: analytic$SLEPTIM2 by analytic$MALE
W = 121370000, p-value < 2.2e-16
alternative hypothesis: true location shift is not equal to 0
```

Importantly, the *p*-value is reported. Not surprisingly, it is a very small *p*-value, and is consistent with what we found with the parametric *t*-tests we conducted.

Next, we will replicate the ANOVA (parametric) and Kruskal–Wallis (nonparametric) tests we ran with the dependent variable as `SLEPTIM2` and the grouping variable, the ordinal `ALCGRP`. For the ANOVA, we will actually make a linear model (`lm`) object named `AlcANOVA`. We will use the `lm` code.

Code:

```
AlcANOVA <- lm(formula = SLEPTIM2 ~ as.factor(ALCGRP), data =
       analytic)
```

Notice we use the `formula` command, then put the dependent variable after the equals sign, followed by the tilde and grouping variable, which in this case is `ALCGRP`. Because we want `ALCGRP` handled as a factor, we will use it in an `as.factor` function. After a comma, we declare the dataset after the equal sign. This creates the object `AlcAnova`. Running a `summary` command on this object will output the statistics we desire.

Code:

```
summary(AlcANOVA)
```

Output:

```
Call:
lm(formula = SLEPTIM2 ~ as.factor(ALCGRP), data = analytic)

Residuals:
    Min      1Q  Median      3Q     Max
-6.1487 -1.0903 -0.0903 0.8739 16.9097

Coefficients:
                    Estimate Std. Error t value Pr(>|t|)
(Intercept)         7.126103   0.009078 785.023  < 2e-16 ***
as.factor(ALCGRP)2 -0.035845   0.013328  -2.690  0.00716 **
as.factor(ALCGRP)3  0.022566   0.017716   1.274  0.20277
---
Signif. codes: 0 '***' 0.001 '**' 0.01 '*' 0.05 '.' 0.1 ' ' 1

Residual standard error: 1.468 on 58128 degrees of freedom
Multiple R-squared: 0.0002203, Adjusted R-squared: 0.0001859
F-statistic: 6.403 on 2 and 58128 DF, p-value: 0.001657
```

The last line is of interest to us, and reports the F-statistic, the degrees of freedom, and the p-value. We observe the p-value to be 0.001657, which would be statistically significant at $\alpha = 0.05$. Let us see what happens when we do the non-parametric version of this test.

For the non-parametric Kruskal–Wallis test, the command is more like `t.test`, in that the command is `kruskal.test`, which uses the argument starting with the dependent variable, followed by a tilde and the grouping variable, `ALCGRP`. In Kruskal–Wallis, "`as.factor`" is assumed so it does not need to be used around `ALCGRP`.

Code:

```
kruskal.test(analytic$SLEPTIM2 ~ analytic$ALCGRP)
```

Output:

```
        Kruskal-Wallis rank sum test

data: analytic$SLEPTIM2 by analytic$ALCGRP
Kruskal-Wallis chi-squared = 22.84, df = 2, p-value = 1.097e-05
```

The results, including the p-value, are reported on the last line. This p-value is very small, and seems to be consistent with what was found in the parametric ANOVA.

This section demonstrated how to develop t-test, Mann–Whitney U-test, ANOVA, and Kruskal–Wallis results that could be used in Table 1 continuous. The test results can be transcribed into Table 1 continuous, and the table will be complete.

The next section describes extra steps that must be taken if conducting a descriptive analysis of a dataset that will later be used in survival analysis.

Descriptive Analysis of Survival Data

In this section, we will focus on our survival analytic dataset developed in Chapter 2 and generate descriptive statistics and plots that are done on time-to-event variables.

Summary Statistics and Plots on Time Variable

To contemplate some descriptive analyses in preparation for regression in survival analysis, we will refer back to our survival analysis dataset we created in Chapter 2, `SurvAnalytic`. Recall that this dataset included all BRFSS respondents who had a valid measure for asthma status (and if yes, age of diagnosis), alcohol status, and veteran status. We intend to use alcohol status as the exposure, being diagnosed with asthma as the event (outcome), and sex and veteran status as candidate confounders. We created three sets of time-to-event variables; the third set corresponded to a study period from birth to age 80, and these variables were called `ASTHMA80` and `TIME80`.

If the analyst were to be performing a survival analysis regression, she would be using a dataset like this and would want to generate summary statistics and plots for the `TIME80` variable as part of a preliminary descriptive analysis. Plots could include histograms and side-by-side box plots, but the analyst must keep in mind that the values for those who do not get asthma during the time period are just their ages. Therefore, box plots would be most meaningful if split first by whether or not `ASTHMA80` = 1, and further plotted. Also, mean and standard deviation of `TIME80` should be presented in descriptive tables (Table 1s) so the reader understands the distribution of this variable, especially with respect to those with the event versus those who are censored.

Generating and Plotting Survival Curves

In Chapter 2, we described a hypothesis that the "survival experience" of being diagnosed with asthma (experiencing the event) will be different in the different alcohol exposure groups. After considering the time variable, as we did earlier in this section, it is important to calculate and plot the survival experience with a Kaplan–Meier plot.

If we turn to SAS, we can use PROC LIFETEST for our descriptive survival analysis and plots. We will start by creating a Kaplan–Meier plot for the entire dataset.

Code:

```
proc lifetest data=r.SurvAnalytic plots = (s) NOTABLE;
        time TIME80 * ASTHMA80(0);
run;
```

We specified NOTABLE in the PROC because otherwise SAS would output a conditional probability table, which can take prohibitively long to run when not using server SAS. We will look at the conditional probability table later, when using R for performing the same tasks.

The code above produces a Kaplan–Meier survival curve plot, and also, reports a summary of censored and uncensored values below.

Plot:

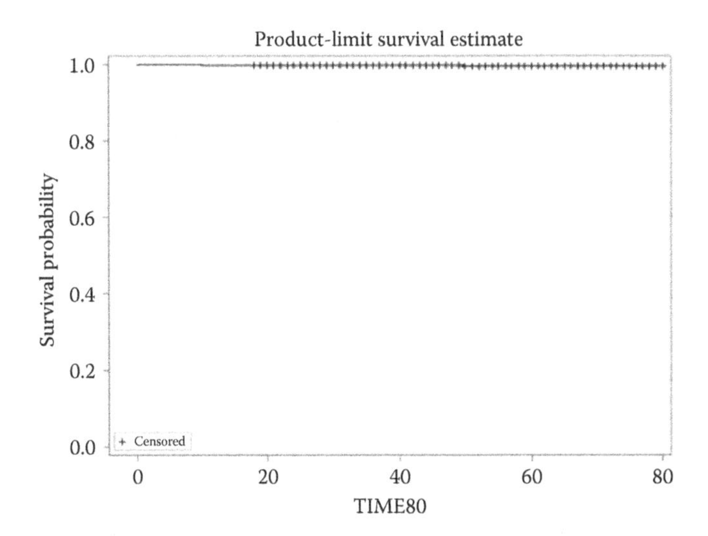

The results on the plot are hard to see on the default output because 97% of the people in this dataset did not get the event, and the survival curve reflects this. It would be nice to adjust the y-axis to have it focus on just the top probabilities, but manipulating this Kaplan–Meier plot in SAS is quite involved, as documented in an extensive white paper by Kuhfeld & So, which explains ways to customize the plot [81].

Next, let us consider our hypothesized exposure, ALCGRP. The following SAS code produces a Kaplan–Meier plot that plots each level of ALCGRP with its own line and provides a legend.

Code:

```
proc lifetest data=r.SurvAnalytic plots = (s) NOTABLE;
        time TIME80 * ASTHMA80(0);
        strata ALCGRP;
run;
```

Plot:

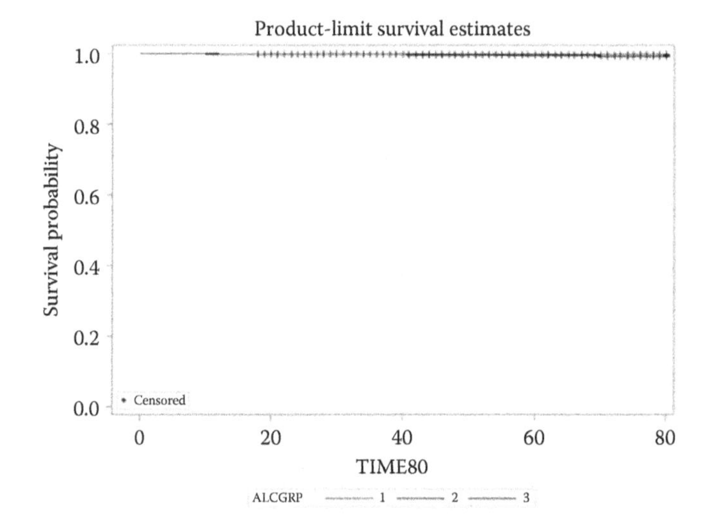

Again, the plot is difficult to interpret, as there are so few events relative to the number of rows in the dataset. However, please notice that when STRATA option was added, it caused a lot more output, including three four tables: Rank Statistics, Covariance Matrix for the Log-Rank Statistics, Covariance Matrix for the Wilcoxon Statistics, and Test of Equality over Strata. We want to direct the reader to notice a set of homogeneity tests in the last table, Test of Equality over Strata, which includes the chi-square, degrees of freedom, and *p*-value for the log–rank test, the Wilcoxon test, and the –2 log likelihood ratio test. We will revisit these tests later, when talking about bivariate tests for survival curves.

In R, we will use the KMSurv package to produce our Kaplan–Meier conditional probability table and plots [2]. We will start by calling up the library survival to invoke the command in the package KMSurv .

```
library(survival)
```

In R, using the KMSurv commands, the strategy is to first create a survival object using the survfit command. This survival object then can have other commands run on it. Let us start by creating a survival object for the entire dataset for TIME80 and ASTHMA80, and we will call the object AllSurv.

```
AllSurv <- survfit(Surv(SurvAnalytic$TIME80,
       SurvAnalytic$ASTHMA80)~ 1, conf.type="none")
```

Notice the arguments in the survfit function. First, Surv is stated, and arguments in Surv are the time variable, TIME80, and the event variable, ASTHMA80. After this, we write ~1. This tells R not to stratify the results by any variable—we are just plotting "one" group. The default option on survfit is to output confidence intervals as well, but because these create problems when plotting the survival object, the option conf.type is set to "none" to tell R not to include confidence intervals in the object.

Next, we can run a summary on AllSurv. Below, the output is collapsed for brevity.

Code:

```
summary(AllSurv)
```

Output:

```
Call: survfit(formula = Surv(SurvAnalytic$TIME80,
  SurvAnalytic$ASTHMA80) ~ 1, conf.type = "none")

time n.risk n.event survival  std.err
  10 380957     688    0.998 6.88e-05
  11 380269      41    0.998 7.08e-05
  12 380228      53    0.998 7.33e-05
  13 380175      29    0.998 7.47e-05
  14 380146      22    0.998 7.57e-05
  15 380124      37    0.998 7.73e-05
  16 380087      22    0.998 7.83e-05
  17 380065      19    0.998 7.91e-05
  18 380046      26    0.998 8.03e-05
  19 377478      22    0.997 8.12e-05
  20 375073      39    0.997 8.29e-05

____________collapsed here ____________
  72  76039       6    0.994 1.60e-04
  73  69191       6    0.994 1.64e-04
  74  63083       2    0.994 1.66e-04
  75  57371       3    0.994 1.68e-04
  76  51676       4    0.994 1.73e-04
  77  46601       4    0.993 1.78e-04
  78  41698       4    0.993 1.84e-04
  80  32819       2    0.993 1.89e-04
```

This is a conditional probability table. This is the table we suppressed with NOTABLE back when using SAS PROC LIFETEST. Under the time column is a list of time intervals when events occurred, n.risk is the number at risk at the beginning of the time interval, and n.event is the number who had the event during the time interval. Under the survival column is the proportion who survived the event in that time period. This proportion is also called the survival probability.

Please observe that the proportion surviving, or survival probability, is higher at the end than 0.97, which is the prevalence of the event in the whole dataset. That is because survival in this table is calculated by interval, taking into account only the people who survived up to the beginning of the interval. Due to censoring as well as having events, people might survive to a particular time interval, but then leave the count in the next interval. For these reasons, from interval to interval, both the numerator and the denominator can change. Many feel that survival analysis therefore is a more honest picture of outcome incidence patterns when compared to overall period prevalence, which is why they prefer to use survival analysis regression rather than logistic regression if time-to-event variables are available [82]. As we found with our severe selection bias with the population of the ASTHMAGE variable, sometimes developing the time variable is too difficult, so we are left with only logistic regression as a choice. However, if time-to-event data that are thought to be valid are available, survival analysis should be considered.

In SAS, when we applied PROC LIFETEST to generate a Kaplan–Meier plot, we did not examine the survival probability table behind it first because we used NOTABLE. We just directly outputted the plot. In R, we need to make the conditional probability table first as part of making our survival object anyway, so we had an opportunity to examine it. This is the same table that SAS made behind the scenes before automatically outputting the Kaplan–Meier plot. In R, we will manually plot this survival object to create our Kaplan–Meier plot.

The code below plots AllSurv to a full screen size. A smaller version is shown in the insert in Figure 3.1a.

Code:

```
plot(AllSurv,
        xlab="Years",
        ylab="Survival Probability",
        firstx=10,
        ymin=0.98,
        col="darkorchid4",
        lwd=2,
        mark.time=FALSE)
text(55, 0.999, "Survival Experience in Entire Dataset")
```

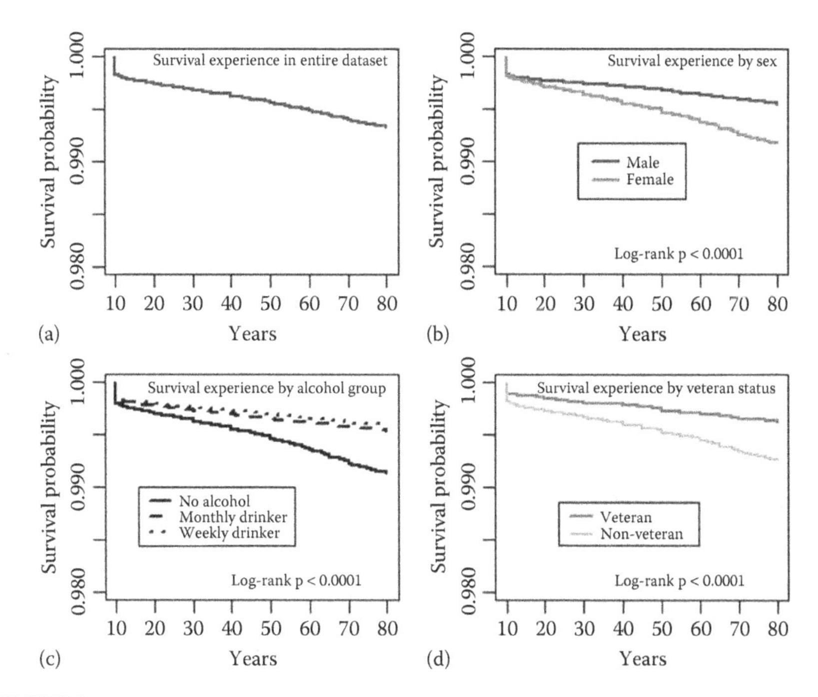

FIGURE 3.1
(See color insert.) Kaplan–Meier plots. (a) Survival experience in entire dataset. (b) Survival experience by sex. (c) Survival experience by alcohol group. (d) Survival experience by veteran status.

There is first a `plot` command, and it is followed by a `text` command to put a title on the plot. In the `plot` command, the first argument is our survival object, `AllSurv`. The options `xlab` and `ylab` place labels on the *x*- and *y*-axis. When we developed `ASTHMAGE2`, which is used in `TIME80` for those who got the event, we truncated the bottom at age 10 because of the way the variable was coded. Therefore, we want our "first x" to be 10, and we set `firstx=10`.

When we plotted the SAS Kaplan–Meier, it was hard to see any action because there were so few events in the dataset. We wanted to focus on the top of the survival curve by starting the *y*-axis higher, but it was not that easy to figure out in SAS. In R, we use the `ymin=` option. Because we observed that the lowest probability at the end of the conditional probability table was still greater than 0.99, to focus in on the action, we set the y minimum, or `ymin`, to 0.98. To make the survival line stand out, we set the color to a dark orchid and set the `lwd`, which stands for "line width," to 2. Up to now, we have been using `lwd=1`, the default, in plots. While the default `lwd=1` tends to work well for box plots and histograms, which plot distinct shapes, it is can be harder to see lines of `lwd=1` on a Kaplan–Meier or a time series plot. Therefore, we will increase the lwd in our plot to 2 to help the lines on the plot stand out. The 2 means it is "twice" as wide as 1, so 1.5 would be one-and-a-half times wide, and so on.

Finally, at the end of the plot command, we set the mark.time option to FALSE. This is because if we do not do that, R will automatically place a vertical mark at the intersection of every event and the survival curve (as we saw on SAS's default plot). This clutters up the plot, so we will turn it off by setting the option to FALSE.

After this, we add a title using a text command which is layered on top of the plot. The 55 says the x-coordinate to center the text around. You will see in the resulting plot that the text is centered around x=55. Next, 0.999 says the y-coordinate to center the text around, and you will see the text positioned as centered around y=0.999.

Next, as we did when generating Table 1s, we want to examine the bivariate relationship between our exposure, ALCGRP, and the survival experience of being diagnosed with asthma. This starts by graphing the survival experience of each group separately on the same Kaplan–Meier plot. In order to do this, we need to start by making a survival object that has these probabilities in it.

Code:

```
AlcSurv <- survfit(Surv(SurvAnalytic$TIME80, SurvAnalytic$
       ASTHMA80)~ SurvAnalytic$ALCGRP, conf.type="none")
```

This code makes the survival object AlcSurv. Notice that the difference between this and the code that made AllSurv is that the ~1 was replaced with the ALCGRP variable. This tells R to calculate stratified conditional probabilities by ALCGRP.

Now that we have this new survival object, we can plot it and compare the survival curves in each ALCGRP.

Code:

```
plot(AlcSurv,
        xlab="Years",
        ylab="Survival Probability",
        firstx=10,
        ymin=0.98,
        lty=1:3,
        lwd=2,
        mark.time=FALSE)
text(55, 0.999,
        "Survival Experience by Alcohol Group")
legend("center",
        c("No Alcohol", "Monthly Drinker", "Weekly Drinker"),
        lty=1:3,
        lwd=2)
```

The code above produces a full screen version of the plot; a smaller version is shown in the insert in Figure 3.1c. As we did with the previous plot, we start with referring to the survival object, AlcSurv, and setting the xlab, ylab, firstx, and ymin options. This time, rather than using color to make the lines distinctive, we will use "line types," or lty. This is appropriate for journals that discourage color figures. The default lty, which we have been using up to now, is 1 for solid line. There are a total of six line types, numbered 1 through 6, that produce different types of dashed and dotted lines. Here, we will set lty as 1:3, meaning we are telling R to use line types 1 (solid), 2, and 3 (two different dashed or dotted lines) to graph the three ALCGRP lines. Again, we set lwd to 2 to increase the line width, and we set mark.time to FALSE. As we did last time, in the next code line, we add our text with the plot title.

Because we were plotting the entire dataset in the last plot, we only had one line and did not need a legend. Now that we are plotting groups, we need to follow up the plot with a legend command. The first argument, "center," says where to place the legend and centers it on the plot. With our plot, putting a legend in the center works because most of the action is at the top of the plot. Other options are "topleft," "topright," "bottomleft," and "bottomright," as well as "top," "bottom," "left," and "right," which centers the legend on those edges.

The problem with using those options is that the border of the legend overlaps with the border of the plot, which may not be desired. Another approach is to set the x- and y-coordinates for the legend for the lower left-hand corner of the legend. Imagine we wanted the lower left corner of the legend to be placed at $x = 20$, $y = 0.985$. We would replace our previous legend code with this code:

Code:

```
legend(x=20,
        y=0.985,
        c("No Alcohol", "Monthly Drinker", "Weekly Drinker"),
        lty=1:3,
        lwd=2)
```

After the argument or arguments instructing R where to place the legend, the next argument in the legend command contains the labels associated with ALCGRP. These get labeled in the numerical order of ALCGRP; because 1 stands for "No Alcohol," it will come first in the list. The next two lines, setting the lty and lwd options in the legend, are very important. They must be copied exactly from the plot, or the legend will be mislabeled.

Viewing the resulting plot in Figure 3.1, it is interesting to notice that the "no alcohol" group apparently had a worse survival experience than the other two groups. While some may interpret this finding as a great reason to have a beer, it is most likely the result of unaddressed confounding, unfortunately. BRFSS is a cross-sectional dataset, and it is reasonable that a person diagnosed with asthma might stop drinking as a result, and that could cause this effect in the plot. In any case, there is a lot of selection bias, and the absolute difference in probabilities is miniscule, so this plot must be taken with a grain of salt.

To demonstrate another stratified plot, let us consider the asthma diagnosis survival experience by sex. The following code produces a full-screen version of the plot; a smaller version is shown in Figure 3.1b. It starts with remaking the survival object stratified by sex, called `SexSurv`, and then plots the object.

Code:

```
SexSurv <- survfit(Surv(SurvAnalytic$TIME80,
     SurvAnalytic$ASTHMA80)~ SurvAnalytic$SEX, conf.type="none")
plot(SexSurv,
       xlab="Years",
       ylab="Survival Probability",
       firstx=10,
       ymin=0.98,
       col=c("brown4","brown1"),
       lwd=2,
       mark.time=FALSE)
text(55, 0.999,
          "Survival Experience by Sex")
legend("center",
       c("Male","Female"),
       col=c("brown4","brown1"),
       lwd=2)
```

The main difference between this code and the code that plotted `AlcSurv` is that the lines are distinguished by color, not line type. In this plot command, we do not set line type as we did when plotting `AlcSurv`. Instead, we include the color command with `col=` and then list the colors. Like with line type, R will graph `SEX` in numerical order, and because 1=Male and 2=Female, the first color will plot males and the second females.

Please also notice that these edits that reformat the lines have been reflected in the `legend` command as well. Like with setting line types, if the analyst sets colors in a plot, she needs to make sure that the legend matches, or the plot will be mislabeled.

This plot shows that females appear to have "worse" survival curve than males, meaning that they were diagnosed earlier with asthma than males. All kinds of philosophical arguments could be thrown at this, but the likely reason is that women have been found to be more likely at all ages to engage the healthcare system than men. If a person engages the healthcare system, then the person has a much higher probability of being diagnosed with asthma if the person has it. Again, confounding is probably responsible for this difference.

But are these curves statistically significantly different? There are tests that can be run to answer this question, which will be covered in the next part of the section.

Bivariate Tests of Survival Curves

Several tests of survival curves have been developed. Two that are commonly used are the log-rank test and the generalized Wilcoxon test (also known as the Gehen/Breslow test) [83]. When we ran PROC LIFETEST in SAS to compare alcohol groups with respect to time-to-asthma diagnosis, we mentioned that the last table output was called Test of Equality over Strata. Let us revisit this table here.

We will focus on the log–rank and Wilcoxon tests, both reporting *p*-values less than 0.0001. What this means is that even though we had very few events in this whole dataset, when stratifying the survival experience by alcohol group, there was a statistically significant difference between survival experiences. Again, this finding is to be taken with a grain of salt, mainly because this is a bivariate analysis and has not been controlled for confounders.

As demonstrated with Table 3.17, SAS outputs the log–rank and Wilcoxon tests as part of PROC LIFETEST. In R, we obtain our bivariate test statistics from running the `survdiff` function on a formula that defines a survival object. Recall that we developed the survival object `AlcSurv` by using a formula in the `survfit` command. Now, we will use that same formula in the `survdiff` command.

Code:

```
survdiff(Surv(SurvAnalytic$TIME80, SurvAnalytic$ASTHMA80)~
    SurvAnalytic$ALCGRP, rho=0)
```

Output:

```
Call:
survdiff(formula = Surv(SurvAnalytic$TIME80, SurvAnalytic$ASTHMA80) ~
    SurvAnalytic$ALCGRP, rho = 0)

                          N Observed Expected (O-E)^2/E (O-E)^2/V
SurvAnalytic$ALCGRP=1 187334     1194      951      62.1     126.8
SurvAnalytic$ALCGRP=2 140377      506      664      37.7      58.6
SurvAnalytic$ALCGRP=3  53246      172      257      28.0      32.5

Chisq= 128 on 2 degrees of freedom, p= 0
```

TABLE 3.17

SAS Table from LIFETEST: Comparison of Time-to-Asthma Diagnosis among Alcohol Groups

Test of Equality over Strata			
Test	**Chi-Square**	**DF**	**Pr > Chi-Square**
Log–rank	128.3614	2	<0.0001
Wilcoxon	96.0477	2	<0.0001
–2 log(LR)	125.4335	2	<0.0001

Please also note the option `rho = 0` in the code. This indicates we are requesting a log–rank test. Note that R's log–rank test results agree with the ones from SAS, with the p-value reported at the bottom of the output as effectively 0.

To request a Wilcoxon, we will rewrite the same code, only this time, setting `rho = 1`.

Code:

```
survdiff(Surv(SurvAnalytic$TIME80, SurvAnalytic$ASTHMA80)~
    SurvAnalytic$ALCGRP, rho=1)
```

Output:

```
Call:
survdiff(formula = Surv(SurvAnalytic$TIME80,
    SurvAnalytic$ASTHMA80) ~ SurvAnalytic$ALCGRP, rho = 1)

                             N Observed Expected (O-E)^2/E (O-E)^2/V
SurvAnalytic$ALCGRP=1 187334     1191      949      61.9     126.6
SurvAnalytic$ALCGRP=2 140377      505      663      37.5      58.4
SurvAnalytic$ALCGRP=3 53246       172      256      27.9      32.5

Chisq= 128 on 2 degrees of freedom, p= 0
```

R's Wilcoxon test produces a p-value that is effectively 0, agreeing with SAS's Wilcoxon test.

A final step in our descriptive survival analysis might be to assemble the results of our descriptive analyses into a series of plots. The following code creates four Kaplan–Meier plots in a matrix: one for the dataset overall and one each for the survival curves stratified by `ALCGRP`, `SEX`, and `VETERAN3`. The results of the log–rank test are added as text on the plots (code for log–rank tests not shown).

Code:

```
##4 plots together

par(mfrow=c(1,1))
layout(matrix(c(1,2,3,4),2,2))

##Overall

plot(AllSurv,
        xlab="Years",
        ylab="Survival Probability",
        firstx=10,
        ymin=0.98,
        col="darkorchid4",
        lwd=2,
        mark.time=FALSE)
```

```
text(55, 0.999,
       "Survival Experience in\n Entire Dataset",
       cex=.75)

##by AlcGrp

AlcSurv <- survfit(Surv(SurvAnalytic$TIME80,
        SurvAnalytic$ ASTHMA80)~ SurvAnalytic$ALCGRP,
        conf.type="none")
plot(AlcSurv,
       xlab="Years",
       ylab="Survival Probability",
       firstx=10,
       ymin=0.98,
       lty=1:3,
       lwd=2,
       mark.time=FALSE)
text(55, 0.999,
       "Survival Experience by Alcohol Group",
       cex=.6)
legend("center",
       c("No Alcohol", "Monthly Drinker", "Weekly Drinker"),
       lty=1:3,
       lwd=2,
       cex=.6)
text(55, 0.981,
       "Log-Rank p<0.0001",
       cex=.6)

##by Sex

SexSurv <- survfit(Surv(SurvAnalytic$TIME80,
        SurvAnalytic$ ASTHMA80)~ SurvAnalytic$SEX,
        conf.type="none")
plot(SexSurv,
       xlab="Years",
       ylab="Survival Probability",
       firstx=10,
       ymin=0.98,
       col=c("brown4","brown1"),
       lwd=2,
       mark.time=FALSE)
text(55, 0.999,
       "Survival Experience by Sex",
       cex=0.75)
legend("center",
       c("Male","Female"),
       col=c("brown4","brown1"),
```

```
        lwd=2,
        cex=0.75)
text(55, 0.981,
        "Log-Rank p<0.0001",
        cex=0.75)

##by Veteran Status

VetSurv <- survfit(Surv(SurvAnalytic$TIME80,
         SurvAnalytic$ ASTHMA80)~ SurvAnalytic$VETERAN3,
         conf.type="none")
plot(VetSurv,
       xlab="Years",
       ylab="Survival Probability",
       firstx=10,
       ymin=0.98,
       col=c("chartreuse4","darkkhaki"),
       lwd=2,
       mark.time=FALSE)
text(55, 0.9995,
       "Survival Experience by \nVeteran Status",
       cex=.5)
legend("center",
       c("Veteran","Non-Veteran"),
       col=c("chartreuse4","darkkhaki"),
       lwd=2,
       cex=.6)
text(55, 0.981,
       "Log-Rank p<0.0001",
       cex=.6)
```

This plot is shown in Figure 3.1. Please observe some features in the code that were used to adjust the plot presentation when put in a matrix. First, notice that some of the title lines are now broken with `\n` to put them on separate lines. Next, notice that the `cex` option is set in `text` commands and the `legend` command. Remember that `cex` scales the item, so when `cex = .6` in a legend, it tells R to make the legend only 60% of its default size. This option was used to adjust text and the legend so that they did not interfere with the clarity of the plot.

To conclude this chapter, the first section reviewed how SAS is used to develop descriptive analyses with a categorical dependent variable and then showed how to use R for the same task. The second section reviewed using SAS to create a descriptive analysis with a continuous dependent variable and then demonstrated how to accomplish the same task in R. The third section explained descriptive survival analysis approaches used in SAS, and demonstrated comparable approaches in R, thus completing our descriptive analysis.

Now that we have completed our descriptive analysis to inform our understanding of relationships in our datasets, we can move on to regression in the next chapter.

Optional Exercises

Section "Making 'Table 1'—Categorical Outcome"

Questions

1. Using R's `table` and `prop.table` commands, using the analytic file, run a crosstab between `ALCGRP` and `SEX` and output row percentages.
2. Using R and building on `Table1Cat`, add the next set of entries after Alcohol Status using `SEX` as the categorical stratification variable.

Answers

1. Possible answer:

   Code:

   ```
   SexAlcFreq <- table(analytic$SEX, analytic$ALCGRP)
   prop.table(SexAlcFreq, 1)
   ```

   Output:

   ```
               1         2         3
     1 0.4458855 0.3897793 0.1643352
     2 0.4941860 0.3874031 0.1184109
   ```

2. Possible answer:

   Code:

   ```
   SexFreq <- table(analytic$SEX, analytic$ASTHMA4)

   Category <- c("Sex", "")
   Level <- c("Male", "Female")
   TotalN <- c("","")
   TotalProp <- c("","")
   HasAsthmaN <- SexFreq[,2]
   HasAsthmaProp <- c("","")
   NoAsthmaN <- SexFreq[,1]
   NoAsthmaProp <- c("","")

   SexTbl <- as.data.frame(cbind(Category, Level, TotalN,
          TotalProp, HasAsthmaN, HasAsthmaProp, NoAsthmaN,
          NoAsthmaProp))

   SexTbl$TotalN <- HasAsthmaN + NoAsthmaN
   SexTbl$TotalProp <- SexTbl$TotalN/TotalObs
   SexTbl$HasAsthmaProp <- SexFreq[,2]/TotalAsthma
   SexTbl$NoAsthmaProp <- SexFreq[,1]/TotalNoAsthma

   Table1Cat <- rbind(Table1Cat, SexTbl)
   ```

Output:

```
         Category            Level TotalN  TotalProp HasAsthmaN HasAsthmaProp
1             All              All  58131 1.00000000       5343    0.09191309
11 Alcohol Status       Nondrinker  26169 0.45017289       2671    0.49990642
2              Monthly Drinker  22646 0.38956839       1897    0.35504398
3               Weekly Drinker   9316 0.16025873        775    0.14504960
12            Sex             Male  52971 0.91123497       4555    0.85251731
21                          Female   5160 0.08876503        788    0.14748269
   NoAsthmaN  NoAsthmaProp
1      52788    0.90808691
11     23498    0.44513905
2      20749    0.39306282
3       8541    0.16179814
12     48416    0.91717815
21      4372    0.08282185
```

Section "Making 'Table 1'—Continuous Outcome"

Questions

1. Using R, copy dataset `BRFSS_a` into a file called `BRFSS_example3`. Using this file, use the `summary` command to find the mean and median of age (`X_AGE80`).
2. Using R and dataset `BRFSS_example 3`, use the `aggregate` command to find the mean ages (`X_AGE80`) by veteran status (`VETERAN3`).
3. Using R and dataset `BRFSS_example 3`, calculate the standard deviation of age (`X_AGE80`).
4. Using R and dataset `BRFSS_example 3`, use the `aggregate` command to find the standard deviation of ages (`X_AGE80`) by veteran status (`VETERAN3`).
5. Using R and the analytic file, add the next set of rows for asthma status (`ASTHMA4`) to `Table1Cont`.
6. Using R and the dataset `BRFSS_example 3`, *t*-test the mean of age (`X_AGE80`) by sex (`SEX`).
7. Using R and the dataset `BRFSS_example3`, run a one-way ANOVA with age (`X_AGE80`) as the dependent variable and veteran status (`VETERAN3`) as the factor.

Answers

1. Answer:

   Code:

```
BRFSS_example3 <- BRFSS_a
summary(BRFSS_example3$X_AGE80)
```

Output:

```
 Min. 1st Qu.  Median    Mean 3rd Qu.    Max.
18.00   44.00   58.00   55.49   69.00   80.00
```

2. Answer:

   Code:

```
aggregate(BRFSS_example3$X_AGE80,
     list(BRFSS_example3$VETERAN3), mean)
```

   Output:

```
  Group.1        x
1       1 63.52864
2       2 54.25074
3       7 58.36000
4       9 53.96939
```

3. Answer:

   Code:

```
sd(BRFSS_example3$X_AGE80)
```

   Output:

```
[1] 16.85709
```

4. Answer:

   Code:

```
aggregate(BRFSS_example3$X_AGE80,
     list(BRFSS_example3$VETERAN3), sd)
```

   Output:

```
  Group.1        x
1       1 14.62773
2       2 16.83744
3       7 16.38275
4       9 14.25256
```

5. Possible answer:

   Code:

```
AsthmaFreq <- as.data.frame(table(analytic$ASTHMA4))
AsthmaMeans <- as.data.frame(aggregate(analytic$SLEPTIM2,
     by=list(analytic$ASTHMA4), mean))
AsthmaSDs <- as.data.frame(aggregate(analytic$SLEPTIM2,
     by=list(analytic$ASTHMA4), sd))
```

```
Category <- c("Asthma Status", "")
Level <- c("No Asthma", "Has Asthma")
TotalN <- AsthmaFreq[,2]
TotalProp <- AsthmaFreq[,2]/TotalObs
SleepMean <- AsthmaMeans[,2]
SleepSD <- AsthmaSDs[,2]

AsthmaTbl <- as.data.frame(cbind(Category, Level, TotalN,
          TotalProp, SleepMean, SleepSD))

Table1Cont <- rbind(Table1Cont, AsthmaTbl)
Table1Cont
```

Output:

```
        Category            Level TotalN           TotalProp          SleepMean
1            All              All  58131                   1   7.1157557929504
2 Alcohol Status       Nondrinker  26169   0.450172885379574  7.12610340479193
3                 Monthly Drinker  22646   0.389568388639452  7.09025876534487
4                  Weekly Drinker   9316   0.160258725980974  7.14866895663375
5  Asthma Status        No Asthma  52788   0.908086907157971  7.12934757899523
6                      Has Asthma   5343 0.0919130928420292  6.98147108366086
           SleepSD
1 1.46860065254059
2 1.59387128199415
3 1.37526185039389
4 1.31219530604596
5 1.43226803362089
6 1.78291979688152
```

6. Answer:

   Code:

```
t.test(BRFSS_example3$X_AGE80 ~ BRFSS_example3$SEX)
```

   Output:

```
        Welch Two Sample t-test

data: BRFSS_example3$X_AGE80 by BRFSS_example3$SEX
t = -47.722, df = 411150, p-value < 2.2e-16
alternative hypothesis: true difference in means is not
    equal to 0
95 percent confidence interval:
-2.494430 -2.297619
sample estimates:
mean in group 1 mean in group 2
       54.09056        56.48659
```

7. Possible answer:

   Code:

```
VetANOVA <- lm(formula = X_AGE80 ~ as.factor(VETERAN3),
     data = BRFSS_example3)
summary(VetANOVA)
```

   Output:

```
Call:
lm(formula = X_AGE80 ~ as.factor(VETERAN3), data =
     BRFSS_example3)


Residuals:
    Min      1Q  Median      3Q     Max
-45.529 -11.529   2.471  12.749  26.031


Coefficients:

                     Estimate Std. Error  t value  Pr(>|t|)
(Intercept)          63.52864    0.06643  956.313   < 2e-16 ***
as.factor(VETERAN3)2 -9.27790    0.07138 -129.971   < 2e-16 ***
as.factor(VETERAN3)7 -5.16864    1.65704   -3.119   0.00181 **
as.factor(VETERAN3)9 -9.55925    0.96791   -9.876   < 2e-16 ***
---
Signif. codes: 0 '***' 0.001 '**' 0.01 '*' 0.05 '.' 0.1 ' ' 1

Residual standard error: 16.56 on 464071 degrees of freedom
  (589 observations deleted due to missingness)
Multiple R-squared: 0.03513, Adjusted R-squared: 0.03513
F-statistic: 5633 on 3 and 464071 DF, p-value: < 2.2e-16
```

Section "Descriptive Analysis of Survival Data"

Questions

1. Using the `SurvAnalytic` dataset in R, develop conditional probability tables and Kaplan–Meier plots for the variables `TIME50` and `ASTHMA50`, overall and stratified by `ALCGRP`. Optionally, change colors, line type, line width, and other formatting to improve readability.
2. Compare the plots resulting from question 1 to the ones demonstrated in the Descriptive Analysis of Survival Data section using

`TIME80` and `ASTHMA80`. What are the differences between the plots (aside from the options you changed)?

3. Using R, conduct a log–rank test on the difference in survival experience between each `ALCGRP` using `TIME50` and `ASTHMA50`.

Answers

1. Possible answer:

   Code:

```
library(survival)

AllSurv <- survfit(Surv(SurvAnalytic$TIME50,
        SurvAnalytic$ASTHMA50)~ 1, conf.type="none")
AlcSurv <- survfit(Surv(SurvAnalytic$TIME50,
        SurvAnalytic$ASTHMA50)~ SurvAnalytic$ALCGRP,
        conf.type="none")

par(mfrow=c(1,1))

plot(AllSurv,
        xlab="Years",
        ylab="Survival Probability",
        firstx=10,
        ymin=0.98,
        col="aquamarine4",
        lty=2,
        lwd=2,
        mark.time=FALSE)
text(35, 0.999, "Survival Experience in Entire Dataset")

plot(AlcSurv,
        xlab="Years",
        ylab="Survival Probability",
        firstx=10,
        ymin=0.98,
        col=rainbow(3),
        lty=4:6,
        lwd=2,
        mark.time=FALSE)
text(35, 0.999,
        "Survival Experience by Alcohol Group")
legend("center",
        c("No Alcohol", "Monthly Drinker", "Weekly
              Drinker"),
        col=rainbow(3),
        lty=4:6,
        lwd=2)
```

   Output not shown.

2. The survival curves look the same as with TIME80 and ASTHMA80, but end at age 50 instead of age 80, as shown on the x-axis.
3. Possible answer:

   Code:

```
survdiff(Surv(SurvAnalytic$TIME50, SurvAnalytic$ASTHMA50)~
    SurvAnalytic$ALCGRP, rho=0)
```

   Output:

```
Call:
survdiff(formula = Surv(SurvAnalytic$TIME50,
    SurvAnalytic$ASTHMA50) ~ SurvAnalytic$ALCGRP, rho = 0)

                           N Observed Expected (O-E)^2/E (O-E)^2/V
SurvAnalytic$ALCGRP=1 187334      956      782      38.8      77.1
SurvAnalytic$ALCGRP=2 140377      462      574      21.7      34.1
SurvAnalytic$ALCGRP=3  53246      157      220      17.9      20.8

Chisq= 78.4 on 2 degrees of freedom, p= 0
```

4

Basic Regression Analysis

In health science analytics, we often use SAS to develop linear, logistic, and survival analysis regression models [84]. These tasks can also be performed in R, and the popularity of analyzing health-related data in R is currently growing [85]. The first section in this chapter will explain the choices the authors made about what approach to regression modeling we will demonstrate in this book. A short review of how SAS linear regression is performed with health data will be provided in the second section, along with an explanation of how to perform the same linear regression tasks in R. In the third section, logistic regression in SAS will be reviewed, along with how to perform comparable operations in R. The fourth section will discuss survival analysis regression. Tasks in survival analysis performed in SAS will also be shown in R. Finally, the chapter will conclude with a section on SAS macros and their analog in R.

This Book's Approach

This section acknowledges there are different approaches to developing regression models to answer prespecified hypotheses. This section first explains the modeling approach we chose to demonstrate in this book, and the rationale for selecting it. Next, it explains why we chose to demonstrate a manual (rather than automated) development of regression models. Third, we describe how we will operationalize the modeling approach we demonstrate later when developing final models. The section will conclude by discussing how this book deals with philosophical issues associated with prespecifying hypotheses before modeling, and avoiding fishing.

Selection of Modeling Approach

This part of the section will present the rationale behind the selection of the modeling process we will demonstrate in this book. In the example scenario, two hypotheses were proposed: one associating the independent variable alcohol consumption with the dependent variable of asthma status, and the second associating the independent variable alcohol consumption with the dependent variable average sleep duration. Hence, it is first necessary to recognize that the purpose of the regression tasks to be demonstrated in this book is to show how to answer hypotheses such as these (hypothesis-driven analysis) and not to simply build a predictive model (exploratory analysis) [86].

Second, it is necessary to recognize that regardless of whether the analyst is building a regression model with or without a hypothesis, there are several ways to approach a model-fitting or model-building strategy. Unfortunately, names and exact definitions of different modeling approaches are not uniform across the healthcare analytics field. This makes it hard to be clear when discussing modeling processes as we will in this book.

Some published papers can give us guidance on terminology we can use to improve our clarity to the reader. Bursac and colleagues performed an interesting simulation to compare several different model-building approaches when conducting an exploratory analysis [52]. This team classified three different approaches as "forward selection" (FS), "backward elimination" (BE), and "stepwise selection" (SS). The authors defined FS as evaluating the chi-square statistic for each independent variable (covariate) in the model after adding it to a model being built, and if the p-value on that covariate was statistically significant, it was kept in the model through all future iterations of model-building [52].

Operationally, in FS, the analyst starts with a blank model, and adds in covariates one at a time in each iteration, making a decision as to whether to retain or drop the new covariate for the next iteration. If the choice is to retain it, it is then retained through the entire modeling process. In contrast, BE is described as starting with a model that includes all proposed covariates, then examining the Wald test for each covariate, and removing the least significant covariate that does not meet the criteria for being retained in the model (e.g., does not have a p-value of 0.05 or less, if $\alpha = 0.05$ is chosen) [52]. Operationally, in BE, after running the first model including all possible independent variables, in each subsequent iteration, the analyst makes the decision as to which covariate to remove, and stops when all the remaining covariates meet the criteria for being retained in the model.

The authors define SS as similar to FS, except that the covariates already in the model do not necessarily need to remain there [52]. They can be removed in later iterations in modeling if they cease to significantly contribute to the model, so there can be an alternation in subsequent iterations between adding covariates to the model, as in FS, and in removing covariates from the model, as in BE [52]. The process of SS terminates when (1) no additional covariate can be added to the model that can meet the criteria to be kept in the model and (2) the last covariate removed from the model was removed due to BE [52].

In two of the simulation studies the authors presented in their article, they designed their analysis to have a binary outcome as the dependent variable and six covariates for potential inclusion in the final model as independent variables [52]. They generated datasets following a logistic regression equation where they purposefully designed the relative impact of these six covariates; this enabled them to set the gold standard or "correct" model [52]. Next, they programmed an automated process to develop models using the same six covariates using either SS, BE, or FS as they defined these processes (described above) [52].

To roughly summarize the results, the authors found that, in 1,000 simulations at the largest sample size they tested (n = 600), the SS and BE processes formed the correct model approximately 70% of the time and FS greatly underperformed and reached the correct model only about 40% of the time [52]. We believe the reason that FS underperformed is that a covariate, once entered and kept in the model, could not be removed from it after other covariates were added, thus limiting the ability to fit the model.

In another article about modeling, Steyerberg and colleagues used different nomenclature, listing several different stepwise approaches, including "forward stepwise," "backward stepwise," and "combined forward-backward stepwise" [87]. "Forward stepwise" in their article means the same thing as FS from the Bursac et al.'s article, "backward stepwise" means the same thing as BE, and "combined forward-backward stepwise" means the same thing as SS. This book will continue to use the terms FS, BE, and SS from the Bursac et al.'s article to refer to these modeling approaches.

With this guidance from the Bursac et al.'s article, we will choose not to demonstrate the FS process as defined by these authors because it underperformed in their analysis. This left us the choice between demonstrating a BE or SS modeling process. We chose to present the demonstration using SS for two reasons. First, it is logistically more effort-intensive to start with all possible covariates in a model and carefully remove the least significant one in each iteration. In our experience, if there is significant collinearity between any of the covariates, they will generate an error when being used together in a model that is already full of other covariates. The risk of this is high in a BE process because the first step is to include all potential covariates in the model. Second, because SS and BE processes can arrive at a similar (or even identical) model, there is no penalty in choosing to demonstrate the SS process rather than the BE process. Further, we have found it easier to understand the model once it is built using the SS process because each introduction of a new covariate in the model can shed light on which covariates may be collinear by changing the behavior of the other covariates in the model.

Selection of Manual Approach

Although Bursac's team approached their simulation using automated processes, these are not uniformly accepted in the statistical community [88,89]. One reason for this is that when the process becomes automated, the analyst is not able to easily direct the software on how to make choices about the optimal format of each covariate to model. As demonstrated in Chapter 2, the continuous variable `ASTHMAGE`, or age at diagnosis of asthma, can be recoded into an ordinal variable as well as a set of indicator variables. If the intention was to include age of asthma diagnosis as an independent variable in our model, decisions would have to be made as to the "correct" way to format this measurement and introduce it into our model, and automating these decisions is not only difficult but open to criticism.

In 1992, David P. Nichols, who worked at SPSS, wrote in a letter of response to an article which included the discussion of automating the introduction of indicator variables into a logistic regression modeling process [89]. Nichols suggested that "software designed to do stepwise regression procedures without explicit facilities for handling categorical regressors is incapable of treating multiple variables as pieces of the same variable without help from the user" [88]. He went on to observe, "This means there is no safe way to automatically perform a stepwise regression analysis" without manually specifying each model in the iterations [88].

Although statistical software capabilities have improved drastically since 1992, and these challenges of choosing the "correct" way to format a measurement for a regression model could likely be solved with advanced programming approaches in SAS, R, or SPSS today, there are still practical reasons to use manual approaches to fitting models. First, they do not involve advanced programming, and second, as Nichols also points out in his letter, it is easy for the programmer to specify the coding of contrasts (choosing which numeric values refer to which categories) [88]. For these reasons, this book will demonstrate a manual model-fitting process.

Operationalizing the Stepwise Selection Process

This book demonstrates how to answer two hypotheses using regression models using the SS approach. Given this intention, this book will operationalize the process this way. First, an outcome, a hypothesized exposure, and a set of potential confounding variables are identified. These are placed in the analytic file we developed in Chapter 2. Next, the SS modeling approach will be applied to develop a final model, and the covariates for the exposure in the final model will be interpreted to answer our hypothesis. Developing and interpreting the final models will be done in this chapter.

The actual process of SS modeling to arrive at a final model will be conducted in two rounds. In both of these rounds, at least one covariate for the exposure will be retained in every iteration of the model, even if it does not meet the criteria to be kept. This is because this is a hypothesis-driven analysis, and a measure of statistical significance of the exposure covariates will need to reside in the final model for interpretation. If the exposure covariates are not statistically significant in the final model, then the hypothesis will be considered not supported (i.e., we will fail to reject the null hypothesis). Conversely, if they are significant, the results of the model will support the hypothesis (i.e., we will reject the null hypothesis).

Also in both modeling rounds, after each iteration, potential confounding covariates that meet the criteria for being kept will be retained in the model, and those that do not meet the criteria for being retained will be discarded, which is consistent with the description of the SS process. The criteria for potential confounding variables being retained in this model in this demonstration are: (1) the covariate's parameter estimate must be associated with a *p*-value < 0.05, or (2) there is an empirical reason to retain the covariate in the model (e.g., the analyst believes from prior experience it should be there).

As mentioned earlier, the SS modeling process will be operationalized into two rounds. In the first round of SS modeling, potential confounding covariates will be tried in the model in the same order they are presented in Table 1. Once all have been tried, those retained in the model will comprise what this book will call the "working model." The second SS round is to "break" the working model. In this round, each discarded covariate is tried again in the model. As with round 1, after each iteration, covariates that do not meet the criteria to be retained are removed. At the end of round 2, the resulting model will be considered the "final model."

The SS process demonstrated in this book will generate many iterations of each regression model. We recommend keeping metadata about these various models because it can make final model selection more informed. Keeping metadata about models will also be demonstrated in this book.

Prespecifying Hypotheses and Avoiding Fishing

In the scientific method, hypotheses must be specified before analyzing the data for them to be considered *a priori,* and only then should the data be loaded into software for analysis. But simply stating a hypothesis before fitting a regression on a dataset with a large number of potential variables might not be good enough to honestly avoid fishing (or at least, the appearance of fishing), which is unethical. Newer terms such as "p-hacking" and "researcher degrees of freedom" have been used to describe what can happen if a hypothesis is declared without much model or data specification, and then a regression model is fit that discards covariates on the basis of their *p*-values and personal opinions of what belongs in the model [90]. Although there is general agreement that these situations should be avoided, the actual line between fitting a model using an SS process and fishing or p-hacking has not been drawn.

How this book will approach this subject is by making the following assumptions. First, the assumption is that using the BRFSS documentation as a guide for selecting variables to include in the analytic dataset is not considered fishing. Working to operationalize the exposure, outcome, and candidate confounders during the process of refining the hypothesis is necessary as a practical matter when analyzing a dataset that has already been collected. If the hypothesis cannot be operationalized to the dataset, then the dataset cannot be used to answer the hypothesis.

A second assumption this book makes is that we are avoiding fishing with respect to the potential confounders because we chose them prior to conducting any analysis. It assumes that by limiting the universe of variables to consider in the model to only hypothesized confounders, we are avoiding fishing. We chose our confounding variables based on the scientific literature and our experiences, and before examining the data (e.g., doing a descriptive analysis).

In Bursac et al.'s article, the authors ran another simulation to develop an exploratory model using the Worcester Heart Attack Study (WHAS) dataset in their example [52]. In their demonstration, they chose 11 covariates as potential independent variables, and a binary dependent variable (vital status: dead or alive) [52]. The authors declined to explain exactly how they chose the 11 covariates to test in the model, but it is reasonable to assume they selected them because they felt the variables in their dataset were potentially confounding [52]. Because this pattern has been standard in the literature, it is hard to argue that our selection of candidate covariates prior to modeling is an example of "researcher degrees of freedom." It seems less logical to include covariates in the analytic dataset that we do not think are confounders in the relationship between the exposure and the outcome.

A third assumption we are making is that including indicator variables for grouping variables in a model independently (meaning without the other indicator variables in the group) when developing a final model is also not fishing or exercising "researcher degrees of freedom." The main debate here is whether or not combining a non-significant level of a grouping variable in with the reference group constitutes fishing. There are opinions on either side of this issue [88,89].

We argue that the problems registered with this assumption are a moot point with large datasets. Imagine a final model developed through SS, which retains only two of the six age indicator variables. By way of the SS process and how we arrived at the final model, adding back non-significant age indicator variables would not improve the model, as they would still not be significant. Therefore, those who do not agree with adding and removing indicator variables for group variables independently in models can simply add back the nonsignificant ones to the final model before presenting it to address this issue.

A final assumption behind our modeling demonstration is that using "empirical reason" to retain a covariate in a model is also not fishing and does not constitute "researcher degrees of freedom." We defend this choice because we are modeling health data, and which can include a lot of human-introduced measurement error as well as other types of biases. Those who believe that we are essentially making an excuse for us to enter our own biases into modeling process will recall Bursac et al.'s paper, wherein the correct model was developed 70% using the SS process [52]. As with the third assumption, at the end of SS modeling, by definition of the SS process, if we try to reintroduce covariates we have already tried that are not already statistically significant, they will still not be statistically significant. They can be included in the final model presentation if the analyst chooses, but we will not be doing that in this book.

To conclude this section, we started by explaining that we are selecting to demonstrate a manual SS modeling approach, and the reasons for using that approach. Next, we described how we will operationalize this approach to SS regression modeling in this book in two defined rounds. Finally, we acknowledged assumptions we made with respect to prespecifying hypotheses *a priori* and laid out the steps we took to avoid fishing, p-hacking, or researcher degrees of freedom. We also acknowledged that other researchers may see it differently, in which case, they are welcome to include different sets of covariates in their final models.

With this introduction complete, we will move on to the next section to demonstrate linear regression and ANOVA.

Linear Regression and ANOVA

We begin this section with a reminder of our linear regression hypothesis, which is that among veterans, after controlling for confounders, alcohol consumption is associated with sleep duration (`SLEPTIM2`). We have been using grouping variable `ALCGRP` up to this point, but in the regression, we will use the indicator variables `DRKMONTHLY` and `DRKWEEKLY` so we can develop independent slopes for each level compared to nondrinkers.

This section will go over the process of preparing to do a linear regression in both SAS and R, and then will walk the reader through one potential process of SS modeling in SAS and R. The section will end with a discussion of linear regression model fit and model presentation.

Preparing to Run Linear Regression

Before running linear regression in any software package, certain considerations are usually made. Typically, a linear regression model with just the hypothesized exposure, called the crude or unadjusted model, is run, and this is used to test for meeting the assumptions behind linear regression. If the unadjusted model does not meet them, different approaches can be taken to "fix" the dependent variable, such as running it through a mathematical operation (e.g., logarithm), calculating an index, or choosing to make it categorical and therefore possibly choosing another type of regression (e.g., logistic). Some of these are demonstrated in Chapter 2.

In SAS, a typical approach to visualizing the dependent variable alone to assess whether or not it meets the linearity assumption is to run `PROC UNIVARIATE` on the dependent variable and request the options "`normal plot`." These options will output not only the summary statistics we expect with `PROC UNIVARIATE` but also a histogram, box plot, and QQ plot of the dependent variable. In Chapter 2, we did this in SAS to produce those plots, and we also used R to develop box plots, histograms, and a QQ plot.

However, to evaluate the assumption of homoscedasticity, we need to run the unadjusted linear regression model, then plot the residuals and evaluate the plot for potential heteroscedasticity. In SAS, this can be done using `PROC REG`.

The model statement is similar to the one used in PROC GLM. We will follow the PROC REG command with a request for SAS to plot the residuals.

Code:

```
proc reg data = r.analytic;
  model SLEPTIM2 = DRKMONTHLY DRKWEEKLY;
plot r.*p.;
run;
```

Plots:

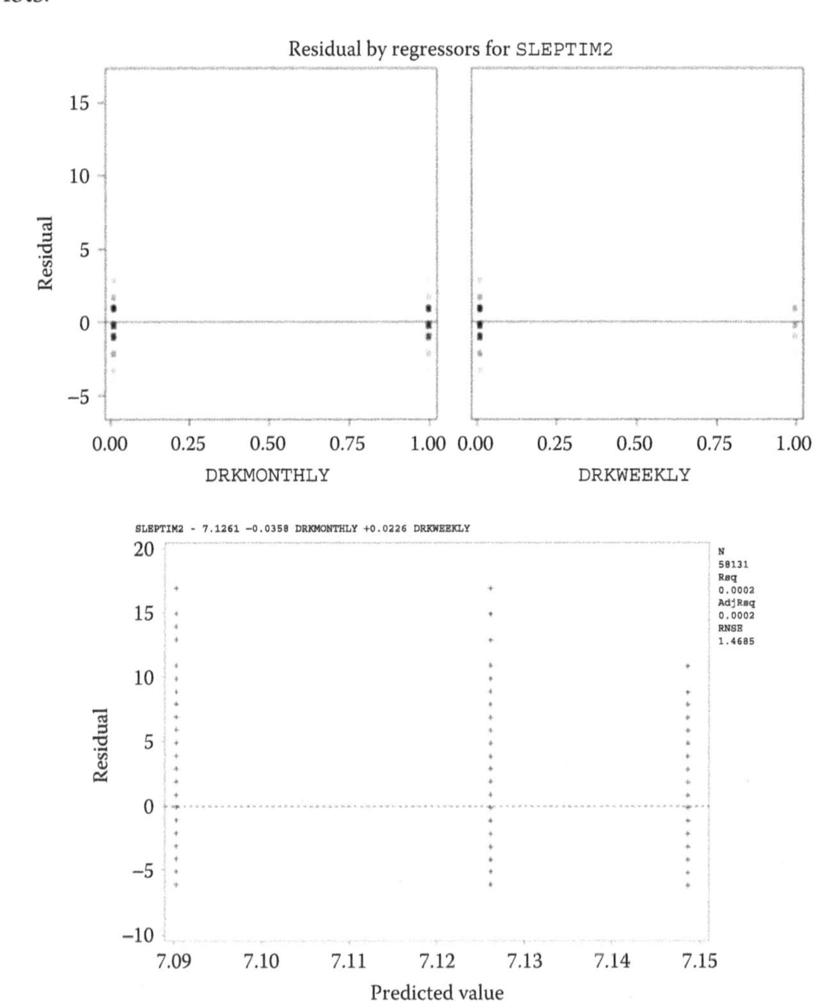

This code produces two plots that are helpful in evaluating heteroscedasticity, but R's defaults provide a better picture. In R, we will use the lm (linear modeling) function we used in Chapter 3 for ANOVAs to create a regression object. We will use the same code as before, but instead of using `ALCGRP`, the grouping variable, we will use `DRKMONTHLY` and `DRKWEEKLY`, the indicator variables. We will call the regression `AlcSleepTimeRegression`.

Code:

```
AlcSleepTimeRegression = lm(SLEPTIM2 ~ DRKMONTHLY + DRKWEEKLY,
data=analytic)
```

Notice that the two variables are separated by a plus. In the next step, we will plot this regression object, but because four default plots come out, we will format them four on a page.

Code:

```
layout(matrix(c(1,2,3,4),2,2))
plot(AlcSleepTimeRegression,
       main = "Alcohol by Sleep Duration")
```

These plots are Figure 4.1 in the color insert and suggest that this regression model violates the assumption of homoscedasticity behind the relationship between the independent variable and the dependent variable. This is because at higher values of sleep duration, there is a different pattern of residuals than at the lower values of sleep duration. In the residuals plots, the first two vertical lines of dots, representing nondrinkers and monthly drinkers, reach up high, with outlier observations, but the third line is much shorter. This effect is mirrored on the QQ plot, where at higher quantiles of sleep duration, the residuals depart from the dotted line.

These plots, as well as our analyses in Chapter 2, suggest that this model does not meet the linearity or homoscedasticity assumptions behind linear regression. Different possibilities exist to address this problem before moving on, including transforming the outcome variable, as we did in Chapter 2. Thomas Lumley and colleagues studied the importance of the normality (linearity) assumption in large public health datasets like the BRFSS by doing a simulation with normal and non-normal data [91]. Their conclusion, which is actually taught in statistics textbooks, is that large samples are valid for any distribution [91]. In the new era of "big data," Lumley's findings should be remembered, so analysts can ease their minds about assumption violations that normally would challenge their analysis if their datasets were smaller.

On that note, we will proceed with developing our linear regression model.

Linear Regression Modeling and Model Fit Statistics

Starting in SAS, let us start the first iteration of our SS round 1 approach by running the unadjusted linear regression model using `PROC GLM`.

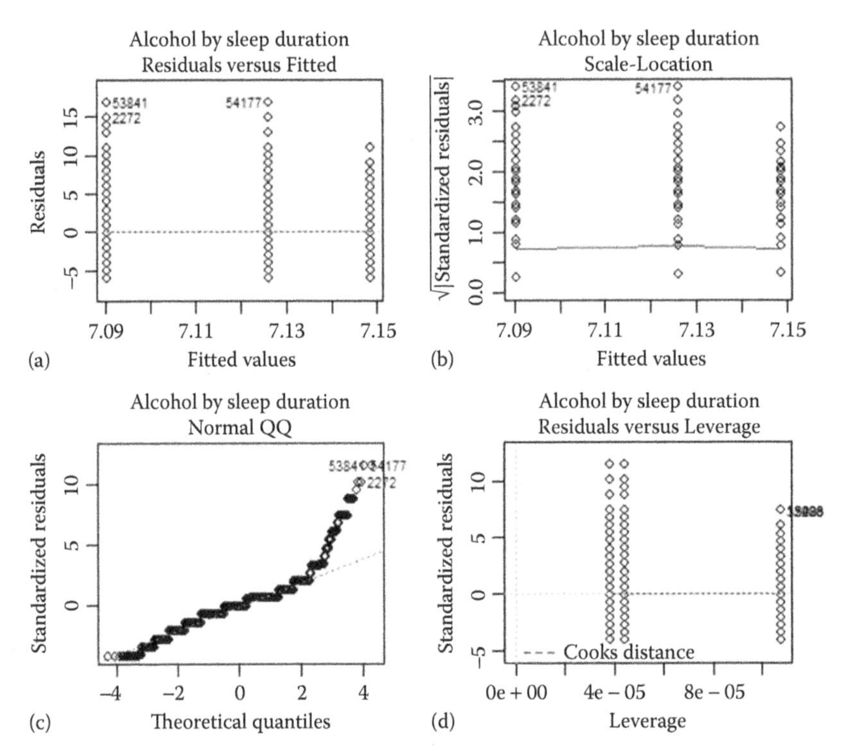

FIGURE 4.1
Diagnostic plots. (a) Alcohol by sleep duration: Residuals versus fitted. (b) Alcohol by sleep duration: Scale-location. (c) Alcohol by sleep duration: Normal QQ. (d) Alcohol by sleep duration: Residuals versus leverage.

Code:

```
proc glm data=r.analytic;
      model SLEPTIM2 = DRKMONTHLY DRKWEEKLY;
run;
```

Several tables are produced as output. Table 4.1 includes the table outputting the parameter estimates from the code above.

The same thing can be done in R by running a `summary` command on the regression object we made earlier in the section that we plotted. However, we

TABLE 4.1
SAS Linear Regression Results of Unadjusted Model

Parameter	Estimate	Standard Error	*t* Value	Pr > |*t*|
`Intercept`	7.126103405	0.00907757	785.02	<.0001
`DRKMONTHLY`	−0.035844639	0.01332756	−2.69	0.0072
`DRKWEEKLY`	0.022565552	0.01771648	1.27	0.2028

will actually choose to remake that regression object and call it `Model1` this time. That way, we can more easily refer to our models in our model metadata.

Code:

```
Model1 = lm(SLEPTIM2 ~ DRKMONTHLY + DRKWEEKLY, data=analytic)
summary(Model1)
```

Output:

```
Call:
lm(formula = SLEPTIM2 ~ DRKMONTHLY + DRKWEEKLY, data = analytic)

Residuals:
    Min      1Q  Median      3Q     Max
-6.1487 -1.0903 -0.0903 0.8739 16.9097

Coefficients:
              Estimate Std.  Error  t value  Pr(>|t|)
(Intercept)   7.126103    0.009078  785.023  < 2e-16   ***
DRKMONTHLY   -0.035845    0.013328   -2.690  0.00716   **
DRKWEEKLY     0.022566    0.017716    1.274  0.20277
---
Signif. codes: 0 '***' 0.001 '**' 0.01 '*' 0.05 '.' 0.1 ' ' 1

Residual standard error: 1.468 on 58128 degrees of freedom
Multiple R-squared: 0.0002203, Adjusted R-squared: 0.0001859
F-statistic: 6.403 on 2 and 58128 DF, p-value: 0.001657
```

Looking at the regression estimates, R helps us by coding covariates with statistically significant slopes with asterisks. We observe that in an unadjusted model, `DRKMONTHLY` but not `DRKWEEKLY` is significant. In Chapter 3, we ran this ANOVA, and saw that the F-test was significant (see last line of output). It is important to remember that linear regression output should not be interpreted unless the F-test is statistically significant. However, it is difficult to have a totally non-significant model using BRFSS because the hugeness of the data confers statistical significance on the most minute differences.

What is particularly useful from this output is the second to the last line, which reports an adjusted R-squared. This is a measure of model fit; the closer to 1, the better the model fit. This adjusted R-squared is very low, but adding covariates will increase it naturally. The aim is to ultimately include the fewest covariates needed to explain the most variation in the dependent variable, which can be estimated by observing changes in the adjusted R-squared from model to model. After trying our many SS iterations of models, the model with the fewest covariates but the highest adjusted R-squared will be selected as the final model. Including the fewest independent variables to explain the behavior of the dependent variable honors the principle of parsimony, and also makes models much easier to interpret [92].

Now that we have run Model1, let us consider what to put in Model2. We will keep both DRKWEEKLY and DRKMONTHLY in all models because they represent our hypothesized exposure. Next in Table 1 is asthma status, but that is not a candidate confounder in this analysis. Instead, asthma status is our outcome for the logistic regression and survival analysis, so we will skip asthma status. After that, we have our age groups, so we can add all the indicator variables we developed in Chapter 2, AGE2 through AGE6, in the model.

Code:

```
Model2 = lm(SLEPTIM2 ~ DRKMONTHLY + DRKWEEKLY +AGE2 + AGE3 +
      AGE4 + AGE5 + AGE6, data=analytic)
summary(Model2)
```

Output:

```
Call:
lm(formula = SLEPTIM2 ~ DRKMONTHLY + DRKWEEKLY + AGE2 + AGE3 +
    AGE4 + AGE5 + AGE6, data = analytic)

Residuals:
    Min       1Q   Median       3Q      Max
-6.4216  -0.7141   0.0780   0.6363  17.4357

Coefficients:
             Estimate Std. Error  t value  Pr(>|t|)
(Intercept)   6.50079    0.04825  134.733   < 2e-16  ***
DRKMONTHLY    0.03603    0.01305    2.760  0.005783  **
DRKWEEKLY     0.05793    0.01727    3.355  0.000795  ***
AGE2         -0.08302    0.05518   -1.505  0.132447
AGE3          0.06353    0.05333    1.191  0.233508
AGE4          0.17732    0.05086    3.487  0.000490  ***
AGE5          0.38516    0.04965    7.757  8.86e-15  ***
AGE6          0.86287    0.04833   17.852   < 2e-16  ***
---
Signif. codes: 0 '***' 0.001 '**' 0.01 '*' 0.05 '.' 0.1 ' ' 1

Residual standard error: 1.43 on 58123 degrees of freedom
Multiple R-squared: 0.05225, Adjusted R-squared: 0.05214
F-statistic: 457.8 on 7 and 58123 DF, p-value: < 2.2e-16
```

This model shows that the adjusted R-squared increased as predicted, but not all of the age indicator variables are performing in the model.

AGE2 and AGE3 are not significant. Let us rerun the model including only the exposure variables and AGE4 through AGE6, and call that Model3.

Code:

```
Model3 = lm(SLEPTIM2 ~ DRKMONTHLY + DRKWEEKLY + AGE4
       + AGE5 + AGE6, data=analytic)
summary(Model3)
```

Output:

```
Call:
lm(formula = SLEPTIM2 ~ DRKMONTHLY + DRKWEEKLY + AGE4 + AGE5 +
      AGE6, data = analytic)

Residuals:
    Min       1Q   Median       3Q      Max
-6.4210  -0.7138  0.0784  0.6358  17.4975

Coefficients:
            Estimate Std. Error  t value  Pr(>|t|)
(Intercept)  6.50245    0.01871  347.531   < 2e-16  ***
DRKMONTHLY   0.03513    0.01305    2.691  0.007121  **
DRKWEEKLY    0.05685    0.01727    3.292  0.000994  ***
AGE4         0.17622    0.02449    7.197  6.24e-13  ***
AGE5         0.38400    0.02190   17.537   < 2e-16  ***
AGE6         0.86170    0.01872   46.032   < 2e-16  ***
---
Signif. codes: 0 '***' 0.001 '**' 0.01 '*' 0.05 '.' 0.1 ' ' 1

Residual standard error: 1.43 on 58125 degrees of freedom
Multiple R-squared: 0.05199, Adjusted R-squared: 0.05191
F-statistic: 637.5 on 5 and 58125 DF, p-value: < 2.2e-16
```

Now, we can look at our Table 1 and see what to add next, which would be our indicator variable MALE. Let us add this in Model4.

Code:

```
Model4 = lm(SLEPTIM2 ~ DRKMONTHLY + DRKWEEKLY + AGE4
       + AGE5 + AGE6 + MALE, data=analytic)
summary(Model4)
```

Output:

```
Call:
lm(formula = SLEPTIM2 ~ DRKMONTHLY + DRKWEEKLY + AGE4 + AGE5 +
    AGE6 + MALE, data = analytic)

Residuals:
    Min       1Q   Median       3Q      Max
-6.4211  -0.7153   0.0862   0.6354  17.4956

Coefficients:
             Estimate Std. Error  t value  Pr(>|t|)
(Intercept)  6.495609   0.025093  258.861   < 2e-16  ***
DRKMONTHLY   0.034925   0.013062    2.674   0.00750  **
DRKWEEKLY    0.056508   0.017287    3.269   0.00108  **
AGE4         0.175950   0.024496    7.183  6.91e-13  ***
AGE5         0.383287   0.021967   17.449   < 2e-16  ***
AGE6         0.860225   0.019063   45.125   < 2e-16  ***
MALE         0.008776   0.021436    0.409   0.68226
---
Signif. codes: 0 '***' 0.001 '**' 0.01 '*' 0.05 '.' 0.1 ' ' 1

Residual standard error: 1.43 on 58124 degrees of freedom
Multiple R-squared: 0.05199, Adjusted R-squared: 0.05189
F-statistic: 531.3 on 6 and 58124 DF, p-value: < 2.2e-16
```

As we can see by the output, `MALE` did not perform in the model. Let us discard it for the next iteration, `Model5`, and put in `HISPANIC`, as this is the next variable in Table 1.

Code:

```
Model5 = lm(SLEPTIM2 ~ DRKMONTHLY + DRKWEEKLY + AGE4
       + AGE5 + AGE6 + HISPANIC, data=analytic)
summary(Model5)
```

Output:

```
Call:
lm(formula = SLEPTIM2 ~ DRKMONTHLY + DRKWEEKLY + AGE4 + AGE5 +
    AGE6 + HISPANIC, data = analytic)

Residuals:
    Min       1Q   Median       3Q      Max
-6.4238  -0.7206   0.0739   0.6322  17.4839
```

```
Coefficients:
             Estimate Std. Error  t value  Pr(>|t|)
(Intercept)   6.51608    0.01898  343.351   < 2e-16  ***
DRKMONTHLY    0.03394    0.01305    2.600   0.00932  **
DRKWEEKLY     0.05603    0.01727    3.245   0.00117  **
AGE4          0.17057    0.02452    6.957  3.52e-12  ***
AGE5          0.37610    0.02197   17.118   < 2e-16  ***
AGE6          0.85169    0.01886   45.152   < 2e-16  ***
HISPANIC     -0.13205    0.03092   -4.271  1.95e-05  ***
---
Signif. codes: 0 '***' 0.001 '**' 0.01 '*' 0.05 '.' 0.1 ' ' 1

Residual standard error: 1.43 on 58124 degrees of freedom
Multiple R-squared: 0.05229, Adjusted R-squared: 0.05219
F-statistic: 534.5 on 6 and 58124 DF, p-value: < 2.2e-16
```

`HISPANIC` was significant in the model, so it would be retained for the next iteration. After `HISPANIC`, all the indicator variables developed should be tried in the model, and either retained or discarded. It is instructive to add sets of indicator variables by topic; for example, adding all the race indicator variables at once in one SS iteration. That way, those that are not significant can be removed in the next iteration, thus moving the group defined by the indicator variable to join the reference group. After round 1 of SS, a working model will have been created.

Next, in round 2 of SS, we would try to break the working model by adding back covariates that were discarded during round 1. This is when discarded covariates such as `AGE2`, `AGE3`, and `MALE` would have their last shot at trying to get into the final model. If they do not fit at that stage, then they are not helping explain the dependent variable better than anything already in the model, so there is no reason to include them. At that point, we would theoretically have our final linear regression model.

Selecting the Final Linear Regression Model

To help in selecting the final model, it is good to record decisions made about modeling iterations in model metadata. Table 4.2 shows an example of a spreadsheet that can be kept about each model run. Notice that the first five models demonstrated, Models 1 through 5, are documented on the sheet.

Under the covariates column, the formula from the R code was copied and pasted. Under the significant covariates column, a list of the only the significant covariates is kept. The adjusted R-squared is filled in as a measure of model fit. Finally, the comments column contains information related to our decisions about what we put in the next model. They reflect the modeling experience described earlier.

At the bottom of Table 4.2 is the final model we selected to answer the hypothesis, `Model31`, which we will present here. Notice the covariates have been ordered in the same order as they are presented in Table 1.

TABLE 4.2

Linear Regression Model Meta-Data

Model	Covariates	Significant Covariates	Adjusted R-squared	Comments
1	DRKMONTHLY + DRKWEEKLY	DRKMONTHLY	0.0002	
2	DRKMONTHLY + DRKWEEKLY + AGE2 + AGE3 + AGE4 + AGE5 + AGE6	DRKMONTHLY, DRKWEEKLY, AGE4 through AGE6	0.0521	Keep AGE4 through AGE6
3	DRKMONTHLY + DRKWEEKLY + AGE4 + AGE5 + AGE6	DRKMONTHLY, DRKWEEKLY, AGE4 through AGE6	0.0519	Add male
4	DRKMONTHLY + DRKWEEKLY + AGE4 + AGE5 + AGE6 + MALE	DRKMONTHLY, DRKWEEKLY, AGE4 through AGE6	0.0519	Remove male, not significant. Add Hispanic.
5	DRKMONTHLY + DRKWEEKLY + AGE4 + AGE5 + AGE6 + HISPANIC	DRKMONTHLY, DRKWEEKLY, AGE4 through AGE6, HISPANIC	0.0522	Keep Hispanic
31	DRKMONTHLY + DRKWEEKLY + AGE3 + AGE4 + AGE5 + AGE6 + HISPANIC + BLACK + ASIAN + OTHRACE + FORMERMAR + NEVERMAR + LOWED + SOMECOLL + INC2 + INC7 + OVWT + OBESE + SMOKER + FAIRHLTH + POORHLTH	Final model	0.0626	

Code:

```
Model31 = lm(SLEPTIM2 ~ DRKMONTHLY + DRKWEEKLY + AGE3 + AGE4 +
        AGE5 + AGE6 + HISPANIC + BLACK + ASIAN + OTHRACE +
        FORMERMAR + NEVERMAR + LOWED + SOMECOLL + INC2 + INC7
        + OVWT + OBESE + SMOKER + FAIRHLTH + POORHLTH,
        data=analytic)
summary(Model31)
```

Output:

```
Call:
lm(formula = SLEPTIM2 ~ DRKMONTHLY + DRKWEEKLY + AGE3 + AGE4 +
      AGE5 + AGE6 + HISPANIC + BLACK + ASIAN + OTHRACE +
      FORMERMAR + NEVERMAR + LOWED + SOMECOLL + INC2 + INC7 +
      OVWT + OBESE + SMOKER + FAIRHLTH + POORHLTH, data =
      analytic)

Residuals:
    Min       1Q  Median      3Q      Max
-6.5588  -0.7379  0.0208  0.6829  18.0720

Coefficients:
             Estimate Std. Error t value   Pr(>|t|)
(Intercept)  6.672289   0.029142  228.957   < 2e-16  ***
DRKMONTHLY   0.002432   0.013262    0.183   0.85449
DRKWEEKLY    0.017829   0.017416    1.024   0.30597
AGE3         0.133870   0.033839    3.956  7.63e-05  ***
AGE4         0.260743   0.029959    8.703   < 2e-16  ***
AGE5         0.470153   0.028043   16.766   < 2e-16  ***
AGE6         0.884061   0.025978   34.031   < 2e-16  ***
HISPANIC    -0.096980   0.031142   -3.114   0.00185  **
BLACK       -0.220159   0.023894   -9.214   < 2e-16  ***
ASIAN       -0.360479   0.060734   -5.935  2.95e-09  ***
OTHRACE     -0.177280   0.026282   -6.745  1.54e-11  ***
FORMERMAR   -0.053547   0.013756   -3.893  9.92e-05  ***
NEVERMAR    -0.282956   0.046288   -6.113  9.84e-10  ***
LOWED        0.024235   0.014693    1.649   0.09907  .
SOMECOLL    -0.027144   0.014671   -1.850   0.06429  .
INC2        -0.074749   0.032316   -2.313   0.02072  *
INC7        -0.030577   0.016000   -1.911   0.05600  .
OVWT        -0.081556   0.014521   -5.616  1.96e-08  ***
OBESE       -0.132287   0.016091   -8.221   < 2e-16  ***
SMOKER      -0.208697   0.017423  -11.978   < 2e-16  ***
FAIRHLTH    -0.151950   0.017314   -8.776   < 2e-16  ***
POORHLTH    -0.179688   0.025370   -7.083  1.43e-12  ***
---
Signif. codes: 0 '***' 0.001 '**' 0.01 '*' 0.05 '.' 0.1 ' ' 1
```

```
Residual standard error: 1.422 on 58109 degrees of freedom
Multiple R-squared: 0.06293, Adjusted R-squared: 0.06259
F-statistic: 185.8 on 21 and 58109 DF, p-value: < 2.2e-16
```

This is just one possible final model of many that could be made using the same analytic dataset and SS linear regression. Observe that in our final model, some of the covariates are less significant than others. It could be argued that different covariates belong in this model. However, it is likely that no matter what other covariates are tried in the model, given this particular analytic dataset, the answer to the hypothesis will not change.

Also note that in this final model, both `DRKMONTHLY` and `DRKWEEKLY` are nowhere near statistical significance. Due to the size of the dataset and the many other covariates present in the model, it is probably not possible that any other reasonable final model could change that finding. Under those conditions, the finding is said to be "robust" [93]. It appears that in veterans in the BRFSS, alcohol consumption is not statistically significantly associated with sleep duration after adjustment for confounders.

Considerations in Improving the Final Model

Our hypothesis is not supported, and some may find this disappointing. In considering this, one can point to the fact that there are many other variables in the BRFSS that we did not even try in this model. The ones we selected were based on the scientific literature and our experience, so we did not have a reason to try any others. But going back to `BRFSS_a` and adding other covariates we did not select to the model after selecting a final model would be risky on a number of counts. First, because we preplanned our hypothesis, we could be accused of a particular type of fishing, which is going back to get covariates to put into the model to "fish" for statistical significance for our hypothesis.

Next, it is necessary that we acknowledge there were sound reasons to select the candidate covariates to include from `BRFSS_a` in our analytic dataset, not to select others. After developing a model with those carefully selected covariates, it is hard to believe that covariates we did not initially select because we did not think they were confounding variables would help us improve the model. The critic who wonders if we should include any of the covariates we excluded can be reminded that through our process, we knew from the beginning that not all of the covariates we tried would be significant when added to this model. This is why we called them potential or candidate confounders.

Considering Collinearity

But it is important to acknowledge that between SS modeling iterations, sometimes it appears covariates are "fighting" each other for significance. The authors have observed this phenomenon between Hispanic ethnicity and education variables in datasets. In early iterations, Hispanic ethnicity will be significant, but when educational variables are added, Hispanic ethnicity is no longer significant. Later in modeling, however, it may show up as significant again. Notice that we removed `AGE3` after running `Model2`, but it showed up in `Model31`, our final model. This means that even though we discarded it early in modeling, when another set of covariates was present in the model and `AGE3` added back, it performed differently, and won its way back in.

When this phenomenon occurs, the covariates that are fighting are collinear in that they are measuring some attribute of the respondent the same way. If for some reason most Hispanics fell in one particular educational group, both the Hispanic and education covariates would be effectively measuring the same thing. This is often seen with multiple indicator variables for different comorbidities. Because many people who have had a stroke also have cardiovascular and other disorders, these variables tend to be collinear. That problem was avoided in our modeling by using the general health variable (`GENHEALTH`). This variable has been found to be a good catchall variable for level of comorbidities. It tends to account for general health status well, which is typically our goal in trying to enter comorbidities into a model to adjust for confounding. In short, in health datasets, collinearity can be a problem even with large samples, and thoughtful design of analytic datasets can reduce the risk of encountering this problem when modeling.

Additionally, the potential for collinearity further dissuades us from the unethical act of fishing in `BRFSS_a` to get more covariates to improve our final model. This is because even if we chose to do this, in a practical sense, we may not be able to improve the model much because our new covariates might be collinear with covariates already in the model.

Adding Interactions

Another way analysts try to improve models after arriving at a final model is to add interaction variables. For example, we could interact the exposure variables, `DRKMONTHLY` and `DRKWEEKLY`, with other covariates in the final model. `Model32` is an example of an interaction model where `HISPANIC` is interacted with `DRKMONTHLY` and `DRKWEEKLY`.

Code:

```
Model32 = lm(SLEPTIM2 ~ DRKMONTHLY + DRKWEEKLY + AGE3 + AGE4 +
        AGE5 + AGE6 + HISPANIC + BLACK + ASIAN + OTHRACE +
        FORMERMAR + NEVERMAR + LOWED + SOMECOLL + INC2 + INC7
        + OVWT + OBESE + SMOKER + FAIRHLTH + POORHLTH +
        (DRKMONTHLY*HISPANIC) + (DRKWEEKLY*HISPANIC),
        data=analytic)
summary(Model32)
```

Output:

```
Call:
lm(formula = SLEPTIM2 ~ DRKMONTHLY + DRKWEEKLY + AGE3 + AGE4 +
      AGE5 + AGE6 + HISPANIC + BLACK + ASIAN + OTHRACE +
      FORMERMAR + NEVERMAR + LOWED + SOMECOLL + INC2 + INC7 +
      OVWT + OBESE + SMOKER + FAIRHLTH + POORHLTH + (DRKMONTHLY
      * HISPANIC) + (DRKWEEKLY * HISPANIC), data = analytic)

Residuals:
    Min      1Q  Median      3Q     Max
-6.5585 -0.7395  0.0213  0.6828 18.0736

Coefficients:
                      Estimate Std. Error t value Pr(>|t|)
(Intercept)            6.67077   0.02916  228.765  < 2e-16 ***
DRKMONTHLY             0.00396   0.01350    0.293 0.769350
DRKWEEKLY              0.02299   0.01775    1.296 0.195103
AGE3                   0.13404   0.03384    3.961 7.48e-05 ***
AGE4                   0.26057   0.02997    8.693  < 2e-16 ***
AGE5                   0.47023   0.02805   16.761  < 2e-16 ***
AGE6                   0.88382   0.02600   34.000  < 2e-16 ***
HISPANIC              -0.06171   0.04491   -1.374 0.169437
BLACK                 -0.22020   0.02389   -9.216  < 2e-16 ***
ASIAN                 -0.36008   0.06073   -5.929 3.07e-09 ***
OTHRACE               -0.17740   0.02628   -6.750 1.50e-11 ***
FORMERMAR             -0.05327   0.01376   -3.872 0.000108 ***
NEVERMAR              -0.28314   0.04629   -6.117 9.60e-10 ***
LOWED                  0.02442   0.01469    1.662 0.096512 .
SOMECOLL              -0.02711   0.01467   -1.848 0.064644 .
INC2                  -0.07530   0.03232   -2.330 0.019808 *
INC7                  -0.03046   0.01600   -1.904 0.056949 .
OVWT                  -0.08145   0.01452   -5.609 2.04e-08 ***
OBESE                 -0.13203   0.01609   -8.204 2.38e-16 ***
SMOKER                -0.20859   0.01742  -11.972  < 2e-16 ***
FAIRHLTH              -0.15222   0.01732   -8.791  < 2e-16 ***
POORHLTH              -0.17974   0.02537   -7.085 1.41e-12 ***
DRKMONTHLY:HISPANIC   -0.03836   0.06682   -0.574 0.565877
DRKWEEKLY:HISPANIC    -0.13539   0.08956   -1.512 0.130618
---
Signif. codes: 0 '***' 0.001 '**' 0.01 '*' 0.05 '.' 0.1 ' ' 1

Residual standard error: 1.422 on 58107 degrees of freedom
Multiple R-squared: 0.06297, Adjusted R-squared: 0.0626
F-statistic: 169.8 on 23 and 58107 DF, p-value: < 2.2e-16
```

Notice in the code, to enter the interaction variables into the model, we use parentheses and an asterisk for the multiplication operation. In this case, both our interaction variables were not significant, so this interaction should not be retained in the model. However, if either of them were significant, an argument could be made that the interaction variable should be retained. Some analysts at this point will try every confounding variable as an interaction with the exposure, hunting for significance, and keeping the interaction terms that are significant [90].

This brings about both a philosophical and a practical problem. The philosophical problem is that our hypothesis was not about Hispanics, or any other confounder in the model. Had we hypothesized that somehow being Hispanic while simultaneously being a consumer of alcohol would have an additive or multiplicative effect on sleep duration, then should not that have been stated in our hypothesis [94]? Some in public health say it is our duty to search out interactions to identify highly vulnerable groups who may be lost in the regular analysis. As an example, Karaca-Mandic and colleagues make this argument for adding interaction terms to nonlinear models [95]. But is it possible that we will only find spurious associations when trying different interactions simply due to the increase in Type I error from what amounts to many *post hoc*, unhypothesized analyses?

The practical problem, however, is probably worse. This problem is that whenever an interaction term is present in a final model, the slope of that term (as well as the slopes of the "lower level" terms, or the terms that make up the interaction) cannot be interpreted alone. They have to be presented as stratum-specific estimates [94,95]. For example, had our interaction terms been significant, then that estimate of drinking's association with sleep duration would have to be calculated separately for Hispanics. For Hispanics who drink monthly, the slopes for `HISPANIC`, `DRKMONTHLY`, and the interaction term would all have to be added together to develop the estimate, and a similar operation would need to be done for Hispanics who drink weekly. On the other hand, for people who were not Hispanic, the slopes for `DRKMONTHLY` and `DRKWEEKLY` could be directly interpreted. It is easy to see how interpretation can be lost if there are multiple interactions with the exposure in the final model [96].

Another way we could try to add interaction terms to our final model is to simply interact confounders together and leave the exposure out of the process. Some argue that trying these interactions can eke out a better model fit [95]. While this may be true, it again sacrifices how interpretable the model is, and how easily its findings can be discerned and applied.

For these reasons, in our demonstration, we will skip fitting interactions and select `Model31` as our final model. This is the model we will present to answer our hypothesis.

Goodness-of-Fit Statistics

Some analysts like to look at goodness-of-fit (GOF) after making their final models. But because after all this modeling, more statistics about our selected final model will mirror what we already know about the model, they will not influence its selection. Even so, some might want to quantify and evaluate the fit of the final model for their own understanding. In those cases, one approach is to run the residual plots on the final model (rather than the unadjusted model, as demonstrated earlier). This can be done in both SAS and R.

R also has a helpful package called `gvlma` [97]. After calling up the library for `gvlma`, we use the `gvlma` command to turn `Model31`, our final model regression object, into the object `GVModel31`, and then run a summary command on it.

Code:

```
library(gvlma)
GVModel31 <- gvlma(Model31)
summary(GVModel31)
```

Output:

(Only the statistics from the bottom of the output are presented below.)

```
ASSESSMENT OF THE LINEAR MODEL ASSUMPTIONS
USING THE GLOBAL TEST ON 4 DEGREES-OF-FREEDOM:
Level of Significance = 0.05

Call:
gvlma(x = Model31)

                        Value     p-value                   Decision
Global Stat         1.068e+05  0.000e+00   Assumptions NOT satisfied!
Skewness            4.926e+03  0.000e+00   Assumptions NOT satisfied!
Kurtosis            1.018e+05  0.000e+00   Assumptions NOT satisfied!
Link Function       3.575e+01  2.239e-09   Assumptions NOT satisfied!
Heteroscedasticity  7.167e+00  7.425e-03   Assumptions NOT satisfied!
```

With smaller samples, the `gvlma` test would be helpful in evaluating a final model. However, with large datasets, the fact that these assumptions are not satisfied should not deter us from interpreting the model.

Linear Regression Model Presentation

There are a variety of ways that final linear regression models are presented in the scientific literature. Table 4.3 is an example of one style of presentation. Notice that even though we only have one final model, three models are actually presented. Under `Model1`, the unadjusted model is presented. In the parameter estimate column, for the Nondrinker category, we put the word Reference to make it clear to the reader that nondrinkers were the reference group. Then, we put the slopes from our unadjusted model

TABLE 4.3

Final Linear Regression Model Presentation

Category	Level	Model 1: Unadjusted		Model 2: Adjusted for Age and Sex		Model 3: Fully Adjusted	
		Parameter Estimate	*p*-value	Parameter Estimate	*p*-value	Parameter Estimate	*p*-value
Alcohol status	Nondrinker	Reference	NA	Reference	NA	Reference	NA
	Monthly drinker	−0.0584	0.0012	−0.0218	0.2168	−0.0154	0.3797
	Weekly drinker	−0.0226	0.2028	−0.0576	0.0009	−0.0178	0.3060
Sex	Male	NA	NA	0.0087	0.6856	NA	NA
	Female	NA	NA	Reference	NA	NA	NA
Age	Age 18 to 24	NA	NA	Reference	NA	Reference	NA
	Age 25 to 34	NA	NA	−0.0828	0.1335	Reference	NA
	Age 35 to 44	NA	NA	0.0637	0.2321	0.1339	<0.0001
	Age 45 to 54	NA	NA	0.1772	0.0005	0.2607	<0.0001
	Age 55 to 64	NA	NA	0.3846	<0.0001	0.4702	<0.0001
	Age 65 or older	NA	NA	0.8616	<0.0001	0.8841	<0.0001
Ethnicity	Hispanic	NA	NA	NA	NA	−0.0970	0.0018
	Non-Hispanic	NA	NA	NA	NA	Reference	NA
	Ethnicity not reported	NA	NA	NA	NA	Reference	NA
Race	White	NA	NA	NA	NA	Reference	NA
	Black/African American	NA	NA	NA	NA	−0.2202	<0.0001
	Asian	NA	NA	NA	NA	−0.3605	<0.0001
	Other race/multi-racial[a]	NA	NA	NA	NA	−0.1773	<0.0001
	Unknown race	NA	NA	NA	NA	Reference	NA

(*Continued*)

TABLE 4.3 (*Continued*)

Final Linear Regression Model Presentation

		Model 1: Unadjusted		Model 2: Adjusted for Age and Sex		Model 3: Fully Adjusted	
Category	**Level**	**Parameter Estimate**	***p*-value**	**Parameter Estimate**	***p*-value**	**Parameter Estimate**	***p*-value**
Marital status	Currently married	NA	NA	NA	NA	Reference	NA
	Divorced, widowed, separated	NA	NA	NA	NA	−0.0535	<0.0001
	Never married	NA	NA	NA	NA	−0.2830	<0.0001
	Not reported	NA	NA	NA	NA	Reference	NA
Highest education level	Less than high school through high school graduate	NA	NA	NA	NA	0.0242	0.0991
	Some college/technical	NA	NA	NA	NA	−0.0271	0.0643
	Four or more years of college	NA	NA	NA	NA	Reference	NA
	Not reported	NA	NA	NA	NA	Reference	NA
Annual household income	<$10k	NA	NA	NA	NA	Reference	NA
	$10k–<$15k	NA	NA	NA	NA	−0.0747	0.0207
	$15k–<$20k	NA	NA	NA	NA	Reference	NA
	$20k–<$25k	NA	NA	NA	NA	Reference	NA
	$25k–<$35k	NA	NA	NA	NA	Reference	NA
	$35k–<$50k	NA	NA	NA	NA	Reference	NA
	$50k–<$75k	NA	NA	NA	NA	−0.0306	0.0560
	$75k or more	NA	NA	NA	NA	Reference	NA
	Not reported	NA	NA	NA	NA	Reference	NA

(Continued)

TABLE 4.3 (*Continued*)

Final Linear Regression Model Presentation

		Model 1: Unadjusted		Model 2: Adjusted for Age and Sex		Model 3: Fully Adjusted	
Category	**Level**	**Parameter Estimate**	***p*-value**	**Parameter Estimate**	***p*-value**	**Parameter Estimate**	***p*-value**
Obesity status	Underweight	NA	NA	NA	NA	Reference	NA
	Normal	NA	NA	NA	NA	Reference	NA
	Overweight	NA	NA	NA	NA	−0.0816	<0.0001
	Obese	NA	NA	NA	NA	−0.1323	<0.0001
	Not reported	NA	NA	NA	NA	Reference	NA
Smoking status	Smoker	NA	NA	NA	NA	−0.2087	<0.0001
	Nonsmoker	NA	NA	NA	NA	Reference	NA
	Not reported	NA	NA	NA	NA	Reference	NA
General health	Excellent	NA	NA	NA	NA	Reference	NA
	Very Good	NA	NA	NA	NA	Reference	NA
	Good	NA	NA	NA	NA	Reference	NA
	Fair	NA	NA	NA	NA	−0.1520	<0.0001
	Poor	NA	NA	NA	NA	−0.1797	<0.0001
	Not reported	NA	NA	NA	NA	Reference	NA

[a] Indicates other race or multiple racial groups.

for the indicator variables for monthly and weekly drinker underneath, with their p-values to the right.* The rest of the rows in the table are for confounders that are in our final model, but not the unadjusted model, so NAs are placed in those cells under Model 1.†

In this case, we chose to present Model 2, which was adjusted for age and sex variables. This was an empirical stylistic choice; age and sex are commonly strong confounders in most analyses, so it is helpful to see how much impact they have on changing the results of the unadjusted analysis. It is interesting to note that between Model 1 and Model 2 as presented in Table 4.3, monthly drinker went from significant to not significant and weekly drinker went from not significant to significant. As we saw in our modeling, Model 2 includes both significant and non-significant covariates. For those in the model, the reference group is noted under the parameter estimate column. The rest of the rows that correspond to variables not given in Model 2 are recorded as NA.

In this table, our final model, `Model31`, is reported as Model 3. In this column, all the values should be filled in and there should be no NAs, except for those variables used in Model 2 that did not survive in Model 3 (such as Male). If an indicator variable among a group of indicator variables did not survive modeling, it is recorded in the reference category, as we see with many of the income indicator variables. Reference variables will have no p-values; those with a parameter estimate will have p-values, and very small ones are recorded as less than 0.0001.

If Table 4.3 is our desired format, then the goal is to take `Model31` and have it exported out in some format that is similar in structure to Table 4.3. That way, as we use Excel to finalize Table 4.3, we benefit from the results having been exported out into a *.csv, from which we can copy and paste estimates directly from the software and avoid transcription errors.

When we turn to SAS, we observe that SAS generates internal tables as part of running each `PROC`, and using the ODS, these can be turned into datasets that are output. We will redo our code in `PROC REG` to take advantage of the ODS to output the parameter estimates to a dataset called "`parms`." These are then exported to *.csv called `SAS_Model31.csv`.

Code:

```
proc reg data=r.analytic;
        model SLEPTIM2 = DRKMONTHLY DRKWEEKLY AGE3 AGE4 AGE5 AGE6
        HISPANIC BLACK ASIAN OTHRACE FORMERMAR NEVERMAR LOWED
        SOMECOLL
        INC2 INC7 OVWT OBESE SMOKER FAIRHLTH POORHLTH /clb;
run;
```

* Some authors may choose to add confidence intervals as well.

† The intercepts may be added to the table for those who want to speak of the linear equation in the narrative of their report.

```
PROC EXPORT DATA= WORK.parms
            OUTFILE= "C:\Users\Monika\Dropbox\R Stats Book\
Analytics\Data\SAS_Model31.csv"
            DBMS=CSV REPLACE;
      PUTNAMES=YES;
RUN;
```

Table 4.4 shows the output from this table.

It is pleasing to see that the slope estimates and the *p*-values are available in this table; these are what are desired for the final table presentation, in Table 4.3. However, there are many other unwanted columns.

We have a tidier option in R. Using the packages `devtools` [98] and `broom` [99], we can output a "`tidy`" model. Basically, these packages take the regression object, `Model31`, and reformat it. Rather than having the table formatted for display in the console, it is now formatted for output into a *.csv.

Let us start by simply looking at the object `Model31` without using the `summary` command.

Code:

```
Model31
```

Output:

```
Coefficients:
(Intercept)  DRKMONTHLY   DRKWEEKLY        AGE3        AGE4        AGE5
   6.672289    0.002432    0.017829    0.133870    0.260743    0.470153
       AGE6    HISPANIC       BLACK       ASIAN    OTHRACE   FORMERMAR
   0.884061   -0.096980   -0.220159   -0.360479   -0.177280   -0.053547
   NEVERMAR       LOWED    SOMECOLL        INC2        INC7        OVWT
  -0.282956    0.024235   -0.027144   -0.074749   -0.030577   -0.081556
      OBESE      SMOKER    FAIRHLTH    POORHLTH
  -0.132287   -0.208697   -0.151950   -0.179688
```

This format is not amenable to being exported into a tabular-formatted *.csv similar in structure to Table 4.3, so we will use the `tidy` command to improve its structure. First, we will copy `Model31` into a `Tidy_Model31` by way of the `tidy` command. Then we will look at `Tidy_Model31` and see the differences in format between that and `Model31`.

Code:

```
Tidy_Model31 <- tidy(Model31)
Tidy_Model31
```

TABLE 4.4

Parameter Estimates Output from PROC REG

Model	Dependent	Variable	DF	Estimate	StdErr	*t*Value	Probt	LowerCL	UpperCL
MODEL1	SLEPTIM2	Intercept	1	6.67229	0.0291	229	<0.0001	6.61517	6.72941
MODEL1	SLEPTIM2	DRKMONTHLY	1	0.00243	0.0133	0.18	0.855	−0.02356	0.02843
MODEL1	SLEPTIM2	DRKWEEKLY	1	0.01783	0.0174	1.02	0.306	−0.01631	0.05196
MODEL1	SLEPTIM2	AGE3	1	0.13387	0.0338	3.96	<0.0001	0.06754	0.2002
MODEL1	SLEPTIM2	AGE4	1	0.26074	0.03	8.7	<0.0001	0.20202	0.31946
MODEL1	SLEPTIM2	AGE5	1	0.47015	0.028	16.77	<0.0001	0.41519	0.52512
MODEL1	SLEPTIM2	AGE6	1	0.88406	0.026	34.03	<0.0001	0.83314	0.93498
MODEL1	SLEPTIM2	HISPANIC	1	−0.09698	0.0311	−3.11	0.002	−0.15802	−0.03594
MODEL1	SLEPTIM2	BLACK	1	−0.22016	0.0239	−9.21	<0.0001	−0.26699	−0.17333
MODEL1	SLEPTIM2	ASIAN	1	−0.36048	0.0607	−5.94	<0.0001	−0.47952	−0.24144
MODEL1	SLEPTIM2	OTHRACE	1	−0.17728	0.0263	−6.75	<0.0001	−0.22879	−0.12577
MODEL1	SLEPTIM2	FORMERMAR	1	−0.05355	0.0138	−3.89	<0.0001	−0.08051	−0.02659
MODEL1	SLEPTIM2	NEVERMAR	1	−0.28296	0.0463	−6.11	<0.0001	−0.37368	−0.19223
MODEL1	SLEPTIM2	LOWED	1	0.02423	0.0147	1.65	0.099	−0.00456	0.05303
MODEL1	SLEPTIM2	SOMECOLL	1	−0.02714	0.0147	−1.85	0.064	−0.0559	0.00161
MODEL1	SLEPTIM2	INC2	1	−0.07475	0.0323	−2.31	0.021	−0.13809	−0.01141
MODEL1	SLEPTIM2	INC7	1	−0.03058	0.016	−1.91	0.056	−0.06194	0.0007831
MODEL1	SLEPTIM2	OVWT	1	−0.08156	0.0145	−5.62	<0.0001	−0.11002	−0.05309
MODEL1	SLEPTIM2	OBESE	1	−0.13229	0.0161	−8.22	<0.0001	−0.16382	−0.10075
MODEL1	SLEPTIM2	SMOKER	1	−0.2087	0.0174	−11.98	<0.0001	−0.24285	−0.17455
MODEL1	SLEPTIM2	FAIRHLTH	1	−0.15195	0.0173	−8.78	<0.0001	−0.18589	−0.11801
MODEL1	SLEPTIM2	POORHLTH	1	−0.17969	0.0254	−7.08	<0.0001	−0.22941	−0.12996

Output:

```
          term     estimate  std.error   statistic        p.value
1  (Intercept)  6.672289153 0.02914212 228.9568630  0.000000e+00
2   DRKMONTHLY  0.002432234 0.01326221   0.1833958  8.544881e-01
3    DRKWEEKLY  0.017828657 0.01741551   1.0237229  3.059704e-01
4         AGE3  0.133870342 0.03383946   3.9560420  7.629216e-05
5         AGE4  0.260743321 0.02995916   8.7032907  3.306610e-18
6         AGE5  0.470153411 0.02804278  16.7655796  6.129524e-63
7         AGE6  0.884060618 0.02597824  34.0308100 2.342882e-251
8     HISPANIC -0.096980061 0.03114193  -3.1141313  1.845770e-03
9        BLACK -0.220159362 0.02389391  -9.2140357  3.242066e-20
10       ASIAN -0.360479358 0.06073382  -5.9353978  2.947909e-09
11    OTHRACE -0.177280101 0.02628158  -6.7454132  1.540163e-11
12  FORMERMAR -0.053546707 0.01375567  -3.8926999  9.924537e-05
13   NEVERMAR -0.282955769 0.04628765  -6.1129866  9.840382e-10
14      LOWED  0.024234905 0.01469331   1.6493833  9.907455e-02
15   SOMECOLL -0.027143908 0.01467058  -1.8502267  6.428595e-02
16       INC2 -0.074748903 0.03231602  -2.3130605  2.072279e-02
17       INC7 -0.030577272 0.01600017  -1.9110596  5.600183e-02
18       OVWT -0.081556088 0.01452135  -5.6162884  1.959920e-08
19      OBESE -0.132286662 0.01609055  -8.2213902  2.052659e-16
20     SMOKER -0.208696762 0.01742319 -11.9781042  5.061890e-33
21   FAIRHLTH -0.151950009 0.01731437  -8.7759457  1.739648e-18
22   POORHLTH -0.179688339 0.02537023  -7.0826462  1.430272e-12
```

This format, when exported to *.csv, presents the results in an easy format to transfer to our desired Excel presentation table format.

In the next code, we export the object `Tidy_Model31`. We name the output model `R_Model31` when exporting it to *.csv so we will not confuse it with our SAS *.csv version of `Model 31`.

Code:

```
write.csv(Tidy_Model31, file = "R_Model31.csv")
```

Table 4.5 displays the tidy model version of `Model31`.

It is indeed much tidier than the parameter output from SAS. Models output like this in *.csv format can be used when formulating a final model presentation table in Excel following the format of Table 4.3.

Plot to Assist Interpretation

After the model presentation tables are done, the models need to be interpreted as the results are written up. Interpretation of a model with so many covariates can be daunting. We have found it useful to create a coefficient plot error bars as a visual guide when interpreting a large final model like `Model31`.

TABLE 4.5
Tidy Model Linear Regression Output from R

	Term	Estimate	Std.error	Statistic	p.value
1	(Intercept)	6.672289153	0.02914212	228.956863	0
2	DRKMONTHLY	0.002432234	0.01326221	0.18339577	0.85448813
3	DRKWEEKLY	0.017828657	0.01741551	1.023722938	0.30597042
4	AGE3	0.133870342	0.03383946	3.956041963	7.6292E-05
5	AGE4	0.260743321	0.02995916	8.703290701	3.3066E-18
6	AGE5	0.470153411	0.02804278	16.76557961	6.1295E-63
7	AGE6	0.884060618	0.02597824	34.03081001	2.343E-251
8	HISPANIC	−0.09698006	0.03114193	−3.11413125	0.00184577
9	BLACK	−0.22015936	0.02389391	−9.21403569	3.2421E-20
10	ASIAN	−0.36047936	0.06073382	−5.93539779	2.9479E-09
11	OTHRACE	−0.1772801	0.02628158	−6.74541321	1.5402E-11
12	FORMERMAR	−0.05354671	0.01375567	−3.89269992	9.9245E-05
13	NEVERMAR	−0.28295577	0.04628765	−6.11298663	9.8404E-10
14	LOWED	0.024234905	0.01469331	1.649383255	0.09907455
15	SOMECOLL	−0.02714391	0.01467058	−1.85022671	0.06428595
16	INC2	−0.0747489	0.03231602	−2.31306048	0.02072279
17	INC7	−0.03057727	0.01600017	−1.91105963	0.05600183
18	OVWT	−0.08155609	0.01452135	−5.61628839	1.9599E-08
19	OBESE	−0.13228666	0.01609055	−8.2213902	2.0527E-16
20	SMOKER	−0.20869676	0.01742319	−11.9781042	5.0619E-33
21	FAIRHLTH	−0.15195001	0.01731437	−8.77594567	1.7396E-18
22	POORHLTH	−0.17968834	0.02537023	−7.08264619	1.4303E-12

While we do not present the plot as a figure in the report, we instead use it as visual support when we are writing.

The package `arm` in R has a command for coefficient plots that will be used for this demonstration [100]; there are other packages for coefficient plots in R, such as one by Jared Lander [101]. The authors could not identify a comparable plot in SAS, so only R will be demonstrated.

The following code creates Figure 4.2 in the color insert.

Code:

```
library(arm)
VarLabels=c("Intercept", "Drink Monthly", "Drink Weekly", "Age
        35-44", "Age 45-54",
        "Age 55-64", "Age 65+", "Hispanic", "Black", "Asian",
        "Other Race",
        "Formerly Married", "Never Married", "Up to HS Educ",
        "Some College",
        "$10k-<$15k Income", "$50k-<$75k Income",
        "Overweight", "Obese",
        "Smoker", "Fair Health", "Poor Health")
```

```
coefplot(Model31,
       vertical=FALSE,
       ylim=c(-0.5, 1),
       main="Model 31 Linear Regression Estimates",
       varnames=VarLabels,
       col=c("darkblue", "darkblue",
              "darkorange", "darkorange", "darkorange",
              "darkorange",
              "blueviolet",
              "darkgreen", "darkgreen", "darkgreen",
              "chocolate", "chocolate",
              "blue4", "blue4",
              "azure4", "azure4",
              "darkgoldenrod2", "darkgoldenrod2",
              "darkred",
              "darkolivegreen4", "darkolivegreen4"))
```

In the code, first, we call up the library "`arm`." Next, we create a vector with variable labels named `VarLabels`. This is done mainly for presentation to others; if this plot was only being used by the analyst, adding these labels would not be necessary. Note that the labels are put in the order of the covariates in `Model31`, including "`intercept`" as the first entry. This will not be printed out, but is necessary to get the command `coefplot` to work.

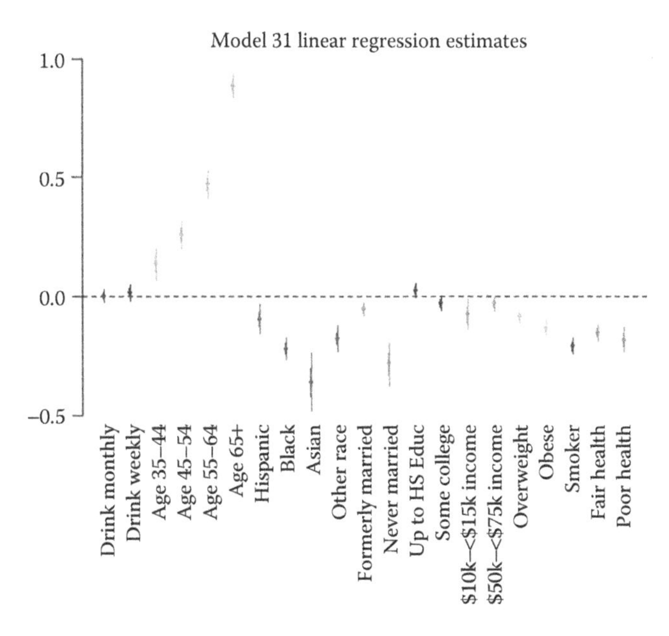

FIGURE 4.2
(See color insert.) Linear regression coefficient plot of final model.

After this, the `coefplot` command produces the plot. The first argument is the regression object, `Model31`. The default plot graphs the parameter estimates vertically, and setting `vertical=FALSE` graphs them horizontally. We use `ylim` to set the lower and upper boundaries of the y-axis to make sure the plot fits in the window properly. We set the `varnames` argument to equal the `VarLabels` vector we made with variable names.

Next, we have a long color argument. Notice how the statements are grouped. The first two "`darkblue`" entries refer to our exposure variables. The next four "`darkorange`" entries refer to the next four variables, which are age indicator variables. By grouping indicators in the same domain by color, the plot can help us easily compare the performance of different concepts in the model.

Let us now look at Figure 4.2, which will help us interpret the model. The line at 0 indicates no association between the covariate and the outcome, sleep duration. Above each covariate label, there is a vertical line with a dot in the middle. The dot is placed at the slope estimate from the parameter estimates. Please notice that the vertical line is actually two lines, a thin, longer one, and a thicker, shorter one. The thicker, shorter one indicates one standard deviation above and below the slope, and the thinner, longer one indicates two standard deviations above and below the slope. Longer lines indicate more error.

As an overall interpretation, it is interesting to note many of the confounders, such as the racial variables, the weight-related variables, the smoker variable, and the fair and poor health variables, serve to reduce sleep duration, as they are plotted entirely below the 0 line. Older age, however, is associated with a dramatic increase in sleep duration. The plot also makes it easy to see that our exposure variables, the education variables, and the income variables have little influence on sleep duration because these lines are plotted near the 0 line.

To conclude, in this section, we used our analytic file and a SS process to develop and interpret a linear regression model to answer our linear regression hypothesis. Approaches in both SAS and R were demonstrated, and the final presentation models were documented in an Excel table, which would be included in a final report or manuscript. Let us move on to the next section, where we use a similar approach to answering our logistic regression hypothesis.

Logistic Regression

In this section, we will move on to answering our logistic regression hypothesis. First, issues in preparation for logistic regression will be examined. Next, we will start the SS modeling process, then discuss issues associated with selecting the final logistic regression model. We will end the section with an examination of logistic regression model presentation.

Estimates Produced by Logistic Regression

To prepare for our logistic regression modelling, let us recall how logistic regression differs from linear regression. First, because we are predicting a binary rather than continuous variable, the slopes reported on the output are log odds of having the outcome. In the health science literature, these are exponentiated and reported as odds ratios (ORs) with their confidence intervals. ORs are very useful for interpretation [102]. An OR of 1 means that the odds of the outcome in the group with the independent variable is the same as the odds of the outcome in the reference group—meaning that there is no association between the independent variable and the outcome. An OR of less than 1 means that the independent variable is associated with a lower odds of the outcome than seen in the reference group, and an OR of greater than 1 means that independent variable is associated with a higher odds of the outcome than the reference group.

To take this further, observe that having the OR and entire 95% confidence interval of the OR either entirely below or entirely above 1 means that the covariate is statistically significant in the model. For this reason, reporting ORs and their 95% confidence intervals is the typical presentation in health literature, even though the parameter estimates output from logistic regression are actually log odds [103]. Also, *p*-values are generally not reported because it is obvious whether or not the covariate is significant in the model by noting whether or not its confidence interval includes 1, and also, the confidence intervals are more informative than *p*-values as to the magnitude of associations [104].

Logistic Regression Considerations

Compared to linear regression, logistic regression is concerned with fewer assumptions [105]. However, there are caveats to using logistic regression for analyses. Carina Mood reports results of a simulation in logistic regression that demonstrates that the results obtained from fitting models in standard ways reported in the literature are generally incorrect because they are affected by omitted (possibly unmeasured) variables, even if these variables are unrelated to the other independent variables in the model [103]. She says the simplest approaches to minimizing this issue in logistic regression include measuring and including unmeasured continuous variables in the model that could affect the outcome (such as a continuous measure of poverty), as well as not categorizing continuous variables already in the dataset [103]. Neither of these options is available when using an already-collected dataset that contains few continuous native variables, such as the BRFSS. Mood also presents more complex solutions to adjust the ORs in the final model to improve their accuracy, and also presents evidence that these adjustments profoundly affect the final model [103]. While it is acknowledged that the approach presented in this book has flaws, because it is standard in the medical literature and there is no obvious alternative, this book will demonstrate SS logistic regression as it is typically reported [52].

The main limitation to using logistic regression is that there need to be enough respondents with the outcome in the dataset to be able to support the model. Peter Peduzzi and colleagues conducted a simulation study, the results of which suggest that the number of rows where the outcome equals 1 (events) divided by the number of predictor variables included in the logistic regression model should equal at least 10 [106]. The reasoning is that the fewer number of events per predictor variable, the greater the chance for regression coefficient estimates to have a lower level of reliability. In our analytic dataset, the number of rows where `ASTHMA4=1` is 5,343. Using the prescribed formula, we should theoretically be able to include up to 534 predictor variables in the logistic regression model we develop. In other words, because most large datasets include enough outcomes to support logistic regression, this limit on the number of independent variables is usually not encountered when modeling.

Peduzzi's team recommended further that the logistic regression model be validated once the final model is determined [106]. Their recommendation is to conduct k-fold cross-validation, which is where the original sample is randomly partitioned into k equal-sized subsamples (such as 5 or 10); one sample is chosen as the validation dataset and the others are considered training datasets. The model is developed using the training datasets and is validated using the validation dataset. This approach has been used in medical science, but the findings of a simulation by Stephenie Lemon and colleagues comparing logistic regression to classification and regression tree (C&RT) analysis using k-fold cross-validation with a health dataset implied that traditional logistic regression does not perform substantially worse without conducting k-fold cross-validation [96]. Further, readers interested in k-fold cross-validation and C&RT approaches are invited to check out the R package `caret` [107].

With BRFSS, external validation, which was also suggested by Peduzzi and colleagues, is perhaps a more reasonable approach to validate a model. That is because BRFSS represents a public health survey that is conducted at regular intervals. External validation means analyzing an external dataset that is somehow related to the study dataset and is meant to provide the same findings, and comparing the final logistic regression models. One of the authors (MMW) did a practical version of this when fitting a BRFSS logistic regression model for publication in the scientific literature [108]. Although the results presented in the paper are from an analysis using the 2014 BRFSS dataset, the 2012 BRFSS dataset was also used to fit a model using the same hypothesis in the early development of the manuscript, before the 2014 dataset was available. The findings reported for the 2014 data in the article were found to be consistent with the unpublished 2012 results, even though both were developed using an SS modeling process, thus assuring the authorship team that their 2014 model was likely valid.

Although validation is desired when developing a logistic regression model, it must be acknowledged that it is generally not done in health science reporting. As an illustration, Steven Bagley and colleagues reviewed 21 published logistic regression analyses from the medical literature, and none of these applied any validation procedures [109]. Hence, we will not demonstrate validating the model we build in this book.

So far, we have established that logistic regression requires a dataset with enough rows where the event variable equals 1 to support a regression model. Another limitation is that these rows also need to make up a large enough proportion of the dataset in a relative sense. In the case of a dataset with very few outcomes—such as a cohort study that collects cancer incidence data in the cohort—a case-control approach might be needed, which entails sampling controls from the non-cases. A case-control study design effectively controls the prevalence of events in the dataset, and would be a way to solve the problem of having too few events, or too small of a proportion of events. In a case–control analysis, where the event can be very rare, exact logistic regression can be used [51]. We are doing a cross-sectional analysis in the demonstration, so a case-control analysis is outside the scope of this book, and we will not be demonstrating exact logistic regression. Readers interested in exact logistic regression are referred to the R package `elrm` [110].

In summary, there are a few dataset-related caveats that must be considered before moving forward with a logistic regression analysis, which were outlined here. Because our analytic dataset will support logistic regression modeling, we will move forward with our model building.

Introduction to Logistic Regression Modeling

Recall our logistic regression hypothesis: Among veterans, after controlling for confounders, alcohol consumption is associated with asthma status. As we did with SS linear regression, to answer this question, we will run iterative models, only this time, all of our models will include the dependent variable `ASTHMA4`. And like with our linear regression modeling, as we have the same exposure in this hypothesis, we will retain `DRKWEEKLY` and `DRKMONTHLY` in all our models.

Also, as we did with linear regression, we will use the SS modeling process by introducing covariates one at a time into iterative models in the order they are reported in Table 1, and keeping track of our decisions in model metadata. After we try each covariate in round 1, we will have a working model and then try to reintroduce covariates removed from the model in the first process in round 2. As with the linear regression process, once we are at the end of round 2, we will have a final logistic regression model.

SS modeling in linear and logistic regression is essentially very similar, but there are a few important differences. During our linear regression models, we paid more attention to the p-values on the slopes rather than the slopes themselves. But when doing logistic regression, it is important to pay attention to the actual values of the ORs and their 95% confidence intervals from model iteration to model iteration. This is why the analyst should actually look at ORs—not the log odds—of each model in between iterations. If small cells occur in a model—which can be possible even in a large dataset when the outcome is binary—it can make the OR unstable and the confidence intervals comically wide. Also, as can be expected, there are different metrics to look at on the output for logistic regression that indicate model-fit parameters, which will be reviewed next.

Logistic Regression Modeling and Model Fitting

SAS offers several methods of running a logistic regression model. One way is to use `PROC LOGISTIC` and designate the value of the event in the formula. We will run the unadjusted model here in SAS. Some SAS users may be familiar with the following code:

Code:

```
proc logistic data=r.analytic ;
     model ASTHMA4 (event='1') = DRKMONTHLY DRKWEEKLY;
run;
```

Others may be more familiar leaving out the `(event='1')` argument, and instead using the `descending` option, and asking for the OR and confidence intervals with the `/risklimits` option [111].

Code:

```
proc logistic data=r.analytic descending;
       model ASTHMA4= DRKMONTHLY DRKWEEKLY /risklimits;
run;
```

Both of these methods of running `PROC LOGISTIC` will produce default output consisting of several tables. We will examine a few of these here. The output table including the parameter estimates is repeated in Table 4.6.

TABLE 4.6

Output from `PROC LOGISTIC`: Parameter Estimates

Analysis of Maximum Likelihood Estimates					
Parameter	**DF**	**Estimate**	**Standard Error**	**Wald Chi-Square**	**Pr > ChiSq**
`Intercept`	1	−2.1744	0.0204	11340.2017	<0.0001
`DRKMONTHLY`	1	−0.2178	0.0315	47.7914	<0.0001
`DRKWEEKLY`	1	−0.2253	0.0427	27.8266	<0.0001

TABLE 4.7

Output from `PROC LOGISTIC`: Odds Ratios

Odds Ratio Estimates			
Effect	**Point Estimate**	**95% Wald Confidence Limits**	
DRKMONTHLY	0.804	0.756	0.856
DRKWEEKLY	0.798	0.734	0.868

TABLE 4.8

Output from `PROC LOGISTIC`: Model Fit Statistics

Model Fit Statistics		
Criterion	**Intercept Only**	**Intercept and Covariates**
AIC	35687.670	35633.106
SC	35696.640	35660.018
–2 Log L	35685.670	35627.106

The default `PROC LOGISTIC` code produces another table that displays the ORs and 95% confidence intervals, shown in Table 4.7. A third important table in the default output for SAS `PROC LOGISTIC` is the one containing model fit statistics, shown in Table 4.8. Notice this table includes the Akaike information criterion (AIC) as well as the –2 log likelihood, which we will revisit later, when we run logistic regression models in R.

R's default logistic regression output is leaner and requires more action from the programmer. First, to make the regression object, we use the same code as we did for linear regression; only for logistic regression, we designate the option for family as "`binomial`." To keep our logistic and linear models uniquely named, we will name the first logistic model `LogModel1` and look at a summary of the regression object.

Code:

```
LogModel1 <- glm(ASTHMA4 ~ DRKMONTHLY + DRKWEEKLY,
          data = analytic, family = "binomial")
summary(LogModel1)
```

Output:

```
Call:
glm(formula = ASTHMA4 ~ DRKMONTHLY + DRKWEEKLY, family = "binomial",
    data = analytic)
```

```
Deviance Residuals:
    Min        1Q    Median        3Q      Max
-0.4640   -0.4640   -0.4183   -0.4183   2.2301

Coefficients:
             Estimate Std.    Error   z value    Pr(>|z|)
(Intercept)    -2.17446      0.02042  -106.490    < 2e-16   ***
DRKMONTHLY     -0.21776      0.03150    -6.913   4.75e-12   ***
DRKWEEKLY      -0.22531      0.04271    -5.275   1.33e-07   ***
---
Signif. codes: 0 '***' 0.001 '**' 0.01 '*' 0.05 '.' 0.1 ' ' 1

(Dispersion parameter for binomial family taken to be 1)

    Null deviance: 35686 on 58130 degrees of freedom
Residual deviance: 35627 on 58128 degrees of freedom
AIC: 35633

Number of Fisher Scoring iterations: 5
```

Note that this default summary output for `LogModel1` includes the AIC at the bottom, but it does not include other model fit statistics, such as the –2 log likelihood. Also, no ORs or 95% confidence intervals are reported. Even so, it is clear from the output from both SAS and R that in the unadjusted model, both alcohol covariates are statistically significant, but it is hard to interpret the actual estimates from the R output because they are on the log odds scale.

With the help of the `devtools` and `broom` packages as demonstrated earlier, we can tidy the model and also add the ORs and confidence intervals manually. First, we will create the object `Tidy_LogModel1` by running the `tidy` command on `LogModel1`.

Code:

```
Tidy_LogModel1 <- tidy(LogModel1)
Tidy_LogModel1
```

Output:

```
         term  estimate  std.error   statistic       p.value
1 (Intercept) -2.174462 0.02041931 -106.490467  0.000000e+00
2  DRKMONTHLY -0.217762 0.03150066   -6.912934  4.747293e-12
3   DRKWEEKLY -0.225308 0.04271244   -5.274996  1.327589e-07
```

Now that the model is in tabular format in the object `Tidy_LogModel1`, we can actually add columns manually with our calculations. We will add the OR by exponentiating the log odds in the estimate column. We will also add the 95% confidence lower limits (LLs) and upper limits (ULs) for each parameter by exponentiating the log odds plus or minus the margin of error.

Code:

```
Tidy_LogModel1$OR <- exp(Tidy_LogModel1$estimate)
Tidy_LogModel1$LL <- exp(Tidy_LogModel1$estimate - (1.96 * Tidy_
      LogModel1$std.error))
Tidy_LogModel1$UL <- exp(Tidy_LogModel1$estimate + (1.96 * Tidy_
      LogModel1$std.error))
Tidy_LogModel1
```

Output:

```
         term  estimate  std.error   statistic      p.value        OR
1 (Intercept) -2.174462 0.02041931 -106.490467 0.000000e+00 0.1136692
2  DRKMONTHLY -0.217762 0.03150066   -6.912934 4.747293e-12 0.8043169
3   DRKWEEKLY -0.225308 0.04271244   -5.274996 1.327589e-07 0.7982703
      LL         UL
1 0.1092098  0.1183108
2 0.7561593  0.8555415
3 0.7341629  0.8679757
```

We observe that both exposure variables are statistically significant in the unadjusted model. Interestingly, both alcohol variables are associated with a significantly lower odds of having asthma compared to the reference group, nondrinkers. Perhaps we should order a beer after all.

As we did with linear regression, let us proceed down our Table 1 and introduce the next covariate. Age groups come next, so we will add them to `LogModel2`. Let us start with a summary of the regression object.

Code:

```
LogModel2 <- glm(ASTHMA4 ~ DRKMONTHLY + DRKWEEKLY +
                       AGE2 + AGE3 + AGE4 + AGE5 + AGE6,
                       data = analytic, family = "binomial")
summary(LogModel2)
```

Output:

```
Call:
glm(formula = ASTHMA4 ~ DRKMONTHLY + DRKWEEKLY + AGE2 + AGE3 +
      AGE4 + AGE5 + AGE6, family = "binomial", data = analytic)

Deviance Residuals:
    Min       1Q   Median       3Q      Max
-0.5045  -0.4458  -0.4421  -0.3992   2.2669
```

```
Coefficients:
            Estimate Std.   Error  z value  Pr(>|z|)
(Intercept) -2.05990      0.11239  -18.328   < 2e-16 ***
DRKMONTHLY  -0.23075      0.03172   -7.275  3.47e-13 ***
DRKWEEKLY   -0.23092      0.04278   -5.398  6.74e-08 ***
AGE2         0.01444      0.12877    0.112    0.9107
AGE3        -0.10272      0.12550   -0.818    0.4131
AGE4        -0.03423      0.11876   -0.288    0.7732
AGE5         0.06254      0.11550    0.541    0.5882
AGE6        -0.19894      0.11293   -1.762    0.0781 .
---
Signif. codes: 0 '***' 0.001 '**' 0.01 '*' 0.05 '.' 0.1 ' ' 1

(Dispersion parameter for binomial family taken to be 1)

    Null deviance: 35686 on 58130 degrees of freedom
Residual deviance: 35569 on 58123 degrees of freedom
AIC: 35585

Number of Fisher Scoring iterations: 5
```

None of the age variables performed in this model, so they would be left out of the next model. Some analysts might choose to keep `AGE6`, as it is approaching statistical significance in this model, with $p = 0.0781$. Instead, we will wait for later, and try to introduce `AGE6` back into a working model in round 2 of modeling. Let us add the covariate `MALE` to the next model, and not include the age variables.

Code:

```
LogModel3 <- glm(ASTHMA4 ~ DRKMONTHLY + DRKWEEKLY +
                     MALE, data=analytic, family = "binomial")
summary(LogModel3)
```

Output:

```
Call:
glm(formula = ASTHMA4 ~ DRKMONTHLY + DRKWEEKLY + MALE, family
    = "binomial",
    data = analytic)

Deviance Residuals:
    Min       1Q    Median       3Q      Max
-0.6033  -0.4471  -0.4062  -0.4041   2.2564
```

```
Coefficients:
             Estimate Std.   Error  z value  Pr(>|z|)
(Intercept)   -1.61155  0.04104  -39.270   < 2e-16 ***
DRKMONTHLY    -0.21149  0.03157   -6.699   2.1e-11 ***
DRKWEEKLY     -0.20094  0.04283   -4.692   2.7e-06 ***
MALE          -0.64106  0.04176  -15.353   < 2e-16 ***
---
Signif. codes: 0 '***' 0.001 '**' 0.01 '*' 0.05 '.' 0.1 ' ' 1

(Dispersion parameter for binomial family taken to be 1)

    Null deviance: 35686  on 58130  degrees of freedom
Residual deviance: 35569  on 58123  degrees of freedom
AIC: 35424

Number of Fisher Scoring iterations: 5
```

MALE is highly significant in this model. Out of curiosity, we may want to see the OR and 95% confidence interval for this estimate. We would have to develop the tidy model to do that.

Code:

```
library (devtools)
library (broom)
Tidy_LogModel3 <- tidy(LogModel3)
Tidy_LogModel3$OR <- exp(Tidy_LogModel3$estimate)
Tidy_LogModel3$LL <- exp(Tidy_LogModel3$estimate - (1.96 * Tidy_LogModel3$std.error))
Tidy_LogModel3$UL <- exp(Tidy_LogModel3$estimate + (1.96 * Tidy_LogModel3$std.error))
Tidy_LogModel3
```

Output:

```
         term   estimate std.error  statistic      p.value        OR        LL        UL
1 (Intercept) -1.6115466 0.04103732 -39.270270 0.000000e+00 0.1995787 0.1841546 0.2162947
2 DRKMONTHLY  -0.2114925 0.03157108  -6.698933 2.099473e-11 0.8093753 0.7608098 0.8610409
3  DRKWEEKLY  -0.2009432 0.04282559  -4.692128 2.703776e-06 0.8179589 0.7521035 0.8895807
4       MALE  -0.6410638 0.04175530 -15.352872 3.388461e-53 0.5267318 0.4853407 0.5716528
```

Like with our alcohol variables, being male is associated with lower odds of asthma compared to being female. Let us retain MALE in the model, and add HISPANIC in the next model.

Code:

```
LogModel4 <- glm(ASTHMA4 ~ DRKMONTHLY + DRKWEEKLY +
          MALE + HISPANIC, data=analytic, family = "binomial")
summary(LogModel4)
```

Output:

```
Call:
glm(formula = ASTHMA4 ~ DRKMONTHLY + DRKWEEKLY + MALE + HISPANIC,
    family = "binomial", data = analytic)

Deviance Residuals:
      Min        1Q    Median        3Q       Max
  -0.6297   -0.4463   -0.4054   -0.4034    2.2579

Coefficients:
             Estimate Std.  Error    z value       Pr(>|z|)
(Intercept)  -1.61816      0.04132    -39.165      < 2e-16 ***
DRKMONTHLY   -0.21113      0.03157     -6.687     2.27e-11 ***
DRKWEEKLY    -0.20066      0.04283     -4.685     2.79e-06 ***
MALE         -0.63848      0.04180    -15.275      < 2e-16 ***
HISPANIC      0.10063      0.07068      1.424        0.154
---
Signif. codes: 0 '***' 0.001 '**' 0.01 '*' 0.05 '.' 0.1 ' ' 1

(Dispersion parameter for binomial family taken to be 1)

    Null deviance: 35686 on 58130 degrees of freedom
Residual deviance: 35414 on 58126 degrees of freedom
AIC: 35424

Number of Fisher Scoring iterations: 5
```

Unlike MALE, HISPANIC does not perform in the model, so we will not retain it for the next iteration. Following the order of covariates in Table 1, let us add the race variables to the next model.

Code:

```
LogModel5 <- glm(ASTHMA4 ~ DRKMONTHLY + DRKWEEKLY +
        MALE + BLACK + ASIAN + OTHRACE, data=analytic, family = "binomial")
summary(LogModel5)
```

Output:

```
Call:
glm(formula = ASTHMA4 ~ DRKMONTHLY + DRKWEEKLY + MALE + BLACK +
    ASIAN + OTHRACE, family = "binomial", data = analytic)

Deviance Residuals:
    Min         1Q     Median        3Q       Max
-0.6998   -0.4398   -0.4014   -0.3991    2.2671
```

```
Coefficients:
              Estimate Std.   Error    z value     Pr(>|z|)
(Intercept)    -1.66564     0.04252   -39.176     < 2e-16 ***
DRKMONTHLY     -0.20307     0.03163    -6.421    1.35e-10 ***
DRKWEEKLY      -0.19115     0.04288    -4.458    8.29e-06 ***
MALE           -0.62148     0.04204   -14.782     < 2e-16 ***
BLACK           0.09428     0.05497     1.715      0.0863 .
ASIAN           0.01738     0.14814     0.117      0.9066
OTHRACE         0.38336     0.05469     7.010    2.39e-12 ***
---
Signif. codes: 0 '***' 0.001 '**' 0.01 '*' 0.05 '.' 0.1 ' ' 1

(Dispersion parameter for binomial family taken to be 1)

    Null deviance: 35686 on 58130 degrees of freedom
Residual deviance: 35370 on 58124 degrees of freedom
AIC: 35384

Number of Fisher Scoring iterations: 5
```

Of the race variables, only the OTHRACE variable was statistically significant. The BLACK variable approaches significance with $p = 0.0863$; it will be up to the analyst as to whether or not to retain or discard this variable at this point. However, ASIAN is clearly not significant, and should not be retained in the model.

Notice that through these first five iterations, our exposure variables remained statistically significant in the model. They produce ORs and associated 95% confidence intervals between 0.7 and 0.9, which describe meaningfully lower odds for the alcohol groups. Some analysts monitor the changes in the estimates for the log odds and the ORs of the exposure variables from model to model, and this guides them as to whether or not to include a confounder. There is a "10% rule," which means that if adding a confounder changes the log odds estimate of the exposure by more than 10%, the confounder should be kept in the model [112]. There is no statistical test for confounding [113]; which covariates to include in a model need to be selected carefully on the basis of the analyst's knowledge and experience, as well as understanding of the data.

Selecting the Final Logistic Regression Model

As with linear regression, it is helpful for model selection to document logistic regression model metadata. Table 4.9 shows an example of a metadata table that documents the model number, covariates in the model, significant covariates, and comments about modeling decisions.

TABLE 4.9

Logistic Regression Model Metadata

Model	Covariates	Significant Covariates	Comments
1	DRKMONTHLY + DRKWEEKLY	DRKMONTHLY and DRKWEEKLY	Add age covariates
2	DRKMONTHLY + DRKWEEKLY + AGE2 + AGE3 + AGE4 + AGE5 + AGE6	DRKMONTHLY and DRKWEEKLY	Remove age covariates, add MALE
3	DRKMONTHLY + DRKWEEKLY + MALE	DRKMONTHLY and DRKWEEKLY, MALE	Retain MALE, add HISPANIC
4	DRKMONTHLY + DRKWEEKLY + MALE + HISPANIC	DRKMONTHLY and DRKWEEKLY, MALE	Remove HISPANIC, add race variables
5	DRKMONTHLY + DRKWEEKLY + MALE + BLACK + ASIAN + OTHRACE	DRKMONTHLY and DRKWEEKLY, MALE, OTHRACE	Remove all race variables except OTHRACE
37	DRKMONTHLY+ DRKWEEKLY + AGE2 + AGE5 + MALE + OTHRACE + NEVERMAR + LOWED + INC1 + INC2 + INC3 + INC4 + OVWT + OBESE + SMOKER + NOEXER + FAIRHLTH + POORHLTH		Final model

As can be seen in Table 4.9, we chose `Model37` as the final model, which is shown below.

Code:

```
LogModel37 <- glm(ASTHMA4 ~ DRKMONTHLY + DRKWEEKLY + AGE2 + AGE5
               + MALE + OTHRACE + NEVERMAR + LOWED + INC1
               + INC2 + INC3 + INC4 + OVWT + OBESE + SMOKER
               + NOEXER + FAIRHLTH + POORHLTH, data=analytic,
               family = "binomial")
summary(LogModel37)
```

Output:

```
Call:
glm(formula = ASTHMA4 ~ DRKMONTHLY + DRKWEEKLY + AGE2 + AGE5 +
    MALE + OTHRACE + NEVERMAR + LOWED + INC1 + INC2 + INC3 +
    INC4 + OVWT + OBESE + SMOKER + NOEXER + FAIRHLTH + POORHLTH,
    family = "binomial", data = analytic)
```

```
Deviance Residuals:
    Min        1Q     Median        3Q       Max
-1.1261   -0.4611   -0.3797   -0.3524   2.4401

Coefficients:
             Estimate Std.   Error      z value     Pr(>|z|)
(Intercept)  -2.01721        0.05779    -34.905      < 2e-16 ***
DRKMONTHLY   -0.05562        0.03288     -1.691     0.090747 .
DRKWEEKLY    -0.01590        0.04398     -0.361     0.717737
AGE2          0.14272        0.06906      2.067     0.038764 *
AGE5          0.09847        0.03649      2.699     0.006961 **
MALE         -0.65587        0.04341    -15.109      < 2e-16 ***
OTHRACE       0.25930        0.05559      4.665     3.09e-06 ***
NEVERMAR      0.21803        0.09672      2.254     0.024190 *
LOWED        -0.11314        0.03254     -3.477     0.000506 ***
INC1          0.40255        0.08505      4.733     2.21e-06 ***
INC2          0.32023        0.06720      4.765     1.88e-06 ***
INC3          0.33256        0.05732      5.802     6.55e-09 ***
INC4          0.13466        0.05136      2.622     0.008742 **
OVWT          0.06397        0.03737      1.712     0.086895 .
OBESE         0.30667        0.03866      7.932     2.16e-15 ***
SMOKER        0.06826        0.04018      1.699     0.089354 .
NOEXER       -0.08294        0.03424     -2.422     0.015431 *
FAIRHLTH      0.61732        0.03775     16.353      < 2e-16 ***
POORHLTH      0.91681        0.05010     18.298      < 2e-16 ***
---
Signif. codes: 0 '***' 0.001 '**' 0.01 '*' 0.05 '.' 0.1 ' ' 1

(Dispersion parameter for binomial family taken to be 1)

    Null deviance: 35686 on 58130 degrees of freedom
Residual deviance: 34537 on 58112 degrees of freedom
AIC: 34575

Number of Fisher Scoring iterations: 5
```

Observing the final model results, we can now interpret the model to answer our hypothesis. Again, our hypothesis that alcohol consumption is associated with asthma status in veterans was not supported. After adjustment for the confounders in the model, neither `DRKWEEKLY` nor `DRKMONTHLY` were statistically significance.

During SS modeling, choices about adding, retaining, or discarding covariates can usually be made based on observing the behavior of the ORs and the levels of significance of the covariates from model to model. However, if there are competing sets of variables, or variables appear to be collinear, model fit statistics may need to be used to split hairs and make final decisions.

An instructive example can be made when trying to figure out the best way to model a continuous independent variable. Imagine the following logistic regression hypothesis: Among veterans, after controlling for confounders, sleep duration will be significantly associated with poor health (POORHLTH). In this case, we could choose to use the same analytic dataset we have, but our exposure would be sleep duration. This means we could use SLEPTIM2 continuously as the exposure-independent variable that is always present in the model, or we could categorize it different ways, such as in quartiles. Comparing nested models is a method that can guide a decision like this.

Let us define Model A as a "base model," with the dependent variable POORHLTH, and the confounding variables AGE2 through AGE6 and MALE. In Model B, we keep all the covariates in Model A, but add SLEPTIM2. We could say that Model A is "nested" in Model B, because Model B contains all the covariates of Model A as well as others. Model C could be the same as Model B, but with indicator variables for sleep quartiles. Again, Model A would be nested in Model C.

The code below uses the quartile code reviewed in Chapter 2 to make a grouping variables for sleep quartiles, called SLEPQUART.

Code:

```
SLEPTIM2Quartiles <- quantile(analytic$SLEPTIM2, na.rm=TRUE, prob = c(0.25, 0.50, 0.75))

analytic$SLEPQUART <- NA
analytic$SLEPQUART[analytic$SLEPTIM2 <= SLEPTIM2Quartiles[1]] <- 1
analytic$SLEPQUART[(analytic$SLEPTIM2 > SLEPTIM2Quartiles[1]) &
        analytic$SLEPTIM2 <= SLEPTIM2Quartiles[2]] <- 2
analytic$SLEPQUART[(analytic$SLEPTIM2 > SLEPTIM2Quartiles[2]) &
        analytic$SLEPTIM2 <= SLEPTIM2Quartiles[3]] <- 3
analytic$SLEPQUART[analytic$SLEPTIM2 > SLEPTIM2Quartiles[3]] <- 4

table(analytic$SLEPTIM2, analytic$SLEPQUART, useNA = c("always"))
```

The top quartile, quartile 4, is assumed to be the healthiest quartile, so it will be chosen for the reference group. The code below adds SLEPQT1, SLEPQT2, and SLEPQT3 for quartiles 1 through 3 of SLEPTIM2.

Code:

```
analytic$SLEPQT1 <- 0
analytic$SLEPQT1[analytic$SLEPQUART == 1] <- 1
analytic$SLEPQT2 <- 0
analytic$SLEPQT2[analytic$SLEPQUART == 2] <- 1
analytic$SLEPQT3 <- 0
analytic$SLEPQT3[analytic$SLEPQUART == 3] <- 1

table(analytic$SLEPQUART, analytic$SLEPQT1, useNA = c("always"))
table(analytic$SLEPQUART, analytic$SLEPQT2, useNA = c("always"))
table(analytic$SLEPQUART, analytic$SLEPQT3, useNA = c("always"))
```

Below is the code that would be used to make all three regressions into objects named `ModelA`, `ModelB`, and `ModelC`, and display them. `ModelB` uses `SLEPTIM2` (sleep duration, continuous) and `ModelC` uses `SLEPQT1`, `SLEPQT2`, and `SLEPQT3` (sleep duration, quartiles).

Model A
Code:

```
ModelA <- glm(POORHLTH ~ AGE2 + AGE3 + AGE4 + AGE5 + AGE6 +
                    MALE, data=analytic, family = "binomial")
summary(ModelA)
```

Output:

```
Call:
glm(formula = POORHLTH ~ AGE2 + AGE3 + AGE4 + AGE5 + AGE6 + MALE,
    family = "binomial", data = analytic)

Deviance Residuals:
    Min        1Q    Median        3Q       Max
-0.4172   -0.3743   -0.3743   -0.2996    3.2343

Coefficients:
            Estimate Std.  Error   z value   Pr(>|z|)
(Intercept) -5.22505      0.45177  -11.566    < 2e-16 ***
AGE2         0.98072      0.47641    2.059     0.0395 *
AGE3         1.32658      0.46340    2.863     0.0042 **
AGE4         2.09669      0.45234    4.635   3.57e-06 ***
AGE5         2.77995      0.44965    6.183   6.31e-10 ***
AGE6         2.55426      0.44889    5.690   1.27e-08 ***
MALE         0.04723      0.06812    0.693     0.4881
---
Signif. codes: 0 '***' 0.001 '**' 0.01 '*' 0.05 '.' 0.1 ' ' 1

(Dispersion parameter for binomial family taken to be 1)

    Null deviance: 26832 on 58130 degrees of freedom
Residual deviance: 26333 on 58124 degrees of freedom
AIC: 26347

Number of Fisher Scoring iterations: 7
```

Model B
Code:

```
ModelB <- glm(POORHLTH ~ AGE2 + AGE3 + AGE4 + AGE5 + AGE6 + MALE +
                    SLEPTIM2, data=analytic, family = "binomial")
summary(ModelB)
```

Output:

```
Call:
glm(formula = POORHLTH ~ AGE2 + AGE3 + AGE4 + AGE5 + AGE6 + MALE +
    SLEPTIM2, family = "binomial", data = analytic)

Deviance Residuals:
    Min       1Q    Median       3Q      Max
-0.5473  -0.3946  -0.3620  -0.2988   3.2675

Coefficients:
              Estimate Std. Error z value Pr(>|z|)
(Intercept)   -4.59690    0.45838 -10.029  < 2e-16 ***
AGE2           0.97466    0.47644   2.046  0.04079 *
AGE3           1.33573    0.46344   2.882  0.00395 **
AGE4           2.11626    0.45238   4.678 2.90e-06 ***
AGE5           2.81983    0.44971   6.270 3.60e-10 ***
AGE6           2.64134    0.44905   5.882 4.05e-09 ***
MALE           0.05271    0.06814   0.773  0.43924
SLEPTIM2      -0.09866    0.01238  -7.972 1.56e-15 ***
---
Signif. codes: 0 '***' 0.001 '**' 0.01 '*' 0.05 '.' 0.1 ' ' 1

(Dispersion parameter for binomial family taken to be 1)

    Null deviance: 26832 on 58130 degrees of freedom
Residual deviance: 26269 on 58123 degrees of freedom
AIC: 26285

Number of Fisher Scoring iterations: 7
```

Model C

Code:

```
ModelC <- glm(POORHLTH ~ AGE2 + AGE3 + AGE4 + AGE5 + AGE6 +
                             MALE + SLEPQT1 + SLEPQT2 +
      SLEPQT3, data=analytic, family = "binomial")
summary(ModelC)
```

Output:

```
Call:
glm(formula = POORHLTH ~ AGE2 + AGE3 + AGE4 + AGE5 + AGE6 + MALE +
   SLEPQT1 + SLEPQT2 + SLEPQT3, family = "binomial", data = analytic)

Deviance Residuals:
    Min       1Q    Median       3Q      Max
-0.5349  -0.4766  -0.3271  -0.2593   3.3544
```

```
Coefficients:
             Estimate Std.   Error z      value     Pr(>|z|)
(Intercept)    -4.82440    0.45423    -10.621     < 2e-16 ***
AGE2            1.00079    0.47670      2.099     0.03578 *
AGE3            1.37564    0.46368      2.967     0.00301 **
AGE4            2.18133    0.45260      4.820    1.44e-06 ***
AGE5            2.89338    0.44991      6.431    1.27e-10 ***
AGE6            2.72102    0.44926      6.057    1.39e-09 ***
MALE            0.05892    0.06863      0.858     0.39064
SLEPQT1        -0.07346    0.05083     -1.445     0.14841
SLEPQT2        -1.33170    0.06269    -21.244     < 2e-16 ***
SLEPQT3        -0.85699    0.05466    -15.680     < 2e-16 ***
---
Signif. codes: 0 '***' 0.001 '**' 0.01 '*' 0.05 '.' 0.1 ' ' 1

(Dispersion parameter for binomial family taken to be 1)

    Null deviance: 26832 on 58130 degrees of freedom
Residual deviance: 25450 on 58121 degrees of freedom
AIC: 25470

Number of Fisher Scoring iterations: 7
```

Notice that in Model B, `SLEPTIM2` is significant, and in Model C, the second and third quartiles of sleep are significant. This means that it is not clear which way sleep duration should be modeled. We can use a nested model comparison to help inform that decision. To do this, we will need the –2 log likelihood of each model.

In SAS, the –2 log likelihood and degrees of freedom for each model are printed on the `PROC LOGISTIC` output, but that is not the case in R. However, R has a package called `nlme`, which has commands we can use on the regression objects that will output this information [114]. We will use the `logLik` command on each model to get the –2 log likelihood and the degrees of freedom.

Code:

```
library(nlme)

logLik(ModelA)
logLik(ModelB)
logLik(ModelC)
```

Output:

```
'log Lik.' -13166.44 (df=7)
'log Lik.' -13134.31 (df=8)
'log Lik.' -12725.08 (df=10)
```

TABLE 4.10

Models to Be Compared

Model	Model Covariates	−2 Log Likelihood	DF	Comment
A	AGE2 + AGE3 + AGE4 + AGE5 + AGE6 + MALE	−13,166	7	Base model
B	AGE2 + AGE3 + AGE4 + AGE5 + AGE6 + MALE + SLEPTIM2	−13,134	8	Includes SLEPTIM2
C	AGE2 + AGE3 + AGE4 + AGE5 + AGE6 + MALE + SLEPQT1 + SLEPQT2 + SLEPQT3	−12,725	10	Includes sleep duration quartiles

Before making our comparisons, we first should assemble a table of our model results. These are displayed in Table 4.10.

Our next step is to compare nested models. To do this, we first find the difference in −2 log likelihood measures between Model B and Model A (nested models), and we also find the difference in the degrees of freedom between them. Next, we do the same for Model C versus Model A, also nested models. These differences are shown in Table 4.11.

As can be seen in Table 4.10, the difference in −2 log likelihood results between Model B and Model 8 is 18, and in Table 4.11, the difference between Model C and Model A is 42. The differences in degrees of freedom are 1 for the first comparison, and 3 for the second comparison (because the quartile indicator variables add degrees of freedom). Our question is—which way, Model B or Model C, gives us the biggest bang for our buck? Which way of putting sleep duration into the model makes the most difference to the base model?

We can answer this question by putting the differences for each model in −2 log likelihoods and degrees of freedom on the chi-square distribution, and see which set of answers gives us the smallest *p*-value. To do this, we can use the `pchisq` command in R. The `pchisq` command takes in the arguments of the value (in this case, of the difference in −2 log likelihoods) and the degrees of freedom value (in this case, of the difference in degrees of freedom between models), and outputs the cumulative distribution function. Because we want the *p*-value, we can get that by subtracting that result from 1.

TABLE 4.11

Model Comparisons

Models in Comparison	−2 Log Likelihood Difference	DF Difference	Chi-Squared P-Value
B versus A	32	1	0.0000
C versus A	441	3	0.0000

Code:

```
1-pchisq(18, df = 1)
1-pchisq(42, df = 3)
```

Output:

```
[1] 2.20905e-05
[1] 4.012127e-09
```

The results show that the second *p*-value is the smallest. This would suggest that quartiles would be a better way to model sleep duration. Further, as shown in Model C's results, `SLEPQT2` was not statistically significant in that model. By having indicator variables for quartiles instead of a continuous variable, if there is a threshold effect—meaning sleep duration has to be at a certain level before any effect is seen—it can be detected.

This type of comparison is used for splitting hairs. Another comparison that can be used for such hairsplitting is the AIC, which comes out on both SAS and R logistic output automatically, and does not require nested models for comparisons. Please note that AIC is a relative comparison between models, meaning that there is no perfect goal AIC number. Contrast this to adjusted R-squared in linear regression, where a perfect score would be 1.0.

A few other issues can come up in final logistic regression model selection. Once in a while, the exposure is so related to the outcome, that there is "partial" or "complete separation of points." Imagine if everyone in our dataset who had asthma was a nondrinker and everyone who did not have asthma was either a weekly or monthly drinker. This would cause complete separation of points, and the model would break and not converge. This would be a shame because, in reality, the exposure is very strongly related to the outcome, and we wish we could reflect that in a model. Therefore, if this happens, we can create a logistic regression using the Firth correction, which adds a little number to the cells that are empty, allowing the model to converge. The Firth correction can be applied by creating the regression object using the `logistf` command in the `logistf` package in R [115].

As with the linear regression demonstration, our logistic regression model showed our hypothesis was not supported. The same issues with risking fishing by adding interaction terms at this point apply to logistic regression as well as linear regression. As with linear regression, if interactions between confounders and exposure variables were introduced into the model at this point, found to be significant, and therefore retained, stratum-specific estimates would need to be presented for each group in the interaction, making presentation complicated. For example, imagine we interacted `MALE` with `DRKWEEKLY` and `DRKMONTHLY`, and both interaction terms were statistically significant. This means that for each variable, `DRKWEEKLY` and `DRKMONTHLY`, we would have to present a separate odds ratio for men and women.

If these concerns are real, one solution is to run logistic regression models separately, one on each group. To carry on with the example, it might be more informative to split the dataset into one for women and one for men, and fit separate models. If biologically, something is very different between the groups, causing each of them to have a unique relationship with the exposure and outcome (making the interaction term significant), then it might be wise to develop a unique model for each group. There may be other relationships between exposure and outcome within the group that need to be dealt with differently.

It is always possible to set up a hypothesis of an interaction, in which case modeling an interaction would be clearly not fishing. Imagine we had indeed hypothesized that not only was asthma associated with alcohol consumption status, but that relationship varied by Hispanic ethnicity. Then the following interaction model could be run:

Code:

```
LogModelExample <- glm(ASTHMA4 ~ DRKMONTHLY + DRKWEEKLY + HISPANIC
       + (HISPANIC*DRKMONTHLY) + (HISPANIC*DRKWEEKLY), data=analytic,
       family = "binomial")
summary(LogModelExample)
```

Output:

```
Call:
glm(formula = ASTHMA4 ~ DRKMONTHLY + DRKWEEKLY + HISPANIC +(HISPANIC *
    DRKMONTHLY) + (HISPANIC * DRKWEEKLY), family = "binomial",
    data = analytic)

Deviance Residuals:
    Min        1Q    Median       3Q      Max
-0.4817   -0.4634   -0.4171   -0.4157   2.2450

Coefficients:
                     Estimate Std.  Error     z value  Pr(>|z|)
(Intercept)          -2.17720       0.02087   -104.319   < 2e-16 ***
DRKMONTHLY           -0.22817       0.03225     -7.076  1.49e-12 ***
DRKWEEKLY            -0.22118       0.04354     -5.080  3.78e-07 ***
HISPANIC              0.06567       0.10092      0.651     0.515
DRKMONTHLY:HISPANIC   0.24426       0.15121      1.615     0.106
DRKWEEKLY:HISPANIC   -0.10341       0.22469     -0.460     0.645
---
Signif. codes: 0 '***' 0.001 '**' 0.01 '*' 0.05 '.' 0.1 ' ' 1

(Dispersion parameter for binomial family taken to be 1)

       Null deviance: 35686 on 58130 degrees of freedom
Residual deviance: 35620 on 58125 degrees of freedom
AIC: 35632

Number of Fisher Scoring iterations: 5
```

Notice how the interaction terms were introduced in the code. They were added as a multiplication equation in parentheses. Notice also how the parameter estimates are labeled on the output. This model shows that the interaction terms were not statistically significant, which means no evidence of interaction.

This part of the section discusses some issues with selecting the final model. As we have already selected `Model37` as our final model, let us move on to presenting the model.

Logistic Regression Model Presentation

As with linear regression, logistic regression models need to be presented, and Table 4.12 shows one presentation style.

As was done with linear regression, an unadjusted model is presented as Model 1 and a model with just age and sex variables is presented as Model 2. The final model (`Model37` from our modeling) is presented as Model 3. This time, for each category and level, under each model column, we record the OR and 95% confidence interval if the set of covariates are in the model, and NA if they are not. We write Reference for every level that ends up in the reference group. As we saw from our output, the confidence intervals for our exposure variables in Model 3 all contain 1, so they are not significant.

To make this table, like we did with linear regression, we would want to output these measurements as a *.csv. In SAS, like we did in linear regression, we can use the ODS to output the parameter estimates from our final model, `Model37`, and then export that as a *.csv.

Code:

```
proc logistic data=r.analytic ;
      model ASTHMA4 (event='1') = DRKMONTHLY DRKWEEKLY AGE2
            AGE5 MALE
            OTHRACE NEVERMAR LOWED INC1 INC2 INC3 INC4
            OVWT OBESE SMOKER NOEXER FAIRHLTH POORHLTH;
      ods output ParameterEstimates = LogModel37;
run;

PROC EXPORT DATA= WORK.LogModel37
          OUTFILE= "C:\Users\Monika\Dropbox\R Stats Book\
                Analytics\Data\SAS_LogModel37.csv"
          DBMS=CSV REPLACE;
     PUTNAMES=YES;
RUN;
```

Table 4.13 shows the resulting format of the *.csv.

The SAS output has the log odds of the estimates. This means that we would have to do some post-processing with these results to get the ORs and

TABLE 4.12

Final Logistic Regression Model Presentation

		Model 1: Unadjusted		Model 2: Adjusted for Age and Sex		Model 3: Fully Adjusted	
Category	**Level**	**Odds Ratio**	**95% Confidence Interval**	**Odds Ratio**	**95% Confidence Interval**	**Odds Ratio**	**95% Confidence Interval**
Alcohol status	Nondrinker	Reference	Reference	Reference	Reference	Reference	Reference
	Monthly drinker	1.01	0.92–1.10	0.99	0.91–1.08	0.96	0.88–1.05
	Weekly drinker	1.25	1.15–1.36	1.22	1.13–1.33	1.02	0.93–1.11
Sex	Male	NA	NA	0.54	0.50–0.59	0.52	0.48–0.57
	Female	NA	NA	Reference	Reference	Reference	Reference
Age	Age 18–24	NA	NA	Reference	Reference	Reference	Reference
	Age 25–34	NA	NA	1.00	0.77–1.29	1.15	1.01–1.32
	Age 35–44	NA	NA	0.89	0.69–1.14	Reference	Reference
	Age 45–54	NA	NA	0.97	0.77–1.23	Reference	Reference
	Age 55–64	NA	NA	1.11	0.89–1.40	1.10	1.03–1.19
	Age 65 or older	NA	NA	0.91	0.73–1.14	Reference	Reference
Race	White	NA	NA	NA	NA	Reference	Reference
	Black/African American	NA	NA	NA	NA	Reference	Reference
	Asian	NA	NA	NA	NA	Reference	Reference
	Other race/multi-racial[a]	NA	NA	NA	NA	1.30	1.16–1.45
	Unknown race	NA	NA	NA	NA	Reference	Reference
Marital status	Currently married	NA	NA	NA	NA	Reference	Reference

(Continued)

TABLE 4.12 (*Continued*)

Final Logistic Regression Model Presentation

		Model 1: Unadjusted		Model 2: Adjusted for Age and Sex		Model 3: Fully Adjusted	
Category	Level	Odds Ratio	95% Confidence Interval	Odds Ratio	95% Confidence Interval	Odds Ratio	95% Confidence Interval
	Divorced, widowed, separated	NA	NA	NA	NA	Reference	Reference
	Never married	NA	NA	NA	NA	1.24	1.03–1.50
	Not reported	NA	NA	NA	NA	Reference	Reference
Highest education level	Less than high school through high school graduate	NA	NA	NA	NA	0.89	0.84–0.95
	Some college/technical	NA	NA	NA	NA	Reference	Reference
	Four or more years of college	NA	NA	NA	NA	Reference	Reference
	Not reported	NA	NA	NA	NA	Reference	Reference
Annual household income	<$10k	NA	NA	NA	NA	1.50	1.27–1.77
	$10k to <$15k	NA	NA	NA	NA	1.38	1.21–1.57
	$15k to <$20k	NA	NA	NA	NA	1.39	1.25–1.56
	$20k to <$25k	NA	NA	NA	NA	1.14	1.03–1.27
	$25k to <$35k	NA	NA	NA	NA	Reference	Reference
	$35k to <$50k	NA	NA	NA	NA	Reference	Reference
	$50k to <$75k	NA	NA	NA	NA	Reference	Reference
	$75k or more	NA	NA	NA	NA	Reference	Reference

(*Continued*)

TABLE 4.12 (*Continued*)

Final Logistic Regression Model Presentation

Category	Level	Model 1: Unadjusted		Model 2: Adjusted for Age and Sex		Model 3: Fully Adjusted	
		Odds Ratio	95% Confidence Interval	Odds Ratio	95% Confidence Interval	Odds Ratio	95% Confidence Interval
	Not reported	NA	NA	NA	NA	Reference	Reference
Obesity status	Underweight	NA	NA	NA	NA	Reference	Reference
	Normal	NA	NA	NA	NA	Reference	Reference
	Overweight	NA	NA	NA	NA	1.07	0.99–1.15
	Obese	NA	NA	NA	NA	1.36	1.26–1.47
	Not reported	NA	NA	NA	NA	Reference	Reference
Smoking status	Smoker	NA	NA	NA	NA	1.07	0.99–1.16
	Nonsmoker	NA	NA	NA	NA	Reference	Reference
	Not reported	NA	NA	NA	NA	Reference	Reference
Exercise status	Exercised in the last month	NA	NA	NA	NA	Reference	Reference
	Did not exercise in the last month	NA	NA	NA	NA	1.09	1.02–1.16
General health	Excellent	NA	NA	NA	NA	Reference	Reference
	Very good	NA	NA	NA	NA	Reference	Reference
	Good	NA	NA	NA	NA	Reference	Reference
	Fair	NA	NA	NA	NA	1.85	1.72–2.00
	Poor	NA	NA	NA	NA	2.50	2.27–2.76
	Not reported	NA	NA	NA	NA	Reference	Reference

[a] Indicates other race or multiple racial groups.

TABLE 4.13

Parameter Estimates Output from `PROC LOGISTIC`

Variable	DF	Estimate	StdErr	WaldChiSq	ProbChiSq	_ESTTYPE_
Intercept	1	−2.0172	0.0578	1218.3568	<0.0001	MLE
DRKMONTHLY	1	−0.0556	0.0329	2.8608	0.0908	MLE
DRKWEEKLY	1	−0.0159	0.044	0.1307	0.7178	MLE
AGE2	1	0.1427	0.0691	4.2709	0.0388	MLE
AGE5	1	0.0985	0.0365	7.2828	0.007	MLE
MALE	1	−0.6559	0.0434	228.309	<0.0001	MLE
OTHRACE	1	0.2593	0.0556	21.7613	<0.0001	MLE
NEVERMAR	1	0.218	0.0967	5.082	0.0242	MLE
LOWED	1	−0.1131	0.0325	12.0915	0.0005	MLE
INC1	1	0.4026	0.085	22.4128	<0.0001	MLE
INC2	1	0.3203	0.0672	22.7141	<0.0001	MLE
INC3	1	0.3326	0.0573	33.6661	<0.0001	MLE
INC4	1	0.1347	0.0514	6.8742	0.0087	MLE
OVWT	1	0.064	0.0374	2.9309	0.0869	MLE
OBESE	1	0.3067	0.0387	62.9119	<0.0001	MLE
SMOKER	1	0.0683	0.0402	2.886	0.0894	MLE
NOEXER	1	−0.0829	0.0342	5.8664	0.0154	MLE
FAIRHLTH	1	0.6173	0.0378	267.4214	<0.0001	MLE
POORHLTH	1	0.9171	0.0501	335.0501	<0.0001	MLE

their 95% confidence intervals for presentation in a format like the one given in Table 4.12. By contrast, in R, we could use tidy model to assemble a table with our ORs and confidence intervals, and write this to a *.csv, as we did with our linear regression final model.

Code:

```
library (devtools)
library (broom)

Tidy_LogModel37 <- tidy(LogModel37)
Tidy_LogModel37$OR <- exp(Tidy_LogModel37$estimate)
Tidy_LogModel37$LL <- exp(Tidy_LogModel37$estimate - (1.96 *
      Tidy_LogModel37$std.error))
Tidy_LogModel37$UL <- exp(Tidy_LogModel37$estimate + (1.96 *
      Tidy_LogModel37$std.error))

write.csv(Tidy_LogModel37, "R_LogModel37.csv")
```

The result is Table 4.14. This format requires less post-processing in Excel to get the results into the format dictated by Table 4.12.

TABLE 4.14

Tidy Model Logistic Regression Output from R

	Term	Estimate	Std.error	Statistic	p.value	OR	LL	UL
1	(Intercept)	−2.01721	0.057791	−34.905	6.25E-267	0.133026	0.11878	0.148981
2	DRKMONTHLY	−0.05562	0.032885	−1.69147	0.090747	0.945895	0.886852	1.00887
3	DRKWEEKLY	−0.0159	0.043979	−0.36149	0.717737	0.984228	0.902942	1.072831
4	AGE2	0.142722	0.069059	2.066681	0.038764	1.153409	1.007394	1.320588
5	AGE5	0.098471	0.036488	2.698705	0.006961	1.103482	1.027321	1.18529
6	MALE	−0.65587	0.043409	−15.1091	1.41E-51	0.51899	0.47666	0.56508
7	OTHRACE	0.259302	0.055587	4.664752	3.09E-06	1.296025	1.162241	1.445208
8	NEVERMAR	0.218027	0.096725	2.254096	0.02419	1.24362	1.028855	1.503216
9	LOWED	−0.11314	0.032536	−3.47736	0.000506	0.893026	0.837855	0.95183
10	INC1	0.402547	0.08505	4.733072	2.21E-06	1.495629	1.265984	1.766932
11	INC2	0.320226	0.067198	4.765422	1.88E-06	1.377439	1.207459	1.571348
12	INC3	0.332564	0.057318	5.80206	6.55E-09	1.394539	1.246351	1.560346
13	INC4	0.134664	0.05136	2.621967	0.008742	1.144152	1.034583	1.265326
14	OVWT	0.063971	0.037366	1.71201	0.086895	1.066062	0.990776	1.147068
15	OBESE	0.306674	0.038664	7.931837	2.16E-15	1.358898	1.259725	1.465879
16	SMOKER	0.068263	0.040183	1.698814	0.089354	1.070647	0.98956	1.158378
17	NOEXER	−0.08294	0.034245	−2.4221	0.015431	0.920402	0.860653	0.9843
18	FAIRHLTH	0.617322	0.037751	16.35265	4.16E-60	1.853957	1.721733	1.996336
19	POORHLTH	0.916807	0.050104	18.29806	8.57E-75	2.501292	2.267331	2.759395

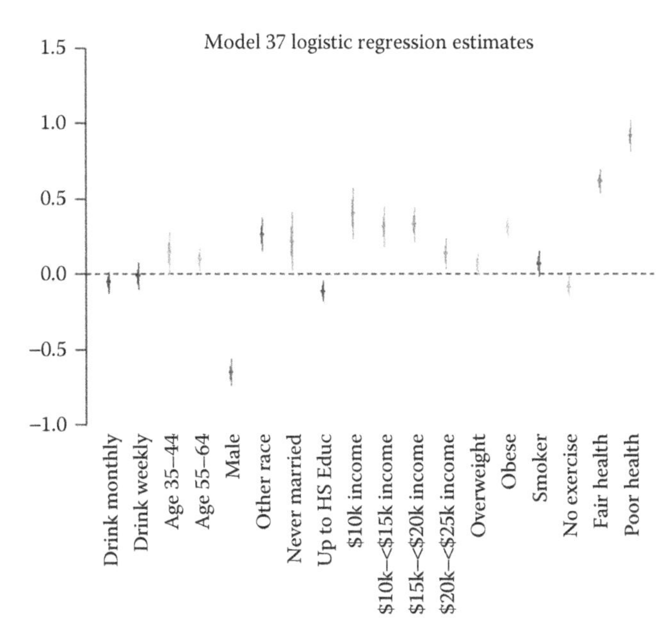

FIGURE 4.3
(See color insert.) Logistic regression coefficient plot of final model.

Plot to Assist Interpretation

As with linear regression, we may want to also create a coefficient plot to help us with interpretation. We will keep the plot on the log odds scale because it would look unbalanced on the OR scale. The following code makes Figure 4.3.

Code:

```
library(arm)
VarLabels=c("Intercept", "Drink Monthly", "Drink Weekly", "Age
35-44", "Age 55-64",
       "Male", "Other Race", "Never Married", "Up to HS Educ",
             "<$10k Income",
       "$10k-<$15k Income", "$15k-<$20k Income", "$20k-<$25k
             Income", "Overweight", "Obese",
       "Smoker", "No Exercise", "Fair Health", "Poor Health")
par(mai=c(1.5,0,0,0))
coefplot(LogModel37,
       vertical=FALSE,
       ylim=c(-1, 1.5),
       main="Model 37 Logistic Regression Estimates",
       varnames=VarLabels,
       col=c("darkblue", "darkblue",
             "darkorange", "darkorange",
```

```
"blueviolet",
"darkgreen",
"chocolate",
"blue4",
"azure4", "azure4", "azure4", "azure4",
"darkgoldenrod2", "darkgoldenrod2",
"darkred",
"cyan3",
"darkolivegreen4", "darkolivegreen4"))
```

Let us review the differences between this coefficient plot code and the code we used for the linear regression coefficient plot. First, our variable labels now reflect the covariates in our logistic model, not our linear model. Next, because some of our variable labels are long, it is helpful to set margins, which is done with the `par` (parameter) command. The `mai` parameter stands for "margins in inches," and the arguments are in the order of bottom, left, top, and right. Because the variable names were being cut off at the bottom of the plot, the margin is adjusted upward, whereas the others are left in the same place. The `ylim` option is adjusted to cover the y limits of where the values are plotted, and the colors are designated so that groups of indicator variables from the same domains are color-coded together.

Like with linear regression, a logistic regression coefficient plot can aid in the interpretation of results. A startling finding in this dataset of veterans is how being male is associated with a dramatically lower log odds of having asthma compared to being female. Another startling finding is how strongly lower income levels are associated with higher log odds of asthma. Obesity, fair health, and poor health also are strongly positively associated with having asthma.

Now that we have completed our linear and logistic regression models, we will turn to survival analysis regression.

Survival Analysis Regression

At this point, let us recall our survival analysis regression hypothesis: In veterans, alcohol consumption is associated with the survival experience of being diagnosed with asthma. Using `SurvAnalytic`, the survival dataset we developed in Chapter 2 will use the time variable `TIME80`, which means our time period is from birth to 80 years old, and the accompanying event variable, `ASTHMA80`, for age of asthma diagnosis, to demonstrate survival analysis regression.

First, we will make some decisions about how to proceed with SS survival analysis regression modeling. Next, SS survival analysis regression modeling will be discussed. How to develop a SS model using survival analysis will be described, along with considerations about final model selection. Finally, model presentation will be discussed.

Selecting a Parametric Distribution in Survival Analysis

In Chapter 3, we generated a Kaplan–Meier plot of the survival probabilities and conducted bivariate statistical tests. These are nonparametric in that they do not assume an underlying distribution. However, they are also descriptive and do not control for confounding variables. To create a multivariate survival analysis regression model that controls for confounders, we have to decide between conducting a parametric analysis (one assuming an underlying distribution) or a semiparametric analysis (Cox proportional hazard model). To help us make this decision, we will plot the survival curve along a parametric distribution and evaluate visually whether or not the survival curve really fits that distribution.

In SAS, as an example, we could plot the exponential distribution of our survival experience by alcohol group with the following `PROC LIFEREG` code.

Code:

```
PROC LIFEREG data=r.SurvAnalytic;
       MODEL TIME80*ASTHMA80(0)= ALCGRP /dist = exponential;
       PROBPLOT Cencolor=red cframe=ligr cfit=blue ppout
            npintervals=simul;
       INSET / cfill = white ctext = blue;
run;
```

Plot:

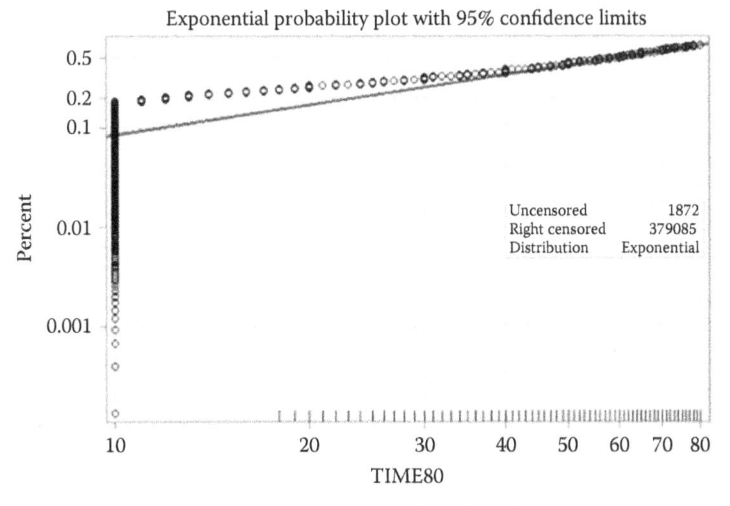

Notice how the circles on the plot represent events and the line on the plot represents a perfect exponential distribution. This plot suggests that data are not exponentially distributed, and so a parametric survival analysis should not be done using the exponential distribution. If we wanted to go on to explore whether the data fit a log-normal distribution in SAS, we could use the same code, but replace "`dist = exponential`" with "`dist = lnormal`." Other common parametric survival distributions to explore in those SAS and R include Weibull, gamma, and log-logistic [116].

In R, there are different options for plotting survival experience assuming a particular distribution; this book will demonstrate the capabilities of a new package, `flexsurv` [117] in making survival plots. We will start as we did above and create an exponential probability survival object in R using the `flexsurv` package.

Code:

```
fit_exp <- flexsurvreg(formula = Surv(TIME80, ASTHMA80) ~
      as.factor(ALCGRP), data = SurvAnalytic , dist="exp")
fit_exp
```

Output:

```
Call:
flexsurvreg(formula = Surv(TIME80, ASTHMA80) ~ as.factor(ALCGRP),
      data = SurvAnalytic, dist = "exp")

Estimates:
                   data mean  est         L95%        U95%        se
rate                      NA   1.10e-04    1.04e-04    1.17e-04    3.19e-06
as.factor(ALCGRP)2  3.68e-01  -4.88e-01   -5.92e-01   -3.84e-01    5.30e-02
as.factor(ALCGRP)3  1.40e-01  -6.22e-01   -7.81e-01   -4.62e-01    8.16e-02
                   exp(est)   L95%        U95%
rate                      NA          NA          NA
as.factor(ALCGRP)2  6.14e-01   5.53e-01    6.81e-01
as.factor(ALCGRP)3  5.37e-01   4.58e-01    6.30e-01

N = 380957, Events: 1872, Censored: 379085
Total time at risk: 21229089
Log-likelihood = -19286.5, df = 3
AIC = 38579
```

As can be seen above, the `fit_exp` survival object output provides parameter estimates. Instead of p-values, it shows 95% confidence intervals both for the estimate (the columns L95% and U95% that immediately follow the column "est") and for the exponentiated estimate (the L95% and U95% columns immediately following "exp(est)"). These results suggest that alcohol consumption is statistically significantly protective of survival without an asthma diagnosis. However, this output is not helpful in trying to decide whether or not to do a parametric survival analysis using the exponential distribution.

If the `summary` command is used on `fit_exp`, the output will be conditional probabilities listed for each `ALCGRP` level (not shown). It would be more informative to develop a plot as we did earlier, in SAS. In SAS, we compared the plotted survival probabilities (i.e., a Kaplan–Meier), compared those to a line representing the exponential distribution, and decided that they did not follow that distribution.

As our intention is to evaluate multiple potential parametric distributions, when we replicate this task in R, let us also include the log-normal distribution on the plot. To do this, we need to start by making a log-normal survival object. We will do that below, and call the object `fit_lnorm`.

Code:

```
library(flexsurv)
fit_lnorm <- flexsurvreg(formula = Surv(TIME80, ASTHMA80) ~
as.factor(ALCGRP), data = SurvAnalytic , dist="lnorm")
fit_lnorm
```

Output:

```
Call:
flexsurvreg(formula = Surv(TIME80, ASTHMA80) ~ as.factor(ALCGRP),
    data = SurvAnalytic, dist = "lnorm")

Estimates:
                     data mean  est      L95%     U95%     se       exp(est)
meanlog                  NA    11.8451  11.5152  12.1750   0.1683       NA
sdlog                    NA     3.1259   3.0001   3.2571   0.0655       NA
as.factor(ALCGRP)2   0.3685     0.5056   0.3931   0.6182   0.0574   1.6580
as.factor(ALCGRP)3   0.1398     0.6387   0.4711   0.8063   0.0855   1.8940
                      L95%      U95%
meanlog                  NA        NA
sdlog                    NA        NA
as.factor(ALCGRP)2   1.4815    1.8556
as.factor(ALCGRP)3   1.6017    2.2397

N = 380957, Events: 1872, Censored: 379085
Total time at risk: 21229089
Log-likelihood = -19240.96, df = 4
AIC = 38489.92
```

Note that the only difference in our code is naming the output object `fit_lnorm` instead of `fit_exp`, and in changing the distribution option to `dist = "lnorm."` As can be seen by the output above, the log-normal distribution model had a lower AIC than the exponential model, and also contradicts the findings from the exponential distribution model in terms of confidence intervals. Each level of alcohol consumption appears significantly risky here.

Now we will make a plot like we did in SAS, only this one will include not only the Kaplan–Meier and lines representing the exponential distribution but also lines representing the log-normal distribution for comparison. The following code visualizes objects `fit_exp` and `fit_lnorm` in a plot using the plot and lines commands from `flexsurv`.

Code:

```
plot(fit_lnorm,
        main="Comparison of Exponential and Log-Normal
                 Distributions\nTIME80 and AGE80",
        xlab="Years",
        ylab="Survival Probability",
        ymin=0.99,
        col="darkcyan",
        lwd=2,
        lty=1:3,
        firstx=10,
        xlim=c(10,80))
lines(fit_exp,
        ymin=0.99,
        col="darkorchid1",
        lwd=2,
        lty=1:3,
        firstx=10,
        xlim=c(10,80))
legend(x = "bottomleft",
        legend = c("Kaplan-Meier", "Log-normal",
        "Exponential"),
        lwd=2,
        col = c("black", "darkcyan", "darkorchid1"))
```

Figure 4.4 shows the results. In the code, note that plot starts by plotting the log-normal line from `fit_lnorm` in dark cyan, but then the "`lines`" command is used to layer on the dark orchid line, plotting the exponential distribution line from `fit_exp` on top of the plot. Regardless of the distribution specified in developing the survival object, the conditional probabilities are present in the object (as we saw when we used the `summary` command), and these are nonparametric. Ultimately, this

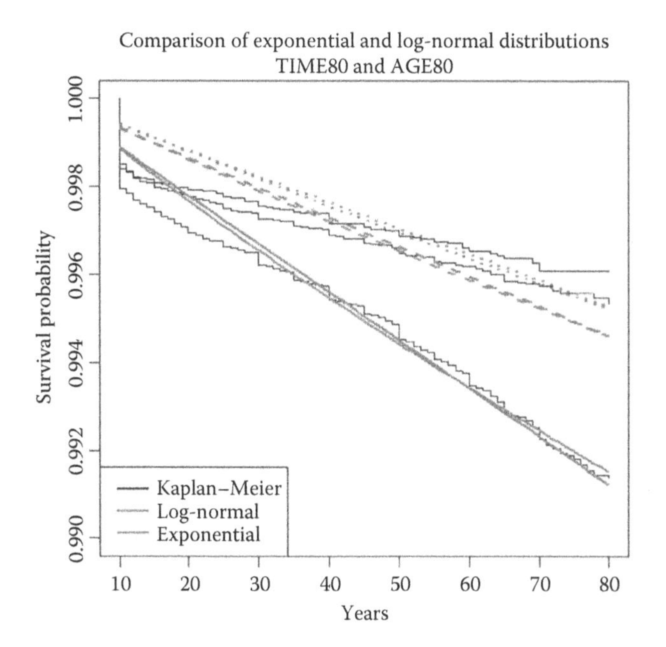

FIGURE 4.4
(See color insert.) Exponential and log-normal fitted survival probability plots.

plot includes a Kaplan–Meier drawn in black using the conditional probabilities from the `fit_lnorm` object, the log-normal fitted distribution drawn in dark cyan, and the exponential fitted distribution drawn in dark orchid, with the different alcohol groups using the same color-coding but drawn in three different line types (notice `lty=1:3` in the plot and `lines` code).

Also note that the legend has been moved to the bottom left through the option `x = "bottomleft"`. For visual simplicity, the different line types are not listed in the legend, but there are three—one for each alcohol consumption group. Because `ALCGRP = 1` is the nondrinkers, their line is solid (`lty=1`), and the other two levels will be two different types of dotted lines (`lty=2:3`). Also, please observe that the option that sets the line width of 2 (`lwd=2`) is required in the legend, even though it is default in the plots and lines commands above it. Without explicitly setting `lwd` (to 1 or another number) in the legend, no lines will print in the legend.

Looking at Figure 4.4, neither of these two distributions is an obvious choice. However, it is also hard to argue that they severely depart from either distribution. This can be a difficult choice for the analyst. But remember, we do not have to choose a distribution, after all. We could use a semiparametric

Cox proportional hazard regression, which will be demonstrated in the next part of this section.

Selecting a Semiparametric Distribution for Survival Analysis

If we wanted to explore using a semiparametric distribution for our survival analysis, we would want to start by graphing the hazards of each alcohol group to make sure they were proportional. Let us use the `survival` package to demonstrate this. Our first step is to call up the `survival` library and make an overall survival curve called `AllSurv`.

Code:

```
library(survival)
AllSurv <- with(SurvAnalytic,Surv(TIME80,ASTHMA80))
```

Next, we will create a proportional hazards survival object called `fit_cox`. We will do this using the `coxph` command from the survival library on the object `AllSurv` and include `as.factor(ALCGRP)`, so we can graph the hazard separated by alcohol groups.

Code:

```
fit_cox <- coxph(AllSurv ~ as.factor(ALCGRP),data=SurvAnalytic)
summary(fit_cox)
```

Output:

```
Call:
coxph(formula = AllSurv ~ as.factor(ALCGRP), data = SurvAnalytic)

  n= 380957, number of events= 1872

                       coef exp(coef)  se(coef)       z  Pr(>|z|)
as.factor(ALCGRP)2 -0.50166   0.60553   0.05313  -9.443   < 2e-16 ***
as.factor(ALCGRP)3 -0.63037   0.53240   0.08159  -7.726  1.11e-14 ***
---
Signif. codes: 0 '***' 0.001 '**' 0.01 '*' 0.05 '.' 0.1 ' ' 1

                   exp(coef)  exp(-coef)  lower .95  upper .95
as.factor(ALCGRP)2    0.6055       1.651     0.5456     0.6720
as.factor(ALCGRP)3    0.5324       1.878     0.4537     0.6247

Concordance= 0.56 (se = 0.006 )
Rsquare= 0 (max possible= 0.117 )
Likelihood ratio test= 130.7 on 2 df, p=0
Wald test = 125.2 on 2 df, p=0
Score (logrank) test = 128.3 on 2 df, p=0
```

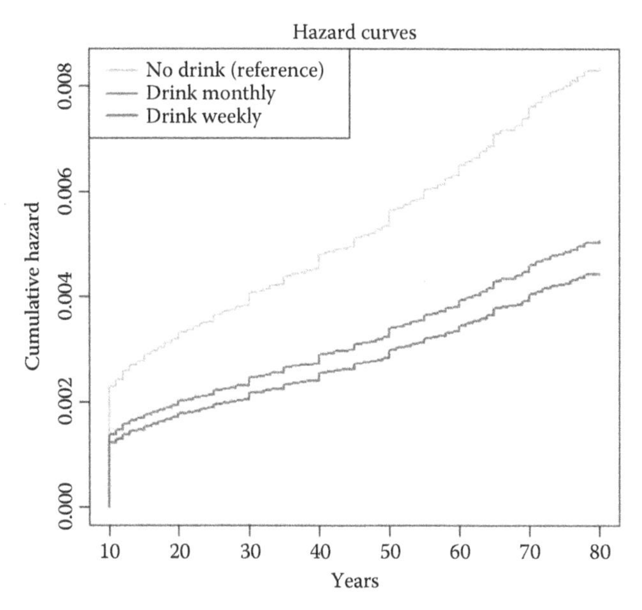

FIGURE 4.5
(See color insert.) Hazard curves.

We can use the plot command on `fit_cox` to plot the cumulative hazard. The code below produces Figure 4.5.

Code:

```
plot(survfit(fit_cox, newdata=data.frame(ALCGRP=1)),
        col="darkgoldenrod1",
        fun="cumhaz",
        main="Hazard Curves",
        xlab="Years",
        ylab="Cumulative Hazard",
        xlim=c(10,80),
        firstx=10,
        conf.int=FALSE,
        lwd=2)
lines(survfit(fit_cox,newdata=data.frame(ALCGRP=2)),
       col="darkcyan",
       fun="cumhaz",
       xlim=c(10,80),
       firstx=10,
       conf.int=FALSE,
       lwd=2)
```

```
lines(survfit(fit_cox,newdata=data.frame(ALCGRP=3)),
       col="darkorchid1",
       fun="cumhaz",
       xlim=c(10,80),
       firstx=10,
       conf.int=FALSE,
       lwd=2)
legend(x = "topleft",
       legend = c("No Drink (Reference)", "Drink Monthly",
       "Drink Weekly"),
       lwd=2,
       col=c("darkgoldenrod1", "darkcyan", "darkorchid1"))
```

Let us look at some features of this code. First, notice that the `lines` command is used similarly to how it was used in the `flexsurv` package—to layer lines onto an established plot. The code first plots the reference group in dark goldenrod and then the next two lines commands add `ALCGRP=2` and `ALCGRP=3` in dark cyan and dark orchid. In the `plot` command, we requested the cumulative hazard rather than the survival probabilities to be plotted through the function option, `fun="cumhaz."` Notice that for the lines to look correct on the plot, the same options need to be set for the lines as well as the plot, so the `fun="cumhaz"` has been added to not only the `plot` command but also to both the `line` commands. The option `conf.int=FALSE` turns off default confidence intervals, as these can clutter up the plot.

Viewing the cumulative hazard plot, we ask ourselves: Are these lines parallel? Does this plot suggest that our approach does not violate the assumption of proportional hazards? The lines look roughly parallel, so no, this plot does not suggest that the assumption of proportional hazards is violated. In this case, it would be reasonable to choose a Cox proportional hazard regression.

Introduction to Survival Analysis Regression Modeling

As with both linear and logistic regression, SS modeling in survival analysis involves two rounds. In the first, each candidate confounder is tried in the model along with the exposure variables, and after each iteration, choices are made as to which variables to discard. The result of round 1 is the working model, and all the discarded variables are tried again in the working model in round 2, and after each iteration, choices are made as to what variables to discard. The result is the final model, which is the one to be interpreted to answer the hypothesis.

Choosing which covariates to retain and discard after every iteration bears similarities to the SS process in linear and logistic regression. After each covariate is introduced, the *p*-values on the slopes of the covariates are reviewed, and decisions are made about inclusion of the variable in future models. For dicey decisions, model fit statistics can be used, as demonstrated with logistic regression and comparing –2 log likelihood measures between nested models, as well as AIC measures between nested or non-nested models.

It is important to notice that in this demonstration, we are taking a big leap in using cross-sectional data for a prospective analysis. We are assuming that the drinking behavior preceded the asthma diagnosis, which probably is not the case, as many people in the dataset were diagnosed as children. However, if we replace the concept of alcohol consumption with a genetic marker, such as the presence of the apolipoprotein ε4 allele, this type of survival analysis would be more defensible, as we can be sure that genetic marker preceded the asthma diagnosis. This dataset is being used only to demonstrate how to do survival analysis using software and not to make a heady comment on survival analysis study design.

Survival Analysis Regression Modeling and Model Fitting

For our linear and logistic regression hypotheses, we developed a full analytic dataset with all hypothesized confounders. For the sake of brevity, we did not do that with `SurvAnalytic`, our survival analysis dataset. In this dataset, we only included the exposure variables, `DRKMONTHLY` and `DRKWEEKLY`, as well as two potential confounders, sex (`MALE`, male=1 and female=0) and veteran status (`VETERAN3`, veteran=1 and nonveteran=0). We will use these variables to demonstrate the principles behind SS survival analysis model fitting without fitting an entire model.

In the beginning of this section, we made plots to try to decide whether or not to do a parametric or semiparametric analysis. We looked at the potential parametric distributions of log-normal and exponential and at the cumulative hazard. The parametric distributions did not fit the data perfectly, but they also were not ruled out. The hazards appeared roughly proportional as well. Therefore, any of the three approaches could be chosen.

Recall that in conducting a parametric or semiparametric survival analysis, our goal is to develop relative risks. Therefore, like we did with logistic regression, we need to exponentiate the slopes into ratios. When we use the parametric models, these exponentiated slopes can be called relative risks. In the Cox proportional hazard model, they are called hazard ratios (HRs).

Parametric Survival Analysis

Imagine we had chosen the parametric exponential distribution. We would then begin our SS survival analysis regression modeling by developing an unadjusted model. In SAS, we could use `PROC LIFEREG` for this.

Code:

```
PROC LIFEREG data=r.SurvAnalytic;
        MODEL TIME80*ASTHMA80(0)= DRKMONTHLY DRKWEEKLY /dist =
        exponential;
run;
```

Notice that we designated `dist=exponential`, and that is how we make sure the regression is using the exponential distribution. The SAS output consists of several tables as usual. Certain tables contain important information. The table titled Fit Statistics, shown here as Table 4.15, includes several measures of model fit, including the –2 log likelihood and the AIC. The parameter estimates are in the table titled Analysis of Maximum Likelihood Parameter Estimates, shown in Table 4.16.

Notice that there is no default output of the exponentiated relative risks or confidence intervals (unlike with the `PROC LOGISTIC` output). Also notice that in this unadjusted model, both exposure indicator variables are significant.

Imagine we want to start our SS process by introducing the `MALE` variable. We would rerun the code with `MALE` added to the formula.

Code:

```
PROC LIFEREG data=r.SurvAnalytic;
       MODEL TIME80*ASTHMA80(0)= DRKMONTHLY DRKWEEKLY MALE/dist
              = exponential;
run;
```

TABLE 4.15

SAS Exponential Model Fit Statistics

Fit Statistics	
–2 log likelihood	27185.38
AIC (smaller is better)	27191.38
AICC (smaller is better)	27191.38
BIC (smaller is better)	27223.93

TABLE 4.16

SAS Exponential Unadjusted Model Parameter Estimates

Parameter	DF	Estimate	Standard Error	95% Confidence Limits		Chi-Square	Pr > ChiSq
Intercept	1	9.1136	0.0289	9.0569	9.1703	99171.0	<0.0001
DRKMONTHLY	1	0.4880	0.0530	0.3840	0.5919	84.62	<0.0001
DRKWEEKLY	1	0.6216	0.0816	0.4618	0.7815	58.09	<0.0001
Scale	0	1.0000	0.0000	1.0000	1.0000		
Weibull Shape	0	1.0000	0.0000	1.0000	1.0000		

TABLE 4.17

SAS Exponential Model Parameter Estimates Adjusted for Sex

Analysis of Maximum Likelihood Parameter Estimates							
Parameter	**DF**	**Estimate**	**Standard Error**	**95% Confidence Limits**		**Chi-Square**	**Pr > ChiSq**
Intercept	1	8.9766	0.0317	8.9144	9.0387	80122.8	<0.0001
DRKMONTHLY	1	0.4338	0.0533	0.3293	0.5384	66.14	<0.0001
DRKWEEKLY	1	0.5518	0.0819	0.3913	0.7123	45.40	<0.0001
MALE	1	0.4556	0.0510	0.3557	0.5555	79.93	<0.0001
Scale	0	1.0000	0.0000	1.0000	1.0000		
Weibull shape	0	1.0000	0.0000	1.0000	1.0000		

Parameter output is shown in Table 4.17. In the table, we see that `MALE` is significant, so we would be likely to keep it for the next iteration.

Let us perform the same tasks in R. We will go back to using the survival package. First, we call up the `survival` library. Next, we make `SurvModel1` our unadjusted exponential `survival` model. Notice, as with the SAS code, we set the option `dist="exp"` to get the exponential distribution.

Code:

```
SurvModel1 <- survreg(formula = Surv(TIME80, ASTHMA80) ~
      DRKMONTHLY + DRKWEEKLY, data = SurvAnalytic , dist="exp")
summary(SurvModel1)
```

Output:

```
Call:
survreg(formula = Surv(TIME80, ASTHMA80) ~ DRKMONTHLY +
DRKWEEKLY,
    data = SurvAnalytic, dist="exp")
               Value Std.  Error       z        p
(Intercept) 9.114        0.0289  314.91  0.00e+00
DRKMONTHLY  0.488        0.0530    9.20  3.61e-20
DRKWEEKLY   0.622        0.0816    7.62  2.50e-14

Scale fixed at 1

Exponential distribution
Loglik(model)= -19286.5 Loglik(intercept only)= -19349.2
        Chisq= 125.43 on 2 degrees of freedom, p= 0
Number of Newton-Raphson Iterations: 9
n= 380957
```

By using the `summary` command on the `SurvModel1` object, we can see that we get the same results as in SAS in terms of the slopes and *p*-values. We also see that R provides us the −2 log likelihood and degrees of freedom.

As with SAS, there is no default output in R containing the exponentiated relative risks and 95% confidence intervals. We can add these in R using the same procedure we did with logistic regression, by using libraries `devtools` and `broom` and the `tidy` command to make a data.frame of the results, then adding the confidence limits as calculations.

Code:

```
library (devtools)
library (broom)

Tidy_SurvModel1 <- tidy(SurvModel1)
Tidy_SurvModel1$RR <- exp(Tidy_SurvModel1$estimate)
Tidy_SurvModel1$LL <- exp(Tidy_SurvModel1$estimate -
       (1.96 * Tidy_SurvModel1$std.error))
Tidy_SurvModel1$UL <- exp(Tidy_SurvModel1$estimate +
       (1.96 * Tidy_SurvModel1$std.error))
Tidy_SurvModel1
```

Output:

```
         term  estimate  std.error  statistic       p.value  conf.low
1 (Intercept) 9.1136068 0.02893995 314.914349 0.000000e+00 9.0568855
2  DRKMONTHLY 0.4879647 0.05304532   9.199015 3.612450e-20 0.3839978
3   DRKWEEKLY 0.6216183 0.08155657   7.621928 2.499151e-14 0.4617703
  conf.high          RR          LL          UL
1 9.1703281  9077.978224  8577.385918  9607.78604
2 0.5919316     1.628997     1.468139     1.80748
3 0.7814662     1.861939     1.586876     2.18468
```

The relative risk of both alcohol groups compared to nondrinkers is significantly high, suggesting that alcohol intake is associated with a higher risk of the event compared to no alcohol intake. Let us introduce `MALE` into the model to make `SurvModel2`, replicating what we did in SAS.

Code:

```
SurvModel2 <- survreg(formula = Surv(TIME80, ASTHMA80) ~
       DRKMONTHLY + DRKWEEKLY + MALE, data = SurvAnalytic ,
       dist="exp")
summary(SurvModel2)
```

Output:

```
Call:
survreg(formula = Surv(TIME80, ASTHMA80) ~ DRKMONTHLY +
      DRKWEEKLY + MALE, data = SurvAnalytic, dist = "exp")
             Value Std.   Error       z         p
(Intercept) 8.977        0.0317  283.06  0.00e+00
DRKMONTHLY  0.434        0.0533    8.13  4.20e-16
DRKWEEKLY   0.552        0.0819    6.74  1.60e-11
MALE        0.456        0.0510    8.94  3.89e-19

Scale fixed at 1

Exponential distribution
Loglik(model)= -19244.4 Loglik(intercept only)= -19349.2
        Chisq= 209.72 on 3 degrees of freedom, p= 0
Number of Newton-Raphson Iterations: 9
n= 380957
```

As we saw in SAS, `MALE` is significant, so we would theoretically retain it as we proceeded with modeling. The following code adds the relative risk in R.

Code:

```
library (devtools)
library (broom)

Tidy_SurvModel2 <- tidy(SurvModel2)
Tidy_SurvModel2$RR <- exp(Tidy_SurvModel2$estimate)
Tidy_SurvModel2$LL <- exp(Tidy_SurvModel2$estimate -
      (1.96 * Tidy_SurvModel2$std.error))
Tidy_SurvModel2$UL <- exp(Tidy_SurvModel2$estimate +
      (1.96 * Tidy_SurvModel2$std.error))

Tidy_SurvModel2
```

Output:

```
         term  estimate   std.error   statistic       p.value   conf.low
1 (Intercept) 8.9765768  0.03171266  283.059739  0.000000e+00  8.9144211
2 DRKMONTHLY  0.4338280  0.05334362    8.132708  4.198065e-16  0.3292765
3   DRKWEEKLY 0.5517621  0.08188506    6.738251  1.603044e-11  0.3912703
4        MALE 0.4556294  0.05096430    8.940168  3.885780e-19  0.3557412
  conf.high           RR          LL          UL
1 9.0387325  7915.489340  7438.466452  8423.103324
2 0.5383796     1.543153     1.389959     1.713232
3 0.7122538     1.736310     1.478854     2.038587
4 0.5555176     1.577166     1.427236     1.742846
```

Like with the alcohol variables, being male is associated with about 1.5 times the risk of the event compared to the other category, female. The relative risk is statistically significant, so we would retain MALE in the next iteration of our exponential model. We could continue our SS modeling in this fashion while keeping model metadata in the format of Table 4.9, which we used for logistic regression metadata.

Semiparametric Survival Analysis

In the case that we do not choose a parametric analysis, and instead choose a semiparametric analysis, we would use different code to fit a Cox proportional hazard model. In SAS, we could use PROC PHREG to construct a proportional hazard regression model. Here is code for the unadjusted model.

Code:

```
PROC PHREG data = r.SurvAnalytic;
model TIME80*ASTHMA80(0)= DRKMONTHLY DRKWEEKLY;
run;
```

Like with PROC LIFEREG, the output is in a series of tables. The one titled Model Fit Statistics which includes the –2 log likelihood and the AIC is shown in Table 4.18.

There is also a table titled Analysis of Maximum Likelihood Estimates, and this holds the parameter estimates and p-values (shown in Table 4.19).

TABLE 4.18

SAS Proportional Hazards Model Fit Statistics

Model Fit Statistics		
Criterion	**Without Covariates**	**With Covariates**
−2 LOG L	47329.507	47198.820
AIC	47329.507	47202.820
SBC	47329.507	47213.889

TABLE 4.19

SAS Proportional Hazard Unadjusted Model Parameter Estimates

Analysis of Maximum Likelihood Estimates						
Parameter	**DF**	**Parameter Estimate**	**Standard Error**	**Chi-Square**	**Pr > ChiSq**	**Hazard Ratio**
DRKMONTHLY	1	−0.50156	0.05313	89.1221	<0.0001	0.606
DRKWEEKLY	1	−0.62957	0.08157	59.5728	<0.0001	0.533

Notice that, as with PROC LIFEREG, the estimates are on the log scale, and are not exponentiated into HRs. We observe that both indicator variables are statistically significant. We can move forward one step in our modeling process by including the MALE variable in the formula.

Code:

```
PROC PHREG data = r.SurvAnalytic;
model TIME80*ASTHMA80(0)= DRKMONTHLY DRKWEEKLY MALE;
run;
```

Table 4.20 shows the parameter estimates.

As shown in Table 4.20, MALE is also significant in this model, and so it would be retained for the next iteration.

Performing the same tasks in R, we will use the coxph command from the package survival. We will use it to make the unadjusted model in object PHModel1, then view a summary of it.

Code:

```
PHModel1 <- coxph(formula = Surv(TIME80, ASTHMA80) ~ DRKMONTHLY
      + DRKWEEKLY, data = SurvAnalytic)
summary(PHModel1)
```

Output:

```
Call:
coxph(formula = Surv(TIME80, ASTHMA80) ~ DRKMONTHLY + DRKWEEKLY,
     data = SurvAnalytic)

  n= 380957, number of events= 1872

                coef exp(coef) se(coef)      z  Pr(>|z|)
DRKMONTHLY  -0.50166   0.60553  0.05313 -9.443  < 2e-16  ***
DRKWEEKLY   -0.63037   0.53240  0.08159 -7.726  1.11e-14 ***
---
```

TABLE 4.20

SAS Proportional Hazards Model Parameter Estimates Adjusted for Sex

Analysis of Maximum Likelihood Estimates						
Parameter	**DF**	**Parameter Estimate**	**Standard Error**	**Chi-Square**	**Pr > ChiSq**	**Hazard Ratio**
DRKMONTHLY	1	−0.44756	0.05342	70.1940	<0.0001	0.639
DRKWEEKLY	1	−0.55929	0.08189	46.6464	<0.0001	0.572
MALE	1	−0.46242	0.05097	82.3147	<0.0001	0.630

```
Signif. codes: 0 '***' 0.001 '**' 0.01 '*' 0.05 '.' 0.1 ' ' 1

             exp(coef) exp(-coef) lower .95 upper .95
DRKMONTHLY      0.6055      1.651    0.5456    0.6720
DRKWEEKLY       0.5324      1.878    0.4537    0.6247

Concordance= 0.56  (se = 0.006 )
Rsquare= 0   (max possible= 0.117 )
Likelihood ratio test    = 130.7 on 2 df, p=0
Wald test                = 125.2 on 2 df, p=0
Score (logrank) test     = 128.3 on 2 df, p=0
```

The summary shows that in R, like in SAS, the estimates are on the log scale. As we did with our exponential analysis, we can fix this using the `tidy` model approach from the `devtools` and `broom` packages (library calls not shown).

Code:

```
Tidy_PHModel1 <- tidy(PHModel1)
Tidy_PHModel1$RR <- exp(Tidy_PHModel1$estimate)
Tidy_PHModel1$LL <- exp(Tidy_PHModel1$estimate - (1.96 *
      Tidy_PHModel1$std.error))
Tidy_PHModel1$UL <- exp(Tidy_PHModel1$estimate + (1.96 *
      Tidy_PHModel1$std.error))

Tidy_PHModel1
```

Output:

```
        term   estimate  std.error statistic      p.value   conf.low
1 DRKMONTHLY -0.5016562 0.05312716 -9.442556 0.000000e+00 -0.6057835
2 DRKWEEKLY  -0.6303659 0.08158981 -7.726038 1.110223e-14 -0.7902790
   conf.high         RR          LL          UL
1 -0.3975289   0.6055270   0.5456457   0.6719798
2 -0.4704529   0.5323969   0.4537168   0.6247211
```

Notice that although both variables are statistically significant, their slopes are in an opposite direction of their slopes in the exponential model. In this model, drinking is associated with protection against the outcome, which mirrors what we found in our Kaplan–Meier analysis, where nondrinkers had a poorer survival experience compared to the drinking groups. Also, notice that other model-fit statistics, including a likelihood ratio test, are present at the bottom of the output.

Next, still using R, we will add the `MALE` variable to make `PHModel2`, and use `tidy` model to develop HRs and 95% confidence intervals.

Code:

```
PHModel2 <- coxph(formula = Surv(TIME80, ASTHMA80) ~
DRKMONTHLY + DRKWEEKLY + MALE,
      data = SurvAnalytic)
summary(PHModel2)

Tidy_PHModel2 <- tidy(PHModel2)
Tidy_PHModel2$RR <- exp(Tidy_PHModel2$estimate)
Tidy_PHModel2$LL <- exp(Tidy_PHModel2$estimate - (1.96 *
      Tidy_PHModel2$std.error))
Tidy_PHModel2$UL <- exp(Tidy_PHModel2$estimate + (1.96 *
      Tidy_PHModel2$std.error))

Tidy_PHModel2
```

Output:

```
Call:
coxph(formula = Surv(TIME80, ASTHMA80) ~ DRKMONTHLY +
DRKWEEKLY +
    MALE, data = SurvAnalytic)

  n= 380957, number of events= 1872

               coef exp(coef) se(coef)      z  Pr(>|z|)
DRKMONTHLY -0.44765   0.63913  0.05342 -8.380   < 2e-16 ***
DRKWEEKLY  -0.56015   0.57112  0.08191 -6.838  8.01e-12 ***
MALE       -0.46268   0.62959  0.05097 -9.077   < 2e-16 ***
---
Signif. codes: 0 '***' 0.001 '**' 0.01 '*' 0.05 '.' 0.1 ' ' 1

           exp(coef) exp(-coef) lower .95 upper .95
DRKMONTHLY    0.6391      1.565    0.5756    0.7097
DRKWEEKLY     0.5711      1.751    0.4864    0.6706
MALE          0.6296      1.588    0.5697    0.6957

Concordance= 0.585 (se = 0.007 )
Rsquare= 0.001  (max possible= 0.117 )
Likelihood ratio test= 217.7 on 3 df, p=0
Wald test            = 205.7 on 3 df, p=0
Score (logrank) test = 211.1 on 3 df, p=0

        term   estimate  std.error statistic      p.value   conf.low
1 DRKMONTHLY -0.4476520 0.05341833 -8.380121 0.000000e+00 -0.5523501
2  DRKWEEKLY -0.5601517 0.08191339 -6.838341 8.011591e-12 -0.7206990
3       MALE -0.4626830 0.05097043 -9.077480 0.000000e+00 -0.5625833
```

```
   conf.high         RR          LL          UL
1 -0.3429540  0.6391270  0.5755944  0.7096722
2 -0.3996044  0.5711224  0.4864107  0.6705873
3 -0.3627828  0.6295922  0.5697343  0.6957388
```

Notice how in R, like in SAS, MALE is statistically significant. Again, the results are the opposite as what we found with the parametric approach, where MALE is associated with protection instead of risk. Please note that, like with a parametric approach, metadata like that for logistic regression shown in Table 4.9 can be kept to aid in final model selection.

Issues to Consider in Survival Analysis

At this point, it is important to reflect on the fact that the results of our exponential analysis seem to be the opposite of the results of our Cox proportional hazards analysis. This is enough to make us worry about the analysis altogether. First, we know we have a lot of limitations with the data and with assumptions we have made about it. But these findings should make us ask—why are we conducting survival analysis of health data anyway?

Do we really believe that modeling the "survival experience" is more accurate or telling than modeling the relationship as a logistic regression? In other words, do we really believe the time variable? Imagine our time variable had to do with a cancer or Alzheimer's diagnosis. Are not these latent conditions that can be diagnosed at later stages [118,119]? And do we not know that ethnic minorities and other populations with low access to healthcare in the United States are more likely to be diagnosed at later stages [120]? And think of all the data entry error that occurs in clinical practice, or all the other measurement errors that can occur in research [121].

Unstable findings like the ones we are getting make it worth asking—are we doing something that we probably should not be doing, when it comes to survival analysis of health data? Survival analysis was invented to study death, and now it is being used for all kinds of things, including stock market applications as well as clinical trials, where luckily there is not much death [122]. Maybe, in the interest of developing intuitively understood and actionable findings, we might want to skip survival analysis beyond plotting a nonparametric Kaplan–Meier and doing a log-rank test.

It is possible that in many instances, there is nothing survival analysis can really add to what we would find in logistic regression. It is always possible to run survival models and logistic regression models and compare them. If the answers are relatively the same, using the more intuitive logistic regression model is warranted, given the caveats with health data described earlier. It generally feels easier for those in public health to formulate a health-related hypothesis as well as an actionable public health goal and plan when thinking of predictors of disease incidence, rather than predictors of a particular survival experience as disease-free.

Notice that the goals of Healthy People 2020 do not talk about survival experience, but rather about prevalence and incidence [123].

Whether using a parametric approach or the semiparametric Cox proportional hazards approach, SS modeling in survival analysis follows the same basic pattern as it does in linear and logistic regression. A working model is developed from trying each covariate one at a time, and then a final model is developed out of trying to reintroduce covariates discarded the first time around. The final model is presented as the answer to the survival analysis hypothesis. The next part of this section will discuss selecting the final survival analysis model.

Selecting the Final Survival Analysis Model

As was apparent in both SAS and R, both parametric and nonparametric survival analyses provide model fit statistics that can be used to help with decisions about final model selection. In both sets of output, for both parametric and semiparametric analyses, the −2 log likelihood and degrees of freedom were available.

Recall how model fit statistics were not very important in terms of SS-related decision-making in logistic regression. In fact, we only used these statistics when we did a nested model comparison to help us decide on how to model independent variable `SLEPTIM2`—continuously or in quartiles. This same approach can be used with survival analysis to answer the same kind of questions. Once the survival distributions have been checked and a model has been developed, it is normally not difficult to use the p-values on covariates to decide what to keep and what not to keep in the model. Comparing nested models is also possible if the analyst needs to split hairs between competing models.

As described under logistic regression, some analysts do not consider adding interaction variables *post hoc* as fishing. Those who feel that way can add interactions to a survival analysis regression model to try to achieve a clearer answer to our hypothesis or a tighter model. The same caveats with interpretation apply, however, meaning that keeping interactions in the model will require an interpretation of stratum-specific estimates, rather than a direct interpretation of relative risk.

Survival Analysis Model Presentation

As shown previously, survival analysis is like logistic regression, in that the relative risks and 95% confidence intervals, rather than slopes and p-values, are presented and interpreted. Like with ORs, relative risks also have the feature that if their confidence intervals contain 1, they are not statistically significant.

For that reason, both parametric and semiparametric survival analysis results can be presented in a similar manner as logistic regression results, as shown in Table 4.12. Unfortunately, the `arm` package's `coefplot` command does not work on survival objects, so it is not possible to use that to make a coefficient plot. Ultimately, the plot is only used to aid with interpretation, and not usually presented, so this is not a serious issue.

As a final note on this topic, the most important choice in survival analysis is whether or not to do it in the first place. Is it really needed to answer a question? Analysts studying events in a cohort with many well-measured variables and a high-level of healthcare contact, such as a cohort of well-characterized patients being followed clinically [124], might find survival analysis particularly meaningful, especially when modeling events such as "becoming tumor free" or "disease going into remission," where the survival experience, not just survival at all, really matters. But if the time variable is iffy, or the survival experience versus survival at all really does not matter, then logistic regression should be used.

A Note about Macros

The elephant in the room throughout this book has been the fact that SAS users regularly build macros, and little mention has been made of R macros in this entire text. That is because the whole approach behind automation in R is different than in SAS. This difference was touched on earlier, in Chapter 3, where a quick example of automation in R was presented. SAS is a procedural language, so macros in SAS represent procedures that are repeated. R is based on functions, so when a SAS user would typically create a macro, an R user would create or use a function.

In SAS, a separate language called macro language is used to build macros. The language is similar to SAS `PROCS` and data steps, but there are some nuances. Macro commands in SAS tend to start with %s, such as the `%MEND` statement that comes at the end of a SAS macro.

In R, there are different alternatives to automation, and one is to make custom functions. The main part of our programming in R consists of preprogrammed functions—the `table` function is an example. To make a custom function in R, we use the `function` command. An example of a custom function is given in Chapter 2, where we describe how to flatten a correlation coefficient matrix so that *p*-values could be more easily readable. The code to build this function is repeated here.

Code:

```
flattenCorrMatrix <- function(cormat, pmat) {
  ut <- upper.tri(cormat)
  data.frame(
    row = rownames(cormat)[row(cormat)[ut]],
    column = rownames(cormat)[col(cormat)[ut]],
    cor =(cormat)[ut],
    p = pmat[ut]
    )
}
```

Notice how the function is named `flattenCorrMatrix`, and is the object being created by this code. The `function` command is used, and the two arguments after it are names of variables to be defined when the function is run. This is similar to SAS macros, where the variables to be defined when the macro is run are also named in the code that makes the macro. The code between the { and the } is all function code, which uses the variables stated in the function argument.

Once the above code is run, the function `flattenCorrMatrix` exists. It can then be reused in other code. Recall how we used it in Chapter 2, by entering the two arguments to define the variables in the function, which were `cormat` and `pmat`. Recall we did this to see the correlation matrix and *p*-values. Repeating the Chapter 2 code below, we enter `res1$r` (rounded to four digits after the decimal) as the first argument, and `res1$P` (rounded to four digits after the decimal) as the second argument.

Code:

```
flattenCorrMatrix(round(res1$r,4), round(res1$P, 4))
```

Although R custom functions are one approach to automation in R, other approaches exist, including the "`apply`" family of functions in R [77], and the "`defmacro`" command in the gtools package for making SAS-like macros in R [49]. However, these are not discussed in detail because they are outside the scope of this book.

In summary, SAS is generally automated using macros, whereas R is automated using a variety of other approaches, including custom functions. An in-depth discussion of automation in R is outside the scope of this book, but we wanted to clarify why we did not discuss macro-building throughout this text, even though we encountered many operations that needed to be repeated. Designing automation for code becomes very different when using R versus using SAS. This is why it can be difficult to rebuild a SAS shop into an R shop because the way code is automated is completely different in the two languages. It is much easier to build either a SAS or R shop from the ground up.

This book presented a toolset of approaches that the health analyst who is fluent in SAS can use to do the same routine analyses in R. It also recommended processes that can improve health analytics, such as model-building suggestions and presentation advice. The authors hope that your use of this book has increased your knowledge and agility with R for conducting analyses of health data. We also hope that what you gain from this book will increase your enjoyment of using R, and will unlock novel, creative ideas that can accompany trying a new software.

Optional Exercises

Section "This Book's Approach"

Questions

1. Why is the FS approach not being demonstrated in this book?
2. Name one step that can be taken when analyzing datasets that are already collected to minimize the appearance of fishing.

Answers

1. In the article described by Bursac et al., FS was compared with BE and SS in a simulation, and was found to perform much worse than BE or SS, so it was not used for demonstration.
2. Answers vary, but could include:
   a. Using dataset documentation to operationalize exposure, outcome, and potential confounding variables before actually examining the data.
   b. Reducing the number of variables eligible to be tried in the model through designing the analytic dataset before proceeding with an analysis.

Section "Linear Regression and ANOVA"

Questions

1. Using R and the analytic dataset, pretend you hypothesize that age group predicts sleep duration. Using the indicator variables developed in Chapter 2 (`AGE2` through `AGE6`), make a regression plot to check the assumptions of linearity and homoscedasticity in this analysis.

2. Do they meet the assumptions or violate them? Explain why you chose that answer. If this were a real analysis, would you proceed with linear regression at this point? Why or why not?
3. In this section, `Model1` through `Model5` began our SS linear regression. Using R and your own approach by making your own SS modeling decisions, complete the linear regression model, and document your decisions in a metadata spreadsheet. What covariates are in your final model? How do they differ from `Model31`, or are they exactly the same? Did you choose to include interactions? Why or why not?
4. Use the model you developed in question 3 to answer the hypothesis. Do you get the same answer as `Model31` did? Why or why not?
5. Prepare a presentation spreadsheet with your final model. You may choose to include `Model1` and `Model2`, as demonstrated, or present other models. If you chose to present other models, why did you make this choice?
6. Using R, make a coefficient plot of your final model. Change the colors and other options to improve readability.

Answers

1. Possible answer:

```
AgeSleepTimeRegression = lm(SLEPTIM2 ~ AGE2 + AGE3 + AGE4
        + AGE5 + AGE6, data=analytic)
layout(matrix(c(1,2,3,4),2,2))
plot(AgeSleepTimeRegression,
        main = "Age Group by Sleep Duration")
```

   Plot not shown.
2. They violate the assumptions. The QQ plot show both the dots departing from the diagonal line both at high levels of the outcome, and at very low levels of the outcome, suggesting linearity is violated. The vertical lines of dots in the residuals plots show different heights across different levels of the outcome and exposure, suggesting a violation of the homoscedasticity assumption. Given Lumley's recommendation, because this is a large public health dataset, I would proceed with linear regression analysis anyway.
3. Answers will vary.
4. Answers will vary.
5. Answers will vary.
6. Answers will vary.

Section "Logistic Regression"

Questions

1. Pretend you had the hypothesis that smoking is associated with obesity in veterans. Using the `SMOKER` variable as the exposure, and the `OBESE` variable as the outcome, in R, create and output the unadjusted logistic regression model called `ModelExp1` with ORs and their 95% confidence intervals.
2. Using a SS modeling process and the analytic dataset, in R, develop a final model for the hypothesis posed in question 1. Create a metadata table to document your decisions. What covariates are in your final model? Which ones are not in it? What difficult choices did you have to make to decide on a final model?
3. Does the model you developed in question 2 support or refute the hypothesis? Interpret it.
4. Using R's `nlme` library and the `loglik` command, find the −2 log likelihood and degrees of freedom for the final model you developed in question 2.
5. Using R, create a model presentation table and a coefficient plot of your final model. Change the colors and other options to improve readability.

Answers

1. Possible answer:

   Code:

```
ModelExp1 <- glm(OBESE ~ SMOKER, data=analytic, family =
"binomial")

library (devtools)
library (broom)

Tidy_ModelExp1 <- tidy(ModelExp1)
Tidy_ModelExp1

Tidy_ModelExp1$OR <- exp(Tidy_ModelExp1$estimate)
Tidy_ModelExp1$LL <- exp(Tidy_ModelExp1$estimate -
      (1.96 * Tidy_ModelExp1$std.error))
Tidy_ModelExp1$UL <- exp(Tidy_ModelExp1$estimate +
      (1.96 * Tidy_ModelExp1$std.error))
Tidy_ModelExp1
```

Output:

```
         term   estimate   std.error statistic      p.value        OR
1 (Intercept)-0.8543218 0.009816052 -87.03315 0.000000e+00 0.4255717
2      SMOKER-0.2862678 0.027055757 -10.58066 3.663573e-26 0.7510614
         LL          UL
1 0.4174622   0.4338387
2 0.7122708   0.7919646
```

2. Answers will vary.
3. Answers will vary.
4. Answers will vary.
5. Answers will vary.

Section "Survival Analysis Regression"

Questions

1. Using R and the `SurvAnalytic` dataset with the `flexsurv` package, fit and plot a log-normal and exponential distribution for `ALGRP` against the survival variables `TIME50` and `ASTHMA50`. Change the colors and other options to improve readability.
2. What are the differences between this plot and the one demonstrated? What do these differences suggest?
3. Using R and the package `flexsurv`, see if you can plot a different distribution other than log-normal and exponential. Which one did you plot? How is it different from log-normal and exponential?
4. Using R and the package survival, plot the cumulative hazard for the survival variables `TIME50` and `ASTHMA50` by `ALCGRP`. Change the colors and other options to improve readability.
5. Using R, continue with the SS parametric survival analysis regression demonstration by developing `SurvModel3`, with the formula on the exponential distribution, including `VETERAN3` in the independent variable list along with `DRKMONTHLY`, `DRKWEEKLY`, and `MALE`.
6. According to the analysis in question 5, is being a veteran positively or negatively associated with survival without an asthma diagnosis until age 50? Is this relationship statistically significant?
7. Using R, continue with the forward stepwise Cox proportional hazard analysis regression demonstration by developing `PHModel3`, including `VETERAN3` in the independent variable list along with `DRKMONTHLY`, `DRKWEEKLY`, and `MALE`.

8. According to the analysis in question 7, is being a veteran positively or negatively associated with survival without an asthma diagnosis until age 50? Is this relationship statistically significant?

Answers

1. Possible answer:

```
fit_lnorm <- flexsurvreg(formula = Surv(TIME50, ASTHMA50)
      ~ as.factor(ALCGRP), data = SurvAnalytic ,
      dist="lnorm")
fit_lnorm

fit_exp <- flexsurvreg(formula = Surv(TIME50, ASTHMA50) ~
      as.factor(ALCGRP), data = SurvAnalytic , dist="exp")
fit_exp

plot(fit_lnorm,
       main="Comparison of Log-normal and Exponential
              Distribution\nTIME50 and AGE50",
       xlab="Years",
       ylab="Survival Probability",
       ymin=0.99,
       col="darkcyan",
       lwd=2,
       lty=1:3)
lines(fit_exp,
       ymin=0.99,
       col="darkorchid1",
       lwd=2,
       lty=1:3)
legend(x = "bottomleft",
      legend = c("Kaplan-Meier", "Log-normal",
      "Exponential"),
       lwd=2,
      col = c("black", "darkcyan", "darkorchid1"))
```

   Plot not shown.

2. This looks the same as the plot demonstrated but ends earlier, at age 50. There is less of a survival experience to graph, so there is less known. This suggests that it is very helpful to have a set of survival data collected over a long period of time relevant to events. The more events in a dataset, the easier it is to characterize the survival experience.
3. Answers will vary.

4. Possible answer:

```
library(survival)
AllSurv <- with(SurvAnalytic,Surv(TIME50,ASTHMA50))

fit_cox <- coxph(AllSurv ~ as.factor(ALCGRP),
data=SurvAnalytic)
summary(fit_cox)

plot(survfit(fit_cox, newdata=data.frame(ALCGRP=1)),
       col="red",
       fun="cumhaz",
       main="Hazard Curves, TIME50 and ASTHMA50",
       xlab="Years",
       ylab="Cumulative Hazard",
       xlim=c(10,50),
       firstx=10,
       conf.int=FALSE,
       lwd=1)
lines(survfit(fit_cox,newdata=data.frame(ALCGRP=2)),
       col="blue",
       fun="cumhaz",
       xlim=c(10,50),
       firstx=10,
       conf.int=FALSE,
       lwd=1)
lines(survfit(fit_cox,newdata=data.frame(ALCGRP=3)),
       col="green",
       fun="cumhaz",
       xlim=c(10,50),
       firstx=10,
       conf.int=FALSE,
       lwd=1)
legend(x = "topleft",
       legend = c("No Drink (Reference)",
       "Drink Monthly", "Drink Weekly"),
       lwd=1,
       col=c("red", "blue", "green"))
```

Plot not shown.

5. Answer:

Code:

```
SurvModel3 <- survreg(formula = Surv(TIME80, ASTHMA80) ~
DRKMONTHLY + DRKWEEKLY
        + MALE + VETERAN3,
        data = SurvAnalytic , dist="exp")
summary(SurvModel3)
```

Output:

```
Call:
survreg(formula = Surv(TIME80, ASTHMA80) ~ DRKMONTHLY +
DRKWEEKLY + MALE + VETERAN3, data = SurvAnalytic, dist =
"exp")
              Value Std.   Error      z        p
(Intercept)    9.804      0.1793  54.68  0.00e+00
DRKMONTHLY     0.438      0.0534   8.20  2.32e-16
DRKWEEKLY      0.555      0.0819   6.78  1.22e-11
MALE           0.330      0.0560   5.88  4.02e-09
VETERAN3      -0.417      0.0889  -4.70  2.66e-06

Scale fixed at 1

Exponential distribution
Loglik(model)= -19232.5 Loglik(intercept only)= -19349.2
      Chisq= 233.34 on 4 degrees of freedom, p= 0
Number of Newton-Raphson Iterations: 9
n= 380957
```

6. Being a veteran is negatively associated with survival without an asthma diagnosis until age 50. This means being veteran is associated with getting diagnosed, and this relationship is statistically significant.

7. Answer:

   Code:

```
PHModel3 <- coxph(formula = Surv(TIME80, ASTHMA80) ~
      DRKMONTHLY + DRKWEEKLY + MALE + VETERAN3,
      data = SurvAnalytic)
summary(PHModel3)
```

Output:

```
Call:
survreg(formula = Surv(TIME80, ASTHMA80) ~ DRKMONTHLY +
      DRKWEEKLY + MALE + VETERAN3, data = SurvAnalytic,
      dist = "exp")
              Value Std.   Error      z        p
(Intercept)    9.804      0.1793  54.68  0.00e+00
DRKMONTHLY     0.438      0.0534   8.20  2.32e-16
DRKWEEKLY      0.555      0.0819   6.78  1.22e-11
MALE           0.330      0.0560   5.88  4.02e-09
VETERAN3      -0.417      0.0889  -4.70  2.66e-06

Scale fixed at 1
```

```
Exponential distribution
Loglik(model)= -19232.5 Loglik(intercept only)= -19349.2
    Chisq= 233.34 on 4 degrees of freedom, p= 0
Number of Newton-Raphson Iterations: 9
n= 380957
```

8. Being a veteran is positively associated with survival without an asthma diagnosis until age 50. This means being veteran is associated with not getting diagnosed, and this relationship is statistically significant.

Section "A Note about Macros"

Questions

1. After completing this book, imagine you were suddenly in charge of building a big data health analytics unit for the United States Veterans Administration for the purposes of studying health in veterans. Would you use SAS in this endeavor? If so, how would you use it? Would you also use R in this endeavor? If so, how would you use it?

Answers

1. Answers will vary.

References

1. R Core Team. The Comprehensive R Archive Network [Internet]. [cited 2016 May 29]. Available from: https://cran.r-project.org/
2. Yan J. Package KMsurv [Internet]. CRAN; 2015 [cited 2016 May 29]. (R Packages). Available from: https://cran.r-project.org/web/packages/KMsurv/KMsurv.pdf
3. RStudio. About RStudio [Internet]. RStudio, 2016 [cited 2016 Dec 25]. Available from: https://www.rstudio.com/about/
4. Brigham Young University Department of Statistics. R and RStudio [Internet]. [cited 2016 Dec 25]. Available from: http://statistics.byu.edu/content/r-and-rstudio
5. Chang W, Cheng J, Allaire JJ, Xie Y, McPherson J, RStudio et al. Shiny: Web Application Framework for R [Internet]. 2016 [cited 2016 Dec 25]. Available from: https://cran.r-project.org/web/packages/shiny/index.html
6. Hull B, Howard R. Useful Tips for Handling and Creating Special Characters in SAS [Internet]. PharmaSUG: SAS Institute; 2013 [cited 2016 May 29]. (PharmaSUG 2013 Conference Proceedings). Report No.: CC30. Available from: http://www.pharmasug.org/proceedings/2013/CC/PharmaSUG-2013-CC30.pdf
7. Mitchell RM. Thumbs Up for ODSgraphics, But Don't Throw Out All Your SAS/GRAPH programs! [Internet]. SUGI 29: SAS Institute; 2004 [cited 2016 May 29]. (SUGI 29 Proceedings). Report No.: 083-29. Available from: http://www2.sas.com/proceedings/sugi29/toc.html
8. Zender CL, Kalt M. At the crossroads: How to decide on your graphics path [Internet]. SAS Global Forum 2012: SAS Institute; 2013 [cited 2016 May 29]. (SAS Global Forum 2012). Report No.: 261–2012. Available from: https://support.sas.com/resources/papers/proceedings12/261-2012.pdf
9. Petersen MR, Deddens JA. 2009. A revised SAS macro for maximum likelihood estimation of prevalence ratios using the COPY method. *Occup Environ Med.* *66*(9):639–639.
10. R Core Team. Contributed Packages [Internet]. [cited 2016 May 29]. Available from: https://cran.r-project.org/web/packages/
11. Updating R for Windows [Internet]. UCLA: Statistical consulting group. [cited 2016 May 29]. Available from: http://www.ats.ucla.edu/stat/r/icu/updating_win.htm
12. Davis CA, Gerick F, Hintermair V, Friedel CC, Fundel K, Kuffner R et al. STABle Model Selection by Optimizing Reliable Classification Performance [Internet]. Lehr-Maximilians Universitat Munchen; 2016 [cited 2016 May 29]. Available from: https://www.bio.ifi.lmu.de/files/Software/stabperf/api/00Index.html
13. Davis CA, Gerick F, Hintermair V, Friedel CC, Fundel K, Kuffner R et al. Reliable Gene Signatures for Microarray Classification: Assessment of Stability and Performance [Internet]. Lehr-Maximilians Universitat Munchen [cited 2016 May 29]. Available from: https://www.bio.ifi.lmu.de/en/download/stabperf/index.html

14. Gilsen B. Date Handling in the SAS system [Internet]. SUGI 28: SAS Institute; 2003. [cited 2016 May 29]. (Seattle SAS Users Group International Proceedings). Report No.: 66–28. Available from: http://www2.sas.com/proceedings/sugi28/066-28.pdf
15. Sun Z, Yang Z. Generalized McNemar's Test for Homogeneity of the Marginal Distributions [Internet]. SAS Institute; 2008 [cited 2016 May 29]. (SAS Global Forum 2008). Report No.: 382.2008. Available from: https://works.bepress.com/zyang/17/
16. Meetup [Internet]. [cited 2016 May 29]. Available from: http://www.meetup.com/
17. Sirosh J. Microsoft Closes Acquisition of Revolution Analytics [Internet]. Cortana Intelligence and Machine Learning Blog; 2015 [cited 2016 May 29]. Available from: https://blogs.technet.microsoft.com/machinelearning/2015/04/06/microsoft-closes-acquisition-of-revolution-analytics/
18. Mango Solutions. EARL - Effective Applications of the R Language [Internet]. [cited 2016 May 29]. Available from: https://earlconf.com/
19. Health.mil. MDR, M2, ICDs Functional References and Specifications [Internet]. [cited 2016 May 30]. Available from: http://www.health.mil/Military-Health-Topics/Technology/Support-Areas/MDR-M2-ICD-Functional-References-and-Specification-Documents
20. Boston Decision LLC. SAS to R: Best Practices in SAS to R Conversion. 2012; Boston, MA.
21. Cassell DL. A Sort of a Mess—Sorting Large Datasets on Multiple Keys [Internet]. SUGI 26: SAS Institute; 2001 [cited 2016 Jun 11]. (SUGI 26 Proceedings). Report No.: 121–26. Available from: http://www2.sas.com/proceedings/sugi26/p121-26.pdf
22. Bellmer T. KanSAS Code: SAS vs SQL Update [Internet]. KanSAS Code; 2015 [cited 2016 May 30]. Available from: http://kansascode.blogspot.com/2015/02/sas-vs-sql-update.html
23. Stroupe J. Nine Steps to Get Started using SAS® Macros [Internet]. SUGI 28: SAS Institute; 2003 [cited 2016 Jun 11]. (SUGI 28 Proceedings). Report No.: 56–28. Available from: http://www2.sas.com/proceedings/sugi28/056-28.pdf
24. Wright WL. PROC TABULATE and the Neat Things You Can Do With It [Internet]. SUGI 28: SAS Institute; 2008 [cited 2016 Jun 11]. (SAS Global Forum 2008). Report No.: 264–2008. Available from: http://www2.sas.com/proceedings/forum2008/264-2008.pdf
25. Centers for Disease Control and Prevention. 2014 BRFSS Survey Data and Documentation [Internet]. 2015 [cited 2016 May 29]. Available from: http://www.cdc.gov/brfss/annual_data/annual_2014.html
26. Oltsik MA. ODS and Output Data Sets: What You Need to Know [Internet]. SAS Institute; 2008 [cited 2016 May 29]. (SAS Global Forum 2008). Report No.: 086–2008. Available from: http://www2.sas.com/proceedings/forum2008/086-2008.pdf
27. Bilenas JV. I Can Do That With PROC FORMAT [Internet]. SAS Institute; 2008 [cited 2016 Jun 11]. (SAS Global Forum 2008). Report No.: 174–2008. Available from: http://www2.sas.com/proceedings/sugi26/p121-26.pdf
28. Harrell FE, Jr. Hmisc: Harrell Miscellaneous [Internet]. 2016 [cited 2016 Jun 13]. Available from: https://cran.r-project.org/web/packages/Hmisc/index.html

29. Hill OT, Kay AB, Wahi MM, McKinnon CJ, Bulathsinhala L, Haley TF. 2012. Rates of knee injury in the U.S. Active Duty Army, 2000–2005. *Mil Med.* *177*(7):840–844.
30. Wallace RF, Wahi MM, Hill OT, Kay AB. 2011. Rates of ankle and foot injuries in active-duty U.S. Army soldiers, 2000–2006. *Mil Med. 176*(3):283–290.
31. Hill OT, Wahi MM, Carter R 3rd, Kay AB, McKinnon CJ, Wallace RF. 2012. Rhabdomyolysis in the US Active Duty Army, 2004–2006. *Med Sci Sports Exerc.* *44*(3):442–449.
32. SAS Institute. SAS surpasses $3 billion in 2013 revenue, growing 5.2% over 2012 results [Internet]. [cited 2016 May 29]. Available from: http://www.sas.com/ro_ro/news/press-releases/2014/january/2013-financials.html
33. Crowley MC. How SAS Became The World's Best Place To Work [Internet]. Fast Company; 2013 [cited 2016 May 29]. Available from: http://www.fastcompany.com/3004953/how-sas-became-worlds-best-place-work
34. Smith D. FDA: R OK for drug trials [Internet]. Revolutions; 2012 [cited 2016 May 29]. Available from: http://blog.revolutionanalytics.com/2012/06/fda-r-ok.html
35. SAS Institute. SAS Global Certification Program [Internet]. [cited 2016 May 29]. Available from: http://support.sas.com/certify/
36. Muenchen RA. The Popularity of Data Analysis Software [Internet]. r4stats.com. 2014 [cited 2016 May 29]. Available from: http://r4stats.com/articles/popularity/
37. Muenchen RA. 2016. *R for SAS and SPSS Users*. Springer Customer Service Center Gmbh: Heidelberg, Germany. 716 p.
38. McQuown G. PROC IMPORT with a Twist [Internet]. SUGI 30: SAS Institute; 2005 [cited 2016 Dec 25]. (SUGI 30 Proceedings). Report No.: 038-30. Available from: http://www2.sas.com/proceedings/sugi26/p121-26.pdf
39. R. Core Team, Bivand R, Carey VJ, DebRoy S, Eglen S, Guha R et al. foreign: Read Data Stored by Minitab, S, SAS, SPSS, Stata, Systat, Weka, dBase,... [Internet]. 2015 [cited 2016 Jul 31]. Available from: https://cran.r-project.org/web/packages/foreign/index.html
40. mrtnj. Using R: common errors in table import [Internet]. R-bloggers; 2014 [cited 2016 August 2]. Available from: http://www.r-bloggers.com/using-r-common-errors-in-table-import/
41. SAS Institute. LENGTH Statement. In: SAS(R) 92 Language Reference: Dictionary [Internet]. Fourth. SAS Institute; 2011 [cited 2016 Dec 25]. Available from: http://support.sas.com/documentation/cdl/en/lrdict/64316/HTML/default/viewer.htm#a000218807.htm
42. R Core Team. R: Count the Number of Characters (or Bytes or Width). In: Documentation for package "base" version 340 [Internet]. 2016 [cited 2016 Dec 25]. Available from: http://stat.ethz.ch/R-manual/R-devel/library/base/html/nchar.html
43. Grosjean P, Ibanez F, Etienne M. Pastecs: Package for Analysis of Space-Time Ecological Series [Internet]. 2014 [cited 2016 Aug 11]. Available from: https://cran.r-project.org/web/packages/pastecs/index.html
44. Revelle W. psych: Procedures for Psychological, Psychometric, and Personality Research [Internet]. 2016 [cited 2016 Aug 11]. Available from: https://cran.r project.org/web/packages/psych/index.html

45. Glynn EF. Chart of R Colors [Internet]. R TechNotes and Graphics Gallery. 2005 [cited 2016 Dec 26]. Available from: http://research.stowers-institute.org/efg/R/Color/Chart/
46. Comtois D. summarytools: Dataframe Summaries, Frequency Tables and Numerical Summaries with Customizable Output [Internet]. 2015 [cited 2016 Aug 11]. Available from: https://cran.r-project.org/web/packages/summarytools/index.html
47. Skau D, Kosara R. 2016. Arcs, angles, or areas: Individual data encodings in pie and donut charts. *Comput Graph Forum*. *35*(3):121–130.
48. C. Color Palettes in R [Internet]. R-bloggers; 2010 [cited 2016 Dec 26]. Available from: https://www.r-bloggers.com/color-palettes-in-r/
49. Warnes GR, Bolker B, Lumley T. gtools: Various R Programming Tools [Internet]. 2015 [cited 2016 Jun 13]. Available from: https://cran.r-project.org/web/packages/gtools/index.html
50. Public Health Knowledge Support Team. Role of chance, bias and confounding in epidemiological studies [Internet]. Health Knowledge; 2010 [cited 2017 Mar 26]. Available from: https://www.healthknowledge.org.uk/e-learning/epidemiology/practitioners/chance-bias-confounding
51. Devika S, Jeyaseelan L, Sebastian G. 2016. Analysis of sparse data in logistic regression in medical research: A newer approach. *J Postgrad Med*. *62*(1): 26–31.
52. Bursac Z, Gauss CH, Williams DK, Hosmer DW. 2008. Purposeful selection of variables in logistic regression. *Source Code Biol Med*. 3:17.
53. Mukamal KJ, Ding EL, Djoussé L. Alcohol consumption, physical activity, and chronic disease risk factors: A population-based cross-sectional survey. *BMC Pub Health*. 6:118.
54. Faestel PM, Littell CT, Vitiello MV, Forsberg CW, Littman AJ. Perceived insufficient rest or sleep among veterans: Behavioral risk factor surveillance system 2009. *J Clin Sleep Med JCSM Off Publ Am Acad Sleep Med*. *9*(6):577–84.
55. Grolemund G, Spinu V, Wickham H, Lyttle J, Constigan I, Law J et al. Lubridate: Make Dealing with Dates a Little Easier [Internet]. 2016 [cited 2016 Aug 18]. Available from: https://cran.r-project.org/web/packages/lubridate/index.html
56. Grolemund G, Wickham H. Dates and Times Made Easy with lubridate. J Stat Softw [Internet]. 2011 [cited 2016 Aug 18];040(i03). Available from: http://econpapers.repec.org/article/jssjstsof/v_3a040_3ai03.htm
57. American Hospital Directory [Internet]. [cited 2013 Apr 22]. Available from: http://www.ahd.com/
58. Bilenas JV. Using PROC RANK and PROC UNIVARIATE to Rank or Decile Variables [Internet]. NESUG 2009: SAS Institute; 2009 [cited 2016 Dec 27]. (Northeast SAS Users Group Proceedings). Report No.: 66–28. Available from: http://www.lexjansen.com/nesug/nesug09/ap/AP01.pdf
59. Wei T, Simko V. Corrplot: Visualization of a Correlation Matrix [Internet]. 2016 [cited 2016 Aug 19]. Available from: https://cran.r-project.org/web/packages/corrplot/index.html
60. Logos T. Two sample Student's t-test #2 [Internet]. R-bloggers. 2009 [cited 2016 Aug 19]. Available from: http://www.r-bloggers.com/two-sample-students-t-test-2/

61. Kadel RP, Kip KE. A SAS Macro to Compute Effect Size (Cohen's d) and its Confidence Interval from Raw Survey Data [Internet]. SESUG 2012: SAS Institute; 2012 [cited 2016 Dec 27]. (Southeast SAS Users Group Proceedings). Report No.: SD-06. Available from: http://analytics.ncsu.edu/sesug/2012/SD-06.pdf
62. Navarro D. lsr: Companion to "Learning Statistics with R" [Internet]. 2015 [cited 2016 Aug 21]. Available from: https://cran.r-project.org/web/packages/lsr/index.html
63. Champely S, Ekstrom C, Dalgaard P, Gill J, Weibelzahl S, Rosario HD. pwr: Basic Functions for Power Analysis [Internet]. 2016 [cited 2016 Aug 21]. Available from: https://cran.r-project.org/web/packages/pwr/index.html
64. Zikmund WG. Basic Data Analysis: Descriptive Statistics [Internet]. Chulalongkorn University; Bangkok, Thailand. Available from: http://pioneer.netserv.chula.ac.th/~ppongsa/2900600/LMRM02.pdf
65. Thompson SR. FREQ Out – Exploring Your Data the Old School Way [Internet]. SAS Institute; 2012 [cited 2016 Nov 4]. (SESUG 2012). Report No.: HW-04. Available from: http://analytics.ncsu.edu/sesug/2012/HW-04.pdf
66. Long S, Abolafia J, Park L. Using SAS® ODS to extract and merge statistics from multiple SAS procedures into a single summary report, a detailed methodology. [Internet]. SAS Institute; 2006 [cited 2016 Nov 4]. (SUGI 31 Proceedings). Report No.: 261–31. Available from: http://www2.sas.com/proceedings/sugi31/261-31.pdf
67. Grubber J, Olsen M, Bosworth H. Creating Journal-Style Tables in an Easy Way (with PROC TABULATE, PROC TEMPLATE, PROC FORMAT and ODS RTF) [Internet]. SAS Institute; 2008 [cited 2016 Nov 4]. (SAS Global Forum 2008). Report No.: 091–2008. Available from: http://www2.sas.com/proceedings/sugi31/261-31.pdf
68. Cochran B. A Gentle Introduction to the Powerful REPORT Procedure [Internet]. SUGI 30: SAS Institute; 2005 [cited 2017 Mar 14]. (SUGI 30 Proceedings). Report No: 259–30. Available from: http://www2.sas.com/proceedings/sugi30/259-30.pdf
69. Kadziola Z. An Easy-to-Use SAS® Table Formatting Macro: Stand-Alone, Flexible, and Quick [Internet]. SUGI 30: SAS Institute; 2005 [cited 2017 Mar 14]. (SUGI 30 Proceedings). Report No.: 164–30. Available from: http://www2.sas.com/proceedings/sugi30/164-30.pdf
70. Porter M. Making journal-quality tables (and other useful hints!) [Internet]. 2006 [cited 2017 Mar 15]; Center for Family and Demographic Research. Available from: https://www.bgsu.edu/content/dam/BGSU/college-of-arts-and-sciences/center-for-family-and-demographic-research/documents/Workshops/2005-workshop-Making-Journal-Quality-Tables-Presentation.pdf
71. Alvira-Hammond M, Bogle RH. Making journal-quality tables [Internet]. CFDR Workshop Series; 2012 [cited 2017 Mar 15]; Center for Family and Demographic Research. Available from: https://www.bgsu.edu/content/dam/BGSU/college-of-arts-and-sciences/center-for-family-and-demographic-research/documents/Help%20Resources%20and%20Tools/Creating%20Journal%20Quality%20Tables/Creating-Journal-Quality-Tables.pdf
72. Winters R. Excellent ways of exporting SAS data to Excel [Internet]. Portland Maine: SAS Institute; 2006 [cited 2017 Mar 12]. (NESUG 17). Available from: http://www.lexjansen.com/nesug/nesug04/io/io09.pdf

73. Hlavac M. Stargazer: Well-Formatted Regression and Summary Statistics Tables [Internet]. 2015 [cited 2017 Mar 15]. Available from: https://cran.r-project.org/web/packages/stargazer/index.html
74. Murdoch D. tables: Formula-Driven Table Generation [Internet]. 2017 [cited 2017 Mar 15]. Available from: https://cran.r-project.org/web/packages/tables/index.html
75. Ceylan Y, Theubl S. Installing R and LaTeX [Internet]. Wirtschafts Universitat Wien Vienna University of Economics and Business. 2014 [cited 2017 Mar 16]. Available from: http://statmath.wu.ac.at/software/R/qfin/
76. R Library Introduction to functions [Internet]. IDRE Stats. [cited 2017 Mar 21]. Available from: http://stats.idre.ucla.edu/r/library/r-library-introduction-to-functions/
77. Kodali T. Using the apply family of Functions in R [Internet]. DataScience+. 2015 [cited 2017 Mar 21]. Available from: https://datascienceplus.com/using-the-apply-family-of-functions-in-r/
78. SAS Institute. About SAS [Internet]. [cited 2017 Apr 2]. Available from: https://www.sas.com/en_us/company-information.html
79. Kabacoff R. Quick-R: Built-in Functions [Internet]. Quick-R. 2017 [cited 2017 Mar 25]. Available from: http://www.statmethods.net/management/functions.html
80. US Department of Commerce. 1.3.5.7. Bartlett's Test [Internet]. Engineering Statistics Handbook. 2013 [cited 2017 Mar 25]. Available from: http://www.itl.nist.gov/div898/handbook/eda/section3/eda357.htm
81. Kuhfeld WF, So Y. Creating and Customizing the Kaplan-Meier Survival Plot in PROC LIFETEST [Internet]. SAS Institute; 2013 [cited 2016 Dec 28]. (SAS Global Forum 2013). Report No.: 427–2013. Available from: https://support.sas.com/resources/papers/proceedings13/427-2013.pdf
82. George B, Seals S, Aban I. 2014. Survival analysis and regression models. *J Nucl Cardiol Off Publ Am Soc Nucl Cardiol. 21*(4):686–694.
83. Allis R. Comparing Kaplan-Meier curves-what are the (SAS) options? [Internet]. PHUse 2009: PHUse; 2009 [cited 2016 Dec 29]. (Pharmaceutical Users Software Exchange). Report No.: SP02. Available from: http://www.lexjansen.com/phuse/2009/sp/SP02.pdf
84. Shen L, Lu J. Healthcare Data Manipulation and Analytics using SAS [Internet]. PharmaSUG: SAS Institute; 2014 [cited 2017 Mar 26]. (PharmaSUG 2014 Conference Proceedings). Report No.: PO17. Available from: http://www.pharmasug.org/proceedings/2014/PO/PharmaSUG-2014-PO17.pdf
85. Strome T. Why you should try R to give your healthcare analytics a serious boost! [Internet]. HealthcareAnalytics.info. 2012 [cited 2017 Mar 26]. Available from: http://healthcareanalytics.info/2012/07/why-you-should-tr-r-to-give-your-healthcare-analytics-a-serious-boost/
86. Schulze MB, Hoffmann K, Kroke A, Boeing H. 2003. Risk of hypertension among women in the EPIC-Potsdam Study: Comparison of relative risk estimates for exploratory and hypothesis-oriented dietary patterns. *Am J Epidemiol. 158*(4):365–373.
87. Steyerberg EW, Eijkemans MJ, Habbema JD. 1999. Stepwise selection in small data sets: A simulation study of bias in logistic regression analysis. *J Clin Epidemiol. 52*(10):935–942.

88. Nichols DP. 1992. Letters: Dummy variables in stepwise regression. *Am Stat. 46*(2):163–165.
89. Cohen A. 1991. Dummy variables in stepwise regression. *Am Stat. 45*(3):226–228.
90. Gelman A, Loken E. The garden of forking paths: Why multiple comparisons can be a problem, even when there is no "fishing expedition" or "p-hacking" and the research hypothesis was posited ahead of time [Internet]. Columbia University; 2013 [cited 2017 Mar 27] p. 17. Available from: http://www.stat.columbia.edu/~gelman/research/unpublished/p_hacking.pdf
91. Lumley T, Diehr P, Emerson S, Chen L. 2002. The importance of the normality assumption in large public health data sets. *Annu Rev Public Health. 23*(1):151–69.
92. Forster MR. Parsimony and Simplicity [Internet]. Department of Philosophy, University of Wisconsin-Madison. 1998 [cited 2017 Mar 28]. Available from: http://philosophy.wisc.edu/forster/220/simplicity.html
93. Ronchetti E. 1985. Robust model selection in regression. *Stat Probab Lett. 3*(1): 21–23.
94. Dallal GE. Interactions in Multiple Regression Models [Internet]. 2012 [cited 2017 Mar 27]. Available from: http://www.jerrydallal.com/lhsp/reginter.htm
95. Karaca-Mandic P, Norton EC, Dowd B. 2012. Interaction terms in nonlinear models. *Health Serv Res. 47*(1 Pt 1):255–274.
96. Lemon SC, Roy J, Clark MA, Friedmann PD, Rakowski W. 2003. Classification and regression tree analysis in public health: methodological review and comparison with logistic regression. *Ann Behav Med Publ Soc Behav Med. 26*(3):172–181.
97. Pena EA, Slate EH. gvlma: Global Validation of Linear Models Assumptions [Internet]. 2014 [cited 2016 Dec 30]. Available from: https://cran.r-project.org/web/packages/gvlma/index.html
98. Wickham H, Chang W, R Core Team. devtools: Tools to Make Developing R Packages Easier [Internet]. 2016 [cited 2016 Dec 30]. Available from: https://cran.r-project.org/web/packages/devtools/index.html
99. Robinson D, Gomez M, Demeshev B, Menne D, Nutter B, Johnston L et al. Broom: Convert Statistical Analysis Objects into Tidy Data Frames [Internet]. 2016 [cited 2016 Dec 30]. Available from: https://cran.r-project.org/web/packages/broom/index.html
100. Gelman A, Su Y-S, Yajima M, Hill J, Pittau MG, Kerman J et al. arm: Data Analysis Using Regression and Multilevel/Hierarchical Models [Internet]. 2016 [cited 2016 Dec 30]. Available from: https://cran.r-project.org/web/packages/arm/index.html
101. Lander JP. Coefplot: Plots Coefficients from Fitted Models [Internet]. 2016 [cited 2016 Dec 30]. Available from: https://cran.r-project.org/web/packages/coefplot/index.html
102. Bush HM. 2011. *Biostatistics: An Applied Introduction for the Public Health Practitioner.* Cengage Learning: Boston, MA. 370 p.
103. Mood C. 2010. Logistic regression: Why we cannot do what we think we can do, and what we can do about it. *Eur Sociol Rev. 26*(1):67–82.
104. Wang EW, Ghogomu N, Voelker CCJ, Rich JT, Paniello RC, Nussenbaum B et al. 2009. A practical guide for understanding confidence intervals and P values. *Otolaryngol—Head Neck Surg Off J Am Acad Otolaryngol-Head Neck Surg. 140*(6):794–799.

105. Long RG. 2008. The crux of the method: Assumptions in ordinary least squares and logistic regression. *Psychol Rep. 103*(2):431–434.
106. Peduzzi P, Concato J, Kemper E, Holford TR, Feinstein AR. 1996. A simulation study of the number of events per variable in logistic regression analysis. *J Clin Epidemiol. 49*(12):1373–1379.
107. Kuhn M, Wing J, Weston S, Williams A, Keefer C, Engelhardt A et al. caret: Classification and Regression Training [Internet]. 2016 [cited 2017 Mar 28]. Available from: https://cran.r-project.org/web/packages/caret/index.html
108. ALHarthi S, Al-Motlag S, Wahi MM. 2017. Is trying to quit associated with tooth loss and delayed yearly dental visit among smokers? Results of the 2014 behavioral risk factor surveillance system (BRFSS). *J Periodontol. 88*(1):34–49.
109. Bagley SC, White H, Golomb BA. 2001. Logistic regression in the medical literature: Standards for use and reporting, with particular attention to one medical domain. *J Clin Epidemiol. 54*(10):979–85.
110. Zamar D, Graham J, McNeney B. R: elrm: exact-like inference in logistic regression models [Internet]. 2015 [cited 2017 Mar 29]. Available from: https://artax.karlin.mff.cuni.cz/r-help/library/elrm/html/elrm.html
111. Karp AH. Getting Started with PROC LOGISTIC [Internet]. SUGI 26: SAS Institute; 2001 [cited 2017 Mar 12]. (SUGI 26 Proceedings). Report No.: 248–26. Available from: http://www2.sas.com/proceedings/sugi26/p248-26.pdf
112. Cueto A, Mesa F, Bravo M, Ocaña-Riola R. 2005. Periodontitis as risk factor for acute myocardial infarction. A case control study of Spanish adults. *J Periodontal Res. 40*(1):36–42.
113. Pearl J. Why there is no statistical test for confounding, why many think there is, and why they are almost right (Technical Report No. R-256). Los Angeles, CA: Department of Computer Science, University of California, Los Angeles; 1998.
114. Pinheiro J, Bates D, DebRoy S, Sarkar D, EISPACK authors, Heisterkamp S et al. nlme: Linear and Nonlinear Mixed Effects Models [Internet]. 2016 [cited 2016 Dec 31]. Available from: https://cran.r-project.org/web/packages/nlme/index.html
115. Heinze G, Ploner M, Dunkler D, Southworth H. logistf: Firth's Bias-Reduced Logistic Regression [Internet]. 2016 [cited 2016 Dec 31]. Available from: https://cran.r-project.org/web/packages/logistf/index.html
116. UCLA: Statistical Consulting Group. Survival Analysis by John P. Klein and Melvin L. Moeschberger Chapter 12: Inference for Parametric Regression Models: SAS Examples [Internet]. IDRE Stats; 2017 [cited 2017 Mar 29]. Available from: http://stats.idre.ucla.edu/sas/examples/sakm/survival-analysis-by-john-p-klein-and-melvin-l-moeschbergerchapter-12-inference-for-parametric-regression-models/
117. Jackson C. flexsurv: Flexible Parametric Survival and Multi-State Models [Internet]. 2016 [cited 2016 Dec 31]. Available from: https://cran.r-project.org/web/packages/flexsurv/index.html
118. Gaugler JE, Hovater M, Roth DL, Johnston JA, Kane RL, Sarsour K. Depressive, Functional Status, and Neuropsychiatric Symptom Trajectories Before an Alzheimer's Disease Diagnosis. Aging Ment Health [Internet]. 2014 [cited 2017 Mar 26];*18*(1). Available from: http://www.ncbi.nlm.nih.gov/pmc/articles/PMC3855584/

119. Song SE, Cho N, Chu A, Shin SU, Yi A, Lee SH et al. 2015. Undiagnosed breast cancer: Features at supplemental screening US. *Radiology. 277*(2):372–380.
120. Iqbal J, Ginsburg O, Rochon PA, Sun P, Narod SA. 2015. Differences in breast cancer stage at diagnosis and cancer-specific survival by race and ethnicity in the United States. *JAMA. 313*(2):165–173.
121. Wahi MM, Parks DV, Skeate RC, Goldin SB. 2008. Reducing errors from the electronic transcription of data collected on paper forms: A research data case study. *J Am Med Inform Assoc JAMIA. 15*(3):386–389.
122. Singh R, Mukhopadhyay K. 2011. Survival analysis in clinical trials: Basics and must know areas. *Perspect Clin Res.* 2(4):145–148.
123. US Office of Disease Prevention and Health Promotion. Healthy People 2020 [Internet]. 2017 [cited 2017 Jan 1]. Available from: https://www.healthypeople.gov/
124. Masini EO, Mansour O, Speer CE, Addona V, Hanson CL, Sitienei JK et al. 2016. Using survival analysis to identify risk factors for treatment interruption among new and retreatment tuberculosis patients in Kenya. *PLOS ONE. 11*(10):e0164172.

Index

Note: Page numbers followed by f and t refer to figures and tables, respectively.